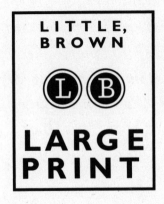

LITTLE,
BROWN

L B

**LARGE
PRINT**

THE
BLOOD
SUGAR
SOLUTION

The UltraHealthy Program for
Losing Weight, Preventing Disease,
and Feeling Great Now!

Mark Hyman, MD

LITTLE, BROWN AND COMPANY

LARGE PRINT EDITION

Little, Brown and Company
Hachette Book Group
237 Park Avenue, New York, NY 10017
www.hachettebookgroup.com

First Edition: February 2012

Little, Brown and Company is a division of Hachette Book Group, Inc., and is celebrating its 175th anniversary in 2012. The Little, Brown name and logo are trademarks of Hachette Book Group, Inc.

The publisher is not responsible for websites (or their content) that are not owned by the publisher.

The Hachette Speakers Bureau provides a wide range of authors for speaking events. To find out more, go to www.hachettespeakersbureau.com or call (866) 376-6591.

Diabesity is a trademark owned by Hyman Enterprises, LLC.

Library of Congress Cataloging-in-Publication Data
Hyman, Mark
    The blood sugar solution : the ultrahealthy program for losing weight, preventing disease, and feeling great now! / Mark Hyman.
       p. cm.
    Includes bibliographical references and index.
    ISBN 978-0-316-12737-0 (hc) / 978-0-316-19617-8 (large print)
    1. Blood sugar—Popular works.   2. Diabetes—Diet therapy—Recipes.   3. Insulin resistance—Popular works.   4. Weight loss—Popular works.   I. Title.
    QP99.3.B5H96 2012
    612.1'2—dc23

2011034644

10 9 8 7 6 5 4 3 2 1

RRD-C

Printed in the United States of America

For the first generation of children in history that will live sicker and die younger than their parents. For their sakes and ours may we all work together to take back our health.

Contents

PART V

TAKE BACK OUR HEALTH

PART VI

THE BLOOD SUGAR SOLUTION MEAL PLAN AND RECIPES

How to Use This Book

You may have picked up this book for many reasons.

You may be interested in understanding the scope and impact of our current global epidemic of obesity and type 2 diabetes or what should be called "diabesity."

You may want to understand the social, political, or economic factors that continue to fuel this epidemic and what we can do about them. You may be a policy maker, health care organization, educator, or religious leader looking for a solution.

You may be a scientifically curious health care consumer or health care practitioner who wants to better understand the biology of obesity and diabetes and why it is so difficult to find an effective solution, despite the advances of modern medicine.

You may want to create or join a group or be part of a grass-roots social movement to change the course of this epidemic.

Or you may simply be looking for a practical solution and program to lose weight and reverse your own type 2 diabetes or pre-diabetes.

Whatever your reasons, this book is for you.

We face a problem that will touch almost everyone on the planet. It is no secret we are in the middle of an explosive epidemic of obesity and type 2 diabetes.

As a physician, scientist, educator, and citizen, I have struggled to find a comprehensive solution. That is what motivated me to write this book, *The Blood Sugar Solution.*

While this book is primarily about obesity and type 2 diabetes, it can be helpful for type 1 diabetics who want to live a healthy blood sugar–balancing lifestyle. Type 1 diabetes is an autoimmune disease that results in damage to the pancreas and **lack of insulin** production. Type 2 diabetes is also an inflammatory disease, but it is a disease of **too much insulin,** where your cells become numb to the insulin produced by the body. This is called **insulin resistance** and often precedes the onset of type 2 diabetes by years or decades. This book is about type 2 diabetes and insulin resistance, so whenever I refer to diabetes in this book, I am referring to type 2 diabetes.

It is about much more than blood sugar. It is about getting to the very root of the problem and providing a solution on a biological, personal, social, and economic level.

The book opens with a simple quiz to help identify if you have "diabesity." Since one in two Americans has this problem, the answer will likely be yes.

In Chapter 1 of Part I, "Understanding the Modern Plague," I explore the scope of the epidemic across the globe and its impact not only on rich Western countries, but also on the developing world. In Chapter 2, we will review the real biologic cause of the epidemic — insulin resistance — and why our current approaches to the problem don't work.

In Chapter 3, I dispel the medical myths that prevent us from effectively addressing the epidemic, for example, that obesity and type 2 diabetes are genetic, or that type 2 diabetes is not reversible, or that medication is effective in preventing or treating diabetes and related diseases.

In Chapter 4, I explore new research on the biology of food addiction and why food cravings and overeating are not your fault. This brings into question our food marketing practices and their impact on children and childhood obesity.

In Chapter 5, I explore how Big Food, Big Farming, and Big Pharma fuel the epidemic of obesity, diabetes, and chronic disease across the globe, creating

> ### *The UltraWellness Quiz: Discover The Root Causes of Weight Gain and Diabetes*
>
> This book will help you understand and treat the underlying causes of weight issues and diabetes and almost any chronic health problem. Inside this book are special quizzes that together make up **The UltraWellness Quiz.** It is the key to discovering the cause and the cure of all your health problems and creating a clear personalized path to health. The science behind this, functional or whole systems medicine, allows you to discover the true source of your health issues through a specific set of quizzes.
>
> **The UltraWellness Quiz** can be filled out in the book, but I encourage you to go to www.bloodsugarsolution.com and fill out the quiz online to get and track your **UltraWellness Score** and start on your road to lifelong health and vitality.

an "obesogenic" environment, and explain what we collectively can do about it.

In Chapter 6, I introduce a new science-based model of whole systems medicine, a road map for addressing chronic disease in the twenty-first century called **functional medicine,** which treats the underlying biologic causes of obesity and diabetes. It applies the advances in personalized medicine, genomics, and systems biology in a practical road map for diagnosing, treating, and reversing disease. It is medicine focused on causes and mechanisms, not location in the body and symptoms. We treat the system and not just the symptoms. We treat the soil or the terrain and not the plant. It is extraordinarily effective for obesity and type 2 diabetes.

In Part II, "The Seven Steps to Treating Diabesity," I explain the latest scientific advances in our understanding of the biology of obesity and diabetes, advances that allow us to discern the root biological causes of the problem. Obesity and diabetes are the result of many different causes, including nutritional, hormonal, immunological, inflammatory, and digestive imbalances, as well as environmental toxins, metabolic dysfunction, and stress. Each of these either separately or collectively may be involved in *your* particular case. Finding out which problems you have through the quizzes in Part II, and personalizing your approach, is critical to healing.

In Part III, "The Blood Sugar Solution: Preparation," you will learn how to prepare your mind, body, and kitchen for the six-week program; how to get together to get healthy by creating or joining a small support group; and finally how to take a measure of your health through *The Blood Sugar Solution* quiz and laboratory tests, which will help you understand the cause and severity of your diabesity.

Part IV, "The Six-Week Action Plan," is a practical six-step, six-week program you can do on your own, or in partnership with your health care provider. It also shows you how to create a community of support for yourself. Support and feedback from a group of people make the program more fun and effective and the change more sustainable.

The six-week action plan outlines:

- How to identify the underlying causes of insulin resistance and diabesity in yourself
- Personalized self-care therapeutic treatments to help you address your unique underlying causes of diabesity
- How to change your diet to reverse the problem and use food as medicine
- A delicious, easy-to-follow menu plan with recipes and shopping lists included
- Which supplements and medication to take in order to improve and optimize insulin function and blood sugar balance
- How to use exercise more effectively and more efficiently
- Stress-reducing tools to reverse diabesity

Note: Following this six-week action plan can radically lower your blood sugar and cause low blood sugar if you are on medication. If you are currently taking medication and wish to follow the program, it's important that you monitor your blood sugar carefully and work with your doctor as needed. It is possible you will need to reduce the amount of medication you are taking. Changes in medication should only be done with the help and supervision of your physician.

- How to address and reduce your exposure to and your body burden of environmental toxins
- Which tests to get to determine whether you have a problem
- How to work with your doctor so you can get the information, tests, and treatments you need to address the problem effectively and use medications intelligently when needed
- Instructions on how to take advantage of our online support tools and community at www .bloodsugarsolution.com
- How to get healthy for life

Part V is a manifesto, a call to action, and a plan for us as individuals, families, communities, schools, workplaces, and faith-based groups to "Take Back

Our Health." A diverse community-based movement is the only way to effectively reverse this epidemic. This will ultimately be necessary if we are to help not only ourselves, but also our children and their children. To paraphrase my friend Hillary Clinton, it takes a village to get healthy.

Join the Blood Sugar Solution Community Today

This book is just the beginning of the resources I have created to help you get healthy for life. The companion website for the book, www.bloodsugar solution.com, also provides an online curriculum, program-enhancing tools, resources, ongoing education, and support.

As you will learn, community is essential, and I have created an entire online web experience to help you get healthy together. The website will help you find others who are on the same journey and offer a way to support each other. Change is often difficult, but sharing your journey and getting support from others are powerful medicines that will ensure your success. I will be part of the community, too, and will do my best to stay in touch and support you along the way.

Visit www.bloodsugarsolution.com and learn more about how to:

1. **Join a Group.** Join a group in our online community, or your local community.
2. **Take Your Quizzes.** Online versions of the Blood Sugar Solution Quizzes have been provided to help you self-diagnose the cause of your problems and get the right treatment.
3. **Take Advantage of *The Blood Sugar Solution* course.** This includes the two-week preparation phase, a six-week program, week-by-week action steps, and ongoing education and support to help you stay healthy for life.
4. **Access Online Checklists.** Use our daily and weekly checklists to help you succeed in the program.
5. **Use Health Trackers.** Access online and mobile weight, height, BMI (body mass index), and lab tests trackers to securely and privately record changes over the course of the program.
6. **Develop Your Personal Journal.** You can record your experience and track your daily diet and exercise securely and privately.
7. **Learn What Supplements to Take.** I provide specific recommendations for the nutrients and supplements you need to succeed in the program.

8. **Access Mind-Body Tools.** I have developed some easy-to-use online exercises for relaxing mind and soul, including breathing exercises and yoga.

9. **Get Tested.** Learn about resources for self-testing and medical testing.

10. **Use Our Health and Nutrition Coaching.** Get personal coaching by trained nutritionists to help you succeed in your program.

11. **Get More Recipes.** With the help of a professional chef, we have developed additional delicious recipes and kid-friendly recipes.

12. **Get Online Cooking Classes.** I developed a set of lessons in simple cooking featuring me— your friendly doctor-chef!

13. **Access Healthy Living Resources.** Information on finding good foods, clean and green products, and tools and resources for fitness and mind-body balance.

14. **View Educational Articles, Videos, and Webinars.** Access videos, webinars, and ongoing education to support you as you move toward health.

15. **Find a Doctor.** Links to functional medicine and integrative medical and health care professionals in your area.

16. **Join a Movement to Take Back Our Health.** Specific action steps for you to take in your family, home, school, workplace, faith-based community, our health care system, and our democracy.

17. Share Your Successes. A place you can post your own stories, and inspire and be inspired by thousands of others.

Visit www.bloodsugarsolution.com to join.

Do You Have Diabesity?

Now let's see if you have diabesity or are at risk for it.

If you answer yes to any of these questions, you may already have diabesity or are headed in that direction. You may not know the answers to all these questions now, but in Part III there is a more extensive quiz with instructions for testing that will help you identify the severity of your diabesity.

- Do you have a family history of diabetes, heart disease, or obesity?   Yes _____ No _____

- Are you of nonwhite ancestry (African, Asian, Native American, Pacific Islander, Hispanic, Indian, Middle Eastern)?   Yes _____ No _____

- Are you overweight (BMI or body mass index over 25)? See page 269 to calculate your BMI based on weight and height. Yes _____ No _____

- Do you have extra belly fat? Is your waist circumference greater than 35 inches for women or greater than 40 inches for men? Yes _____ No _____

- Do you have sugar and refined carbohydrate cravings? Yes _____ No _____

- Do you have trouble losing weight on a low-fat diet? Yes _____ No _____

- Has your doctor told you your fasting blood sugar is a little high (greater than 100mg/dl) or have you actually been diagnosed with insulin resistance, pre-diabetes, or diabetes? Yes _____ No _____

- Do you have high levels of triglycerides (over 100 mg/dl) or low

HDL (good) cholesterol
(less than 50 mg/dl)?   Yes _____ No _____

- Do you have heart disease? Yes _____ No _____

- Do you have high blood
  pressure?   Yes _____ No _____

- Are you inactive
  (less than 30 minutes of
  exercise 4 times a week)?   Yes _____ No _____

- Have you had gestational
  diabetes or polycystic
  ovarian syndrome?   Yes _____ No _____

- Do you suffer from infertility,
  low sex drive, or sexual
  dysfunction?   Yes _____ No _____

THE
BLOOD
SUGAR
SOLUTION

Diabesity: What You Don't Know May Kill You

What's in a name: insulin resistance, metabolic syndrome, syndrome X, obesity, pre-diabetes, adult-onset diabetes, type 2 diabetes. These are all essentially one problem; some vary by severity but *all* can have deadly consequences. The diagnosis and treatment of the underlying causes that drive all these conditions are actually the same.

Diabesity is a more comprehensive term to describe the continuum from optimal blood sugar balance toward insulin resistance and full-blown diabetes. If you answered yes to any of the questions in the quiz on page xxiii, you may already have diabesity.

Nearly all people who are overweight (over 70 percent of adult Americans) already have "pre-diabetes" and have significant risks of disease and death. They just don't know it. Even worse, while the word "diabesity" is made up of the concepts of obesity and diabetes, even those who aren't over-weight can have this problem. These are the "skinny fat" people. They are "underlean" (not enough mus-cle) instead of "overweight" and have a little extra weight around the middle, or "belly fat." Currently there are no national screening recommendations, no treatment guidelines, no approved medications, and no reimbursement to health care providers for diagnosing and treating anything other than full-blown diabetes. Think about that. **Doctors are not expected, trained, or paid to diagnose and treat the single biggest chronic disease in America,** which, along with smoking, causes nearly all the major health care burdens of the twenty-first cen-tury, including heart disease, stroke, dementia, and even cancer. But here is the good news—there is a scientifically proven solution that I have mapped out for you in this book.

Our current medical practice has not caught up with our knowledge. In 2008, the American College of Endocrinology and the American Association of Clinical Endocrinologists gathered twenty-two experts and reviewed all the scientific data on pre-diabetes and diabetes. They heralded a wake-up clarion call for individuals, the health care commu-nity, and governments around the world.[1] Their con-clusions were as follows:

1. The diagnosis of pre-diabetes and diabetes is arbitrary. A fasting blood sugar over 100 mg/dl is considered pre-diabetes, and a blood sugar over 126 mg/dl is considered diabetes. **However, they found these cutoffs don't reflect the whole spectrum of risk—including heart disease, cancer, dementia, stroke, and even kidney and nerve damage—which starts at *much* lower numbers, numbers most people consider normal.**

2. The DECODE study of 22,000 people[2] examined the continuum of risk measured not by fasting blood sugar, but by blood sugar after a big sugar drink (the best way to diagnose the problem). The study found that even starting at blood sugar levels that were perfectly normal (95 mg/dl), there was a steady and significant risk of heart disease and complications well below the accepted abnormal of less than 140 mg/dl for pre-diabetes and long before people reached the diabetic cutoff of 200 mg/dl.

Bottom line: Even if you have perfectly normal blood sugar, you may be sitting on a hidden time bomb of disease called diabesity, which prevents you from losing weight and living a long healthy life. Insulin resistance is the major cause of aging and death in the developed and most of the developing world.

This book will help you identify and reverse this explosive situation for yourself. It also lays out a comprehensive action plan for greater collective action to solve this problem individually and collectively by getting healthy together.

PART I

UNDERSTANDING THE MODERN PLAGUE

For this we must make automatic and habitual, as early as possible, as many useful actions as we can, and guard against the growing into ways that are likely to be disadvantageous to us, as we should guard against the plague.

— William James,
"The Laws of Habit," *The Popular Science Monthly* (February 1887)

It ain't what you don't know that gets you into trouble. It's what you know for sure that just ain't so.

— Mark Twain

1

A Hidden Epidemic:
The United States of Diabetes

Diabesity, the continuum of health problems rang-
ing from mild insulin resistance and overweight to
obesity and diabetes, is the single biggest global
health epidemic of our time. It is one of the leading
causes of heart disease, dementia, cancer, and premature death in the world and is almost entirely
caused by environmental and lifestyle factors. This
means that it is almost 100 percent preventable and
curable.

Diabesity affects over 1.7 billion people worldwide. Scientists conservatively estimate it will affect
1 in 2 Americans by 2020, 90 percent of whom **will
not be diagnosed.** I believe it *already* affects more
than 1 in 2 Americans and up to 70–80 percent of
some populations.

Obesity (almost always related to diabesity) is the

leading cause of preventable death in the United States and around the world. Gaining just 11–16 pounds doubles the risk of type 2 diabetes, while gaining 17–24 pounds triples the risk. **Despite this, there are no national recommendations from government or key organizations advising screening or treatment for pre-diabetes.** We are becoming the United States of Diabetes.

The prevalence of type 2 diabetes in America has tripled since the 1980s. In 2010 there were 27 million Americans with diabetes (25 percent of whom were not diagnosed) and 67 million with pre-diabetes (90 percent of whom were not diagnosed). African-Americans, Latin Americans, and Asians have dramatically higher rates of diabesity than Caucasians do.[1] By 2015, 2.3 billion people worldwide will be overweight and 700 million will be obese. The number of diabetics will increase from 1 in 10 Americans today to 1 in 3 by the middle of this century.

A CHILDHOOD PROBLEM

Perhaps most disturbing, our children are increasingly affected by this epidemic. We are raising the first generation of Americans to live sicker and die younger than their parents. Life expectancy is actually declining for the first time in human history.

Here are some startling statistics:

- One in three children is overweight in America.
- Childhood obesity has tripled from 1980 to 2010.
- There are now more than 2 million morbidly obese children above the 99th percentile in weight.
- In New York City, 40 percent of the children are overweight or obese.
- One in three children born today will have diabetes in their lifetime.
- Childhood obesity will have more impact on the life expectancy of children than all childhood cancers combined.

A GLOBAL PROBLEM

Diabetes is just as widespread in other parts of the world: In 2007, it was estimated that 240 million people worldwide had diabetes. It is projected to affect 380 million by the year 2030, about 10 times the number of people affected by HIV/AIDS.[2] Sadly this is a gross underestimate. Estimates in 2011 put the worldwide total at 350 million. In China alone, rates of diabetes were almost zero 25 years ago. In 2007, there were 24 million diabetics in China, and scientists projected that by 2030 there would be 42 million diabetics in China. However, by 2010, there were 93 million diabetics and 148 million pre-diabetics

Special Note: Childhood Obesity and Diabetes—The Blood Sugar Solution for Children

The biggest tragedy is the global spread of childhood obesity and "adult"-onset or type 2 diabetes in little children. We are now seeing eight-year-old children with diabetes, fifteen-year-olds with strokes, and twenty-five-year-olds who need cardiac bypass. While *The Blood Sugar Solution* is a program mostly for adults, it is also powerful and effective for children. The whole family must be part of the solution, and we have to make our homes, communities, and schools safe for our children.

The Blood Sugar Solution includes many child-friendly recipes. And when it comes to supplements, there is something for everyone, even infants and children. In fact, any child over twelve years of age with diabesity can follow the basic Blood Sugar Solution plan. Children younger than twelve or those who qualify for the Advanced Plan should work with an experienced functional medicine practitioner. See www .bloodsugarsolution.com for how best to support your children's health if they are overweight or have type 2 diabetes.

in China, almost all of whom were previously undiagnosed. Imagine if we had 148 million new cases of AIDS overnight in one country.

Sixty percent of the world's diabetics will eventually come from Asia because it is the world's most populous region. The number of individuals with impaired glucose tolerance or pre-diabetes will increase substantially because of increased genetic susceptibility to the harmful effects of sugar and processed foods. Interestingly, people in this Asian population (who are uniquely susceptible to diabetes even though they may not be obese) are increasingly affected as they adopt a more Western diet. Weaker environmental laws and regulations also expose them to increasing levels of toxins, which, as we will see later, are a significant cause of diabesity.[3]

Ponder this: From 1983 to 2008, the number of people in the world with diabetes increased sevenfold, from 35 to 240 million. In just three years, from 2008 to 2011, we added another 110 million diabetics to our global population. Shouldn't the main question we ask be *why is this happening?* instead of *what new drug can we find to treat it?* Our approach must be novel, innovative, and widely applicable at low cost across all borders. Billions and billions have been wasted trying to find the "drug cure," while the solution lies right under our nose. This is a lifestyle and environmental disease and won't be cured by a medication.

DIABESITY: THE MAJOR CAUSE OF CHRONIC DISEASE AND DECREASED LIFE EXPECTANCY

Diabesity is one of the leading causes of chronic disease in the twenty-first century, including heart disease, stroke, dementia, and cancer.[4]

Consider the following:

- One-third of all diabetics have documented heart disease.[5]
- It is estimated that nearly everyone else with type 2 diabetes has undiagnosed cardiovascular disease.
- People with diabetes are four times more likely to die from heart disease, and the rate of stroke is three to four times higher in this population.
- Those with pre-diabetes are also four times more likely to die of heart disease.[6] So having pre-diabetes isn't really "pre" anything in terms of risk.
- There is a fourfold increased risk for dementia in diabetics.[7] And pre-diabetes is a leading cause of "pre-dementia," also known as mild cognitive impairment.
- The link between obesity and cancer is well documented and is driven by insulin resistance.[8]
- Diabesity is the leading cause of high blood pressure in our society. Seventy-five percent of those with diabetes have high blood pressure.

- Diabesity is also the leading cause of liver failure from NASH (nonalcoholic steatohepatitis), also known as fatty liver. It affects 30 percent of our general population (about 90 million) and 70–90 percent of those who have diabesity. Those with fatty liver are at much greater risk of heart attack and death.[9]
- Diabesity is an important cause of depression and mood disorders. Women with diabetes are 29 percent more likely to develop depression, and women who took insulin are 53 percent more likely to develop depression.[10]
- Nervous system damage affects 60–70 percent of people with diabetes, leading to a loss of sensation in the hands and feet, slow digestion, carpal tunnel syndrome, sexual dysfunction, and other problems. Almost 30 percent of people age forty or older with diabetes have impaired sensation in their feet, and this frequently leads to amputations.
- Diabesity is also the leading cause of blindness among people ages twenty to seventy-four.
- Diabesity is the leading cause of kidney failure — accounting for 44 percent of new cases each year.
- People with poorly controlled diabetes are three times more likely to have periodontal or severe gum disease.

A recent remarkable study published in the *New England Journal of Medicine* examining 123,205 deaths in 820,900 people found that diabetics died an average of six years earlier than nondiabetics and 40 percent of those did not die from heart disease or the usual diabetes-related causes.[11] They died from other complications not obviously related to diabetes, complications most wouldn't necessarily correlate with the disease. Yet it makes perfect sense given that diabesity is the underlying cause that drives most chronic illnesses.

DIABESITY: A MAJOR GLOBAL THREAT TO ECONOMIC DEVELOPMENT

Direct health care costs in the United States over the next decade attributable to diabetes and pre-diabetes will be $3.4 trillion, or one in every ten health care dollars spent. Obese citizens cost the U.S. health care system 40 percent more than normal-weight citizens. In a sample of 10 million commercial health plan members, those without diabetes cost $4,000 a year compared to $11,700 for those with diabetes, and $20,700 for those with complications from diabetes.

Diabesity places a large economic burden on our society. The direct and indirect costs of diabetes in America in 2007 amounted to $174 billion. The cost of obesity is also significant, and amounts to $113 billion every year. From 2000 to 2010, these two conditions have already cost us a total of $3 trillion. That's three times the estimated cost of fixing our entire health care system![12]

Are we getting our money's worth? Is our current approach winning the battle against these completely preventable and curable diseases? Clearly the answer is *no!*

The Impact of Diabesity on Developing Nations

Diabetes is not just a problem for rich countries with too much food; it is also a disease of poverty[13] that is increasing in developing countries as well.[14] In India, diabetes carries a greater risk of death than infectious disease. In the Middle East, nearly 20–25 percent of the population is diabetic. When I helped in Haiti (the poorest country in the Western hemisphere) after the earthquake in 2010, I asked the director of Haiti's main public hospital what the major medical problems were prior to the earthquake. His answer surprised me: heart disease, high blood pressure, and diabetes—all caused by diabesity.

By 2020, there will be fewer than 20 million deaths worldwide from infectious disease, but more than 50 million deaths from chronic preventable lifestyle diseases—heart disease, diabetes, and cancer. These are all fueled by the same preventable risk factors: high blood pressure, overweight, physical inactivity, high blood sugar, high cholesterol, and smoking. But strikingly, 95 percent of private and public efforts and funding focus almost exclusively on combating communicable or infectious disease.[15]

THE SOLUTION: TAKE BACK OUR HEALTH

There is a solution available, one that is accessible and scalable, one that is available to everyone and prevents, treats, and reverses diabesity at a fraction of the cost. This book provides that solution for individuals, communities, and nations. It will require significant change at all levels, but each of us has the power to transform this problem.

In addition to curing diabesity on an individual level, we need a movement. I call it *Take Back Our Health,* and in Part V, I explain how we can all join this movement so we can get healthy together. It starts with the individual, but moves into families, communities, workplaces, schools, and faith-based organizations and filters through us to government and corporations.

In the next chapter, we will look at the true causes of diabesity, and why current treatments aren't working.

2

The Real Causes of Diabesity

As a former emergency room doctor, I know that for acute illness and trauma, there is nothing better than conventional medicine's current tools and knowledge. However, when it comes to chronic disease and to the diabesity epidemic, we clearly have a massive global problem on our hands. We know that our current approach to prevention and treatment is not working because millions more are affected every year. Treating diabetes with medications or insulin is like mopping up the floor while the faucet continues to overflow. That is exactly how my patient, Jane, a fifty-three-year-old African-American corporate executive was being treated until she came to see me.

Reversing Diabetes: A Patient's Story

Being smart and accomplished, Jane had the time and resources to fix her out-of-control diabetes, except for one thing. No one gave her the knowledge and tools necessary to avoid going on insulin (which was the next step her doctor recommended), or to actually reverse her problems. In fact, when diabetics start taking insulin shots, they usually gain weight and their blood pressure and cholesterol begin to rise and they get more depressed. That is because too much insulin is the problem, not the solution. It will help the blood sugar come down, but the real causes of diabetes are never addressed.

Jane developed a whole list of conditions, including high blood pressure, low HDL (good) cholesterol, high triglycerides, and sleep apnea. By the time I saw her, Jane had had diabetes for ten years, and despite taking maximum doses of diabetes medication such as metformin and glyburide, her blood sugar was over 300 mg/dl (normal is less than 90 mg/dl), and her hemoglobin A1c, which measures the average blood sugar over the last six–eight weeks, was 10.3 (ideal is less than 5.5; diabetes is over 6.0).

She did her best to eat well. She had oatmeal for breakfast, and chicken and salads for lunch and dinner. By nighttime, however, her appetite was out of control and she craved sugar, candy, and ice cream. Most nights, she came home from work too tired to cook or exercise. In fact, she was so exhausted, she was going to take early retirement because she couldn't focus or keep up with her work.

Doctors prescribed a beta-blocker for high blood pressure and Lipitor for high cholesterol (both of which make diabetes and insulin resistance worse). Of course, she had some predisposing factors for diabetes—her father had died at fifty-five from a stroke (and most likely had pre-diabetes), and her mother and aunts all had type 2 diabetes.

Jane was obese; she was 5-foot-2, weighed 190 pounds, and had a BMI of 34. Her blood pressure was very high—164/104—despite the fact that she was on blood pressure medication.

She had a fatty liver from diabetes. Her cholesterol looked normal on Lipitor, with an LDL of 100 mg/dl, but no one checked what was most important about her cholesterol—the size of her cholesterol particles. Small particles are caused by insulin resistance, are very harmful, and don't improve with statin drugs. A good number is fewer than 600 small particles; Jane had 1,320. Her vitamin D was also very low at 17 ng/dl (normal > 45 ng/dl), which also contributes to diabesity, because she worked inside, had dark skin, and lived in the Northeast.

She also had many problems with her mitochondria, the factories that produce energy in the cells. This is a major factor in insulin resistance (see Chapter 13), indicating the need for coenzyme Q10, alpha lipoic acid, and B vitamins including biotin. She had low levels of minerals, including magnesium and chromium, which are important in blood sugar control. She also had oxidative stress and high levels of lipid peroxides, indicating rancid fats in her blood— all linked to diabetes.

The first thing we had her do was get her appetite under control and her energy back by teaching her to eat only real, whole food (nothing packaged or processed) and to eliminate all flour and sugar. To curb her cravings and reduce her appetite, we had her eat protein with every meal (including breakfast), have a protein snack in the morning and afternoon, and not eat three hours or less before bed. Jane's diet became primarily organic with cleaner sources of protein (lean meats, fish, eggs, and protein powder), low-glycemic (low sugar) snack bars, nuts, seeds, legumes, fresh fruit, vegetables, and some whole grains. When she started the program, she was inspired to clean out her kitchen cabinets of all unhealthy foods. She then stocked up at the natural foods market, buying a greater variety of foods.

Jane admitted that she followed the diet perfectly for one week, and then began to cheat.

When she did, she noticed that certain foods caused symptoms. In particular, she thought that dairy and sugary foods significantly worsened her afternoon fatigue.

She went back on *The Blood Sugar Solution* food plan and very quickly started feeling better. She finally felt she could start to exercise. Eventually I had her do interval and resistance strength training, which also helps reverse diabetes.

We corrected her nutritional deficiencies of B vitamins, vitamin D, chromium, and magnesium, and added fish oil. And we gave her support for her energy and calorie burning in her cells with alpha lipoic acid and coenzyme Q10. We also gave her a special super fiber known as PGX before every meal, which slows absorption of sugar and fat and makes you feel full so you eat less. Instead of sugary oatmeal to start the day, she had a medicinal protein shake. All these things have been shown to improve blood sugar control and correct insulin resistance.

We had her start high-dose niacin (vitamin B3) to increase her cholesterol particle size and took her off the beta-blocker and the diabetes drug glyberide, which pushes insulin higher. This type of drug, called an oral hypoglycemic, actually makes things worse over time by pushing the pancreas to pump out more insulin. The drug even has a black box warning that it *increases* the risk of heart attacks, which is exactly what you are trying to prevent by taking the drug to lower blood sugar.

After four months, Jane's energy was dramatically increased. Her blood sugar decreased from over 300 mg/dl to about 90 mg/dl. Her blood pressure went from 164/104 to 127/79. Her skin was clearer, and her cravings were gone. She had exercised every day, lost 20 pounds, and her sleep apnea went away.

After a few more months she lost a total of 30 pounds. Her blood sugar, hemoglobin A1c, liver, cholesterol, and vitamin D tests all returned to normal. Even her small dense cholesterol particles got light and big and fluffy and went from 1,320 to 615, and her mitochondrial and calorie burning increased to normal. She went from being so sick she almost had to retire to feeling empowered in life and health and "at a magical point, happy and enjoying life."

GETTING TO THE ROOT OF THE PROBLEM

Jane didn't need insulin. She needed the right knowledge and plan. As physicians, we are trained to offer medication or surgery to solve diabetes (and disease in general), when the real causes include poor-quality diet, nutritional deficiencies, hormonal imbalances, allergens, microbes, digestive imbalances, toxins, cellular energy problems, and stress. We think that treating the risk factors, such as high blood sugar, cholesterol, and blood pressure, with medications will help. But we don't learn how to identify and treat the *real* causes of disease.

Doctors (and patients) never ask the most important question: Why is your blood sugar, blood pressure, or blood cholesterol too high, and why is your blood too sticky and likely to clot?

In truth, diabetes and elevated blood sugar, blood pressure, and cholesterol are simply symptoms that result from problems with diet, lifestyle, and environmental toxins interacting with our unique genetic susceptibilities.

WHY LOWERING YOUR BLOOD SUGAR CAN KILL YOU

Shocking new findings should make us question our outdated approach to treating diabetes by simply lowering blood sugar with medication or insulin. The ACCORD study published in the *New England Journal of Medicine* in 2008 involved 10,000 patients with diabetes who were designated to receive intensive or regular therapy to lower blood sugar.[1] These patients were monitored and their risks of heart attack, stroke, and death were evaluated.

Surprisingly, the patients who had their blood sugar lowered the most had a higher risk of death. In fact, the National Institutes of Health stopped the study after three and a half years, because it was evident that the aggressive blood sugar lowering led to more deaths and heart attacks.

How could this happen if, as we believe, elevated blood sugar is the cause of all the evils of diabetes? Why would *lowering* blood sugar lead to worse outcomes?

This may surprise you, but *many* of the methods used to lower blood sugar, such as insulin or oral hypoglycemic drugs, actually make the problem worse by increasing insulin levels. Contrary to what most people think, type 2 diabetes and diabesity are diseases of too much, not too little, insulin. Insulin is the real driver of problems with diabesity.

INSULIN RESISTANCE: THE REAL CAUSE OF DIABESITY

When your diet is full of empty calories and an abundance of quickly absorbed sugars, liquid calories (sodas, juices, sports drinks, or vitamin waters),[2] and refined carbohydrates (bread, pasta, rice, and potatoes), your cells slowly become resistant or numb to the effects of insulin, and need more and more of it to keep your blood sugar levels balanced. This problem is known as **insulin resistance.** A high insulin level is the first sign of a problem. Unfortunately, most doctors never test this. The higher your insulin levels are, the worse your insulin resistance. As the problem worsens, your body starts to lose muscle, gain fat, become inflamed, and you rapidly age and deteriorate. In fact, insulin resistance is the single most important phenomenon that leads to rapid and premature aging and all its resultant diseases, including heart disease, stroke, dementia, and cancer.[3, 4]

High levels of insulin tell your body to gain weight around the belly, and you become more apple-shaped over time. Insulin, the fat storage hormone, also drives more inflammation and oxidative stress, and myriad downstream effects including high blood pressure, high cholesterol, low HDL, high triglycerides,[5] poor sex drive, infertility, thickening of the blood, and increased risk of cancer, Alzheimer's, and depression.

Hypoglycemia (low blood sugar) is often an early symptom of insulin resistance. If you skip meals or eat too much sugar or refined carbs, you will experience swings in blood sugar that make you feel anxious, irritable, tired, and can even cause palpitations and panic attacks. Stuffing down a big cinnamon bun or swigging a 20-ounce soda will cause big spikes in sugar and insulin and a quick surge in energy, followed by the inevitable crash as your blood sugar plummets. Eventually your cells become so resistant to insulin that your blood sugar stays up and your pancreas can't produce enough insulin to fight against the high blood sugar and your numb cells. That's when you cross the line to diabetes.

Diabesity can be prevented, treated, and reversed. But new and better drugs or procedures are *not* the solution. Diabesity will not be cured by a pill or surgery. Blockbuster drugs such as Avandia fail in their promise and often cause harm. Gastric bypass surgery has increased from 10,000 to 200,000 per year in the last decade. But how many of the 1.7 billion overweight citizens of the world can undergo gastric bypass? And how many of those will gain back most of the weight they lost?

Our current problem-solving tools, methods of diagnosis, and way of treating patients are still based on nineteenth- and twentieth-century ideas about the origins of disease and overlook the complex web of biology as well as the social, political, and economic conditions at the root of our current chronic disease epidemic.

Chronic disease results from imbalances in our biology that occur as a result of the interactions between our genes and our environment. We first must focus on the causes (poor diet, stress, toxins, microbes, allergens) that disturb our whole system. We must understand and work with the network of our biological systems that become imbalanced because of the effects of the environment in which we live. We must use a new map to navigate chronic disease, one that is based on a new model of treating chronic illness. This map is called **functional medicine** (www.functionalmedicine.org). It is a way of treating the causes, not just the risk factors; of treating the whole system, not just the symptoms; of creating health, not just treating disease. In fact, if you focus on creating health rather than treating disease, the disease often takes care of itself. Disease goes away as a side effect of getting healthy.

3

Seven Myths About Obesity
and Diabetes That Keep Us Sick

Many of the notions we hold to be true about disease
are, in fact, misconceptions or falsehoods. This is
especially true of diabetes and obesity. Before we can
go beyond simply treating symptoms and risk factors,
we must examine and give up the myths of diabetes.

MYTH 1: DIABETES IS GENETIC

We have been led to believe that diabetes is a genetic
disorder, that if we have a family history of diabetes
we are more likely to get it, and that diabetes is essentially a random genetic event over which we have no
control.

The truth is quite different.

As I mentioned earlier, from 1983 to 2008 the number of people in the world with diabetes increased sev-

enfold, from 35 million to 240 million (and I believe this is actually a serious underestimate). Change of this magnitude could not happen with a purely genetic or inherited disorder in such a short time. The genetic code of the human population changes only 0.2 percent every 20,000 years. It is not altered from generation to generation. What many people don't realize is that our genes *are* affected by our environment. Our genetic code itself may not change, but the way those genes are *expressed* is highly influenced by the world around us. And our environment has changed more in the last hundred years than in all of previous human history.

In truth, diabetes is almost entirely induced by environmental and lifestyle factors. While there are some predisposing genes, those genes get turned on (or "expressed") only under conditions of poor diet, sedentary lifestyle, stress, and exposure to environmental toxins. Therefore, a search for the diabetes gene and the magic bullet drug or gene therapy to treat it will lead us nowhere. Scientists who have examined the human genome for the obesity and diabetes gene have been disappointed.[1] While understanding our genes and the predispositions they give us can help us personalize our approach to metabolism and weight loss, they can shift our focus away from the most important target: the modifiable lifestyle and environmental factors that are driving this epidemic. **How we eat, how much we exercise, how we manage stress, our exposure to environmental and food-based toxins, and the structural violence or "obesogenic environment" that influences these factors are what is truly driving our diabesity epidemic.**

The collection of environmental, dietary, and lifestyle exposures we each experience has been called the "exposome."[2] The exposome, which affects our genetic expression, in the end may be much more important in determining health or disease than our actual genome. It is becoming increasingly clear that 90 percent of our disease risks are due to differences in environment, not genes.[3] Looking at the things that wash over our genes from outside sources (air, water, diet, drugs, organic pollutants, heavy metals, radiation, and physical or psychological stressors) and from internal processes (inflammation, free radical production and oxidative stress, allergens, infections, and even gut flora) gives us insight into the origins of and the cure for our chronic disease epidemic. Changing your exposome is the foundation of *The Blood Sugar Solution*.

The exposome directly influences our genes, resulting in changes in gene function or expression that lead to the disordered biological state of diabesity. The genetic code itself doesn't change, but which parts of this code are expressed *does* change.

This is an important idea. We can't change our genes, but we can change their function and expression. The collective experience of our lives—our intrauterine environment, diet, toxins, microbes, allergens, stresses, social connections, thoughts, and beliefs—controls which genes are turned on or off. It also controls the quality and type of proteins produced by our DNA, as well as what happens to those proteins and how they function once they are produced.

More striking is that if your DNA is tagged by an environmental factor, those alterations in genetic expression can be passed down through generations. The way in which our genes are tagged or turned on or off by our exposome is called "epigenetics." The "epigenome" becomes inheritable. If your grandmother ate too much sugar, or smoked, or was exposed to mercury from too much sushi, she may have "turned on" genes that lead to diabesity. Her epigenome, which carries increased risk of disease, would then be passed down from generation to generation. This does mean your risk is increased, but it's far from being a death sentence.

Your genes provide the instruction book for all the proteins in your body, which control your physiology and biology. You may have a genetic predisposition to diabetes or obesity, but you are not predestined. Every moment, you have the power to transform your gene expression and reverse disease by changing the messages and instructions you send to your DNA. You can "turn off" the genes your grandmother "turned on" generations ago.

For those who are still not convinced and believe that diabetes is genetic, let me tell you the story of the Pima Indians of Arizona. After living for centuries in a harsh desert environment, in the early 1900s they were plunged into a Western culture and food environment. Their traditional diet was essentially plant-based—whole grains, squash, melons, legumes, beans, and chilies—supplemented by gathered foods, including mesquite, acorns, cacti, chia, herbs, and fish. Although the diet was high in carbohydrates, they were low-glycemic carbs—which means they converted into sugar in their bodies relatively slowly and did not lead to high blood sugar levels. Within one generation, the Pimas switched to a diet rich in sugar, sodas, white flour, trans fats, and processed foods. This is a diet I call the "white menace"—white sugar, white flour, and white fat (shortening). They went from being thin and fit with no obesity, diabetes, or heart disease in their population to being the second most obese population in the world. Eighty percent of Arizona Pimas have diabetes by the time they are thirty years old, and they are lucky to live to age forty-six. Pima children as young as three or four are getting adult-onset diabetes and need cardiac bypass surgery by the time they are twenty.

The diabesity epidemic in the Pimas is not due to a recent genetic mutation. They sent their ancient, desert-dwelling genes a different set of instructions. **Food is not just calories. It is information,** and the typical American high-glycemic-load diet turned on the Pimas' diabesity genes.

They didn't have much of a choice about this. You do. This affects not only the poor or Native American populations, but all of us. Obesity takes nine years off the life of the average person,[4] and obesity in adolescents creates the same risk of premature death as heavy smoking.[5]

Have no doubt: Diabesity is not a genetic disorder in the strictest sense. While it's true that the genes you inherited from your parents or grandparents may put you at greater risk, that doesn't necessarily mean you *must* get diabesity. The condition is a *direct* outcome of dietary, lifestyle, and environmental factors turning on all the wrong genes. It is about a bad "exposome," not bad genes. You can turn these genes off, and *The Blood Sugar Solution* will show you how.

MYTH 2: DIABETES IS NOT REVERSIBLE

Most of us are taught that diabetes is not reversible and that we are destined to suffer progressive decline in function, including heart disease, kidney failure, blindness, amputation, strokes, and dementia. We also believe that it is nearly impossible to treat obesity or to be able to maintain long-term weight loss. We think that the only treatment options are to limit the consequences and reduce the complications.

However, there is clear evidence from the scientific literature that diabetes *is* reversible, especially if it is caught in the early stages and treated aggressively through lifestyle intervention and nutritional support, and occasionally with medications.[6] Even most later-stage diabetes can be reversed with very intensive lifestyle changes, medications, and supplements.

A groundbreaking study[7] showed unequivocally that even people with advanced type 2 diabetes, when the pancreas has pooped out and the insulin-producing (beta) cells are damaged, can recover and diabetes can be reversed in just *one week* through dramatic changes in diet (a very low-glycemic, low-calorie, plant-based diet). In the study, patients' blood sugars plummeted, triglyceride levels fell, and the pancreas recovered (measured by sophisticated MRI techniques). After just one week, they were taken off their medication, proving that diabetes is not a progressive, incurable condition. And the diet was more powerful than medication; yes, it may take a lot of work to reverse diabetes, but your body can heal given the right conditions. In *The Blood Sugar Solution,* I will show you how to do this.

But most doctors don't catch diabetes in the early stages. Doctors typically measure a person's fasting blood sugar — the level of glucose present in a blood sample drawn a minimum of eight hours after the last meal. A recent study showed that anyone with a fasting blood sugar of over 87 mg/dl was at increased risk of diabetes. Yet most doctors are not concerned until the blood sugar is over 110 mg/dl or, worse, 126 mg/dl, the level that technically signals diabetes. But diagnosing problems with insulin resistance and blood sugar control at this point occurs too late in the game. In fact, your **blood sugar is the last thing to go up.** Your **insulin spikes first,** and despite being the simplest way to detect problems early, doctors rarely order the two-hour glucose tolerance test, which measures not only glucose but also insulin levels at fasting and one and two hours after a sugar drink — a much more effective way to catch problems before the onset of disease. (See the online guide *How to Work with Your Doctor to Get What You Need* at www.bloodsugarsolution.com to learn what tests to ask for and how to interpret them.)

I recommend early testing for anyone who has a family history of type 2 diabetes, belly fat or increased waist size, or abnormal cholesterol. The blood sugar quiz at the beginning of the book, and the more detailed diabesity quiz in Part III, can help you understand your risk and act early. Don't wait until your sugar is high. That would be too late.

If you have already reached the very late stage of type 2 diabetes when your pancreas has been damaged, you can still experience extraordinary gains in health and vitality if you treat the problem with a whole-systems approach like the one outlined in this book. Remember: Diabetes can be reversed.[8]

MYTH 3: PRE-DIABETES ISN'T A PROBLEM UNTIL IT TURNS INTO FULL-BLOWN DIABETES

The most important idea in this book is that **pre-diabetes is *not* "pre" anything.** It is a deadly disease driving our biggest killers—heart attacks, strokes, cancer, dementia, and more.

A Heart Attack Is Not "Pre" Anything: A Patient's Story

John learned the truth about pre-diabetes the hard way. He was a forty-nine-year-old salesman who had spent his career going from job site to job site. One day, after ten years of eating fast food on the run, John experienced that dreaded crushing chest and left arm pain. The heart attack got his attention, along with the angiogram and the need for two stents to open his clogged arteries. He came to me wondering what had happened. He thought he was healthy, albeit a little overweight. He didn't have high blood pressure or diabetes and his cholesterol was normal at 173. What he didn't know was that he had pre-diabetes, and his doctor had not picked it up in his yearly physical.

His diet was pretty typical for an American male—fast food, burgers, fries, sodas, and chips, and he drank at least two beers a day. The only green things he ate were green M&Ms. Over ten years, during which he suffered a stressful relationship and the death of his mother, he gained 50 pounds and his waist went from 32 to 36 inches. His blood tests showed normal blood sugar and cholesterol, but a very low good cholesterol, or HDL, of 34 mg/dl (ideal is greater than 60 mg/dl). He also had a fatty liver caused by his sugary processed diet. When we looked a little deeper, we found that after a sugar drink (which is the best way to test for pre-diabetes and diabetes), his insulin and blood sugar skyrocketed—a clear sign of pre-diabetes. We also found he had dangerous small, dense cholesterol particles, even on Lipitor, and high levels of mercury (he lived on the Gulf and ate a lot of fish). His omega-3 fats (EPA and DHA), which help normalize blood sugar, improve insulin sensitivity, and reduce the risk of heart disease, were low even though he ate fish.

By the time I saw him, he was on a cabinetful of medication, including a beta-blocker (which made him tired), and a whopping 80 mg, or eight times the starting dose, of Lipitor (which can cause more insulin resistance and increase the risk of diabetes). Statins such as Lipitor also lower coenzyme Q10, which is needed for cells to make energy and burn calories. He was put on a blood pressure pill (ACE inhibitor) and two blood thinners (Plavix and aspirin). He lost a few pounds right after his heart attack but still had a long way to go.

I put him on *The Blood Sugar Solution*. Over the course of a year, he went from a fast-food-eating, soda-drinking, pill-popping, big-bellied guy to a thin, fit, healthy man. He lost 62 pounds and gained 30 years of life. He took up running and got healthier and healthier. We gave him special nutrients to improve insulin sensitivity, including chromium, biotin, alpha lipoic acid, vitamin D3, PGX (a special fiber to lower blood sugar, insulin, and cholesterol levels), and fish oil. I also gave him high-dose niacin (vitamin B3) to raise his good cholesterol and turn his dangerous small, dense LDL particles into light, large, fluffy ones. I corrected the deficiency of coenzyme Q10. We boosted his liver detoxification with n-acetyl-cysteine and helped his body get rid of the mercury. We helped him thin his blood with natural blood thinners.

After a year, he was no longer on any of the medication he'd started on — no Lipitor, no blood pressure meds, no blood thinners — and all his numbers were better than when he was actually on the medication. His blood sugar was 93, his total cholesterol went from 173 mg/dl on the Lipitor to 137 mg/dl off the Lipitor, while his good cholesterol went from 34 mg/dl to 58 mg/dl and all his particles were light and fluffy. These are better results than any medication can achieve. His fatty liver was healed, and at fifty years old, he was healthier than ever.

John's heart attack happened because of his pre-diabetes. In fact, one study found that about two-thirds of all patients admitted to the emergency room with heart attacks had pre-diabetes or undiagnosed diabetes.[9] Another important study found that the risk of heart attack increases with any increase in average blood sugar, even for those who don't have diabetes.[10] Taking statins and beta-blockers, which actually cause insulin resistance, would not have corrected John's pre-diabetes.

Many people believe that pre-diabetes isn't a problem until it becomes full-blown diabetes, that it is just a warning sign. Nothing could be farther from the truth. It is an earlier stage of diabesity that carries with it nearly all the risks of diabetes. Pre-diabetes can kill you before you ever get to diabetes, through heart attacks, strokes, and even cancer.

Pre-diabetes can even cause "pre-dementia" or mild cognitive impairment—think of it as early Alzheimer's.[11] Recent studies have shown that diabetics have a fourfold increased risk of developing Alzheimer's, and patients with pre-diabetes or metabolic syndrome have a dramatically increased risk of pre-dementia or mild cognitive impairment (MCI). You don't even have to have diabetes to have brain damage and memory loss from high insulin levels and insulin resistance. Just having pre-diabetes can give you pre-dementia. Alzheimer's disease is actually being called type 3 diabetes today.[12] Recent studies have found that as your waist size goes up, the size of your brain goes down.[13] Your brain function is also impaired. One extraordinary brain imaging study by Dr. Daniel Amen and his colleagues found that obesity was associated with decreased blood flow in your frontal cortex (the portion of your brain that controls executive decision making—"should I have that doughnut right now or not?").

And if that isn't bad enough, pre-diabetes can cause impotence in men and infertility in women (it can be related to polycystic ovarian syndrome).

So if your doctor has diagnosed you with pre-diabetes or metabolic syndrome, don't think that you are only at risk for something "in the future," such as diabetes or heart attack. The problems are happening right now.

MYTH 4: ONCE YOU START ON INSULIN, THERE IS NO GOING BACK

Insulin treatment in diabetes is a slippery slope, because increased insulin dosage often leads to increased weight gain, higher blood pressure, and elevated cholesterol. Remember, insulin is a fat storage hormone that also drives appetite and inflammation. Blood sugar improves, but overall risk of heart disease does not. That is why insulin should be the last resort in managing blood sugar and diabetes. And if you have to be on insulin, get on the lowest dose possible. Eating whole, real, fresh food and exercising vigorously will keep your blood sugar low and your insulin needs down.

The good news is that, with aggressive lifestyle

intervention and dietary change, you can reverse diabetes and stop insulin therapy under your doctor's supervision.[14] Many of my patients and my colleagues' patients have successfully gotten off insulin. By understanding and treating *all* the underlying causes of diabetes, the possibility exists of not only eliminating insulin treatment, but also reversing diabetes and insulin resistance.

This is not seen as much in conventional medical care, because the type of diet and lifestyle intervention advice is not adequate or properly designed to create a reversal of diabetes. It is possible with the right treatment approach, based on functional medicine, and new models of group care and community support that teach sustainable behavior change and nutritional life skills (including cooking, shopping, exercise, and mind-body skills).

MYTH 5: LOWERING BLOOD SUGAR WITH MEDICATION PREVENTS DEATH AND HEART ATTACKS IN DIABETICS

Avandia, the world's number one blockbuster diabetes drug, contributed to the deaths of 47,000 people from heart disease in the first eleven years of its use (this data was hidden from the government and the public most of that time). We have to give up on the hope for the magic pill that will fix our problems.

Large drug trials have attempted to prove that targeting risk factors such as cholesterol or blood sugar levels with drugs reduces the risk of heart disease, diabetes, and death. Despite hundreds of millions of research dollars spent over many decades, aggressive risk factor treatment of the two most important targets—cholesterol and blood sugar—has consistently failed to show benefit in preventing disease (although treatment may be helpful if you have already had a heart attack).

Recent large trials published in the *New England Journal of Medicine*[15, 16, 17, 18] have confirmed that by treating risk factors with drugs, not only may we be ineffective in preventing heart attacks, diabetes, and death, but we may also be creating harm by ignoring the root causes of disease. Chronic disease is not due to a drug deficiency. High cholesterol is not a Lipitor deficiency. High blood sugar is not an Avandia deficiency. Isolating one risk factor, or even separately treating multiple risk factors, will fail until it is done in the context of addressing the upstream drivers of disease.

Everyone loves the idea of popping a pill to fix the problem. Cardiologists advocate handing out statins at fast-food restaurants. Taking Lipitor at the same time you're consuming a cheeseburger, fries, and soda misses the point. Those foods kill you in ways that have nothing to do with your cholesterol—they make you insulin resistant, and they don't give you the fiber, vitamins, minerals, and antioxidants that real food does. What's worse, new research shows that statins don't work for prevention, even though over 75 percent of prescriptions are given to prevent heart disease. They do work to prevent a second heart attack, but not the first one. The independent Cochrane Collaboration[19] performed a comprehensive review of the research using statins to prevent heart disease by examining fourteen major studies involving 34,000 patients at low risk for a heart attack. They found little or no benefit. If you haven't already had a heart attack, these drugs won't help you prevent one, despite misleading drug ads or doctors' advice.

In addition to the Cochrane Review, many other studies also support this and point out the frequent and significant side effects that come with taking these drugs.[20] In 10–15 percent of the patients who take them, they cause muscle damage, cramps, weakness, and aches; exercise intolerance[21] (even in the absence of pain and elevated CPK, or muscle enzymes); sexual dysfunction; liver and nerve damage; and other problems.[22] They also can cause significant cellular, muscle, and nerve injury and cell death in the *absence* of symptoms.[23]

A study published in the *Journal of the American*

Medical Association examined five major clinical trials on statins including 32,752 nondiabetics over 4.9 years. During the study period, 2,749 patients (or 8.4 percent) developed diabetes.[24] Those on the highest doses of statins (which are increasingly prescribed by physicians) were at the highest risk of developing diabetes. If all doctors followed the latest cholesterol treatment guidelines, and all their patients took their prescribed statin medication, there would be 3.5 million more diabetics in America. Oops.

There is no lack of research calling into question the benefits of statins. Unfortunately, that research doesn't get the benefit of the billions of dollars of marketing and advertising that statins do.

Should diabetics not try to control their blood sugar? Yes, they should. It is clear that elevated blood sugar causes small vessel injury leading to blindness, kidney damage, nerve damage, and cataracts. And the major causes of death in diabetics are heart disease, heart attacks, and strokes. But these problems are best addressed not through medication, but by treating the root causes.

It is the elevated levels of insulin that cause high blood pressure, abnormal cholesterol, and inflammation, not high blood sugars.

Lowering your blood sugar without addressing

the underlying causes gives you a false sense of security and leads you to believe that you are doing something good to prevent heart attacks and early death. Unfortunately, the evidence shows otherwise.

Tragically, insurance doesn't usually pay for the right treatment—intensive lifestyle therapy (although I believe this soon will change). No one profits from lifestyle medicine, so it is not part of medical education or practice. It should be the foundation of our health care system, but doctors ignore it because they get paid to dispense medication and perform surgery. They should be paid to develop and conduct practice-based and community programs in sustainable lifestyle change.

The future of medical care must be to transform general lifestyle guidance—the mandates to eat a healthy diet and get regular exercise that many physicians try to provide to their patients—into individually tailored lifestyle prescriptions for both the prevention and the treatment of chronic diseases.

And delivering lifestyle interventions through small groups is the most powerful way to create sustainable behavior change. Remember, it is easier to get healthy together. Lifestyle is often the best medicine when applied correctly, and it is the only thing that will get us started on the road to reversing this global health crisis.

MYTH 6: HEART SURGERY AND ANGIOPLASTY ARE GOOD TREATMENTS FOR DIABETICS WITH HEART DISEASE

A study in the *New England Journal of Medicine* showed that surgery and angioplasty for diabetics with heart disease work no better than medication in reducing heart attacks and death, and have higher risks.[25]

How Unproven Treatments Can Kill: A Patient's Story

Dan's dad was diabetic. He had the best medical, pharmaceutical, and surgical care available. Nevertheless, he suffered from very poor health. He went to the emergency room with chest pain and was quickly shuttled into the cath lab for an angiogram. He was told he needed a cardiac bypass operation, even though research evidence has shown no reduced mortality for cardiac bypass or angioplasty in diabetics. Not providing effective treatment is one thing, but providing harmful, costly, and ineffective treatment like this is unethical.

After the bypass, Dan's father developed a postoperative infection of MRSA (an antibiotic-resistant killer staph bacteria) in his sternum, which led to a month in the intensive care unit; plastic surgery to repair the chest defect left after surgeons removed his infected sternum; and "ministrokes," which led to pre-dementia[26] and a protracted recovery from hospitalization, requiring months of home care.

The surgery and subsequent therapy with blood thinners and cholesterol and blood-pressure-lowering medications did not enhance the quality of his health and life. In fact, he declined rapidly physically and mentally and died of a stroke.

Dan's father was not offered the treatment that would have cost less than 2 percent of the $400,000 his care cost, and would have likely created an infinitely enhanced quality of life by actually reversing the underlying causes of his diabetes and heart disease. If he were simply provided the choice of a different treatment—an individual or group program for sustainable and comprehensive lifestyle change, based on the principles in *The Blood Sugar Solution*—perhaps he would still be alive and our national debt would have been reduced by $400,000. It should be our right to have access to proven treatments that provide better value for the individual and for the health care system.

MYTH 7: WEIGHT LOSS IS NECESSARY FOR THE REVERSAL OF DIABETES

At an American Diabetes Association convention in New York City, the main booth front and center in the convention hall presented a breakthrough "cure" for diabetes—the surgical treatment of diabetes with gastric bypass surgery. Unfortunately, I have seen many patients who gained back all the weight they lost, and more, after gastric bypass. My patient Alan, for instance, had been overweight since he was six years old and never experienced a day without ravenous hunger. At forty years old, he had a gastric bypass and went from 450 pounds to 250 pounds, but then gained back 100 pounds. At sixty years old, Alan was sick and tired, and he had to deal with all the complications of gastric bypass surgery.

Gastric bypass is touted as a solution for obesity; in fact, the number of gastric bypass surgeries performed each year has increased tenfold in 10 years to about 230,000 a year—at $30,000 a pop. While this approach works for some, clearly it's not the answer for our epidemic of diabesity. It often fails, and it can cause many complications, including vomiting and nutritional deficiencies.

Shrinking someone's stomach to the size of a walnut with surgery is one way to battle obesity and may be lifesaving for a few, but it doesn't address the underlying causes. And many will regain the weight because they didn't change their understanding of their bodies or relationship to food.

Clearly, weight loss is critical and important for obtaining optimal health. However, what we are finding in patients who have gastric bypass surgery is that even a dramatic change in diet in a short period of time creates dramatic metabolic changes. All the parameters that we thought were related to obesity, such as high blood sugar, high cholesterol, high blood pressure, inflammation, and clotting, are dramatically reduced even *without* significant weight loss because of the rapid effects of dietary changes that control which genes get turned on or off.[27] This is called *nutrigenomics*—the way food talks to your genes. While weight loss is important, what's *more* important is the quality of food you put in your body—food is information that quickly changes your metabolism and genes.

The converse is also true, as we learned in a study in the *New England Journal of Medicine* that discussed a woman who had 20 kilos (more than 40 pounds) of abdominal fat removed by liposuction.[28] She showed no changes in any of her metabolic markers of obesity, including blood sugar, cholesterol, blood pressure, and inflammation. Despite losing 20 kilos, she was still sick.

The take-home message is that the *quality of the*

food we put in our bodies drives our gene function, metabolism, and health. It is not simply a matter of your weight, or calories in/calories out. Eating powerful, gene-altering, whole, real, fresh food that you cook yourself can rapidly change your biology. You will lose weight, by getting your systems in balance, not by starving yourself. *The Blood Sugar Solution* is like getting a gastric bypass without the pain of surgery, vomiting, and malnutrition.

4

Food Addiction: Fixing Your Brain Chemistry

Whatever happened to old-fashioned willpower? Everybody knows that the obesity epidemic is a matter of personal responsibility. People should exercise more self-control. They should avoid overeating and reduce their intake of sugar-sweetened drinks and processed food. There are no good foods or bad foods; it's everything in moderation. Right?

This sounds good in theory, except for one thing...

New discoveries in science prove that processed, sugar-, fat-, and salt-laden food — food that is made in a plant rather than grown on a plant (as Michael Pollan, author of *In Defense of Food,* would say) — is biologically addictive.

Remember the old potato chip commercial with the tag line "Bet you can't eat just one"? Bet you can't imagine that kind of commercial for broccoli or apples. No one binges on those foods. Yet it's easy to imagine a mountain of potato chips, a whole bag of cookies, or a pint of ice cream vanishing quickly in an unconscious, reptilian-brain eating frenzy. Broccoli is not addictive, but chips, cookies, ice cream, and soda can become as addictive as any drug.

In the 1980s, First Lady Nancy Reagan championed the "just say no" approach to drug addiction. Unfortunately, that approach hasn't fared too well — and it won't work for our industrial food addiction either. There are specific biological mechanisms that drive addictive behavior. Nobody chooses to be a heroin addict, cokehead, or drunk. Nobody chooses to have a food addiction either. These behaviors arise from primitive neurochemical reward centers in the brain that override normal willpower and, in the case of food addictions, overwhelm the ordinary biological signals that control hunger.

Why is it so hard for obese people to lose weight despite the social stigma, despite the health consequences such as high blood pressure, diabetes, heart disease, arthritis, and even cancer, and despite their intense desire to lose weight? It is not because they *want* to be fat.

It is because in the vast majority of cases, certain types of food — processed foods made of sugar, fat, and salt combined in ways kept secret by the food industry—are addictive. We are biologically wired to crave these foods and eat as much of them as possible.

ARE YOU ADDICTED?

While some of us may be more genetically predisposed to the addictive properties of food (or heroin or alcohol), if you examine your own behavior and your relationship to sugar in particular, you will likely find that your behavior around sugar matches up perfectly with why you can't control your diabesity. Use the scale below, developed by researchers from Yale's Rudd Center for Food Policy and Obesity,[1] to determine if you have a food addiction.

If you find yourself scoring 3 or higher, or answering yes to more than two of the questions, you may be suffering from food addiction.

Based on these psychological criteria and new neurological research, many of us, including most obese children, are "addicted" to industrial food.[2]

Let's review some of the scientific findings confirming that food can, indeed, be addictive:

1. Sugar stimulates the brain's pleasure or reward centers through the neurotransmitter dopamine exactly like other addictive drugs.[3]

2. Brain imaging (PET scans) shows that high-sugar and high-fat foods work just like heroin, opium, or morphine in the brain.[4]

Circle the number that best matches the level of your behavior: 0 = never, 1 = once a month, 2 = two to four times a month, 3 = two to three times a week, and 4 = all the time.

1. I find that when I start eating certain foods, I end up eating much more than planned.	0 1 2 3 4
2. I find myself continuing to consume certain foods even though I am no longer hungry.	0 1 2 3 4
3. Not eating certain types of food or cutting down on certain types of food is something I worry about.	0 1 2 3 4
4. I find that when certain foods are not available, I will go out of my way to obtain them. For example, I will drive to the store to purchase certain foods even though I have other options available to me at home.	0 1 2 3 4

(Continued)

5. There have been times when I consumed certain foods so often or in such large quantities that I started to eat food instead of working, spending time with my family or friends, or engaging in other important activities or recreational activities I enjoy.	0 1 2 3 4
6. I have had withdrawal symptoms such as agitation, anxiety, or other physical symptoms when I cut down or stopped eating certain foods. (Please do not include withdrawal symptoms caused by cutting down on caffeinated beverages such as soda pop, coffee, tea, energy drinks, etc.)	0 1 2 3 4
7. I have consumed certain foods to prevent feelings of anxiety, agitation, or other physical symptoms that were developing. (Please do not include consumption of caffeinated beverages such as soda pop, coffee, tea, energy drinks, etc.)	0 1 2 3 4

8. My behavior with respect to food and eating causes significant distress.	0 1 2 3 4
9. I experience significant problems in my ability to function effectively (daily routine, job/school, social activities, family activities, health difficulties) because of food and eating.	0 1 2 3 4

IN THE PAST 12 MONTHS	No	Yes
10. My food consumption has caused significant psychological problems such as depression, anxiety, self-loathing, or guilt.	0	1
11. My food consumption has caused significant physical problems or made a physical problem worse.	0	1
12. Over time, I have found that I need to eat more and more to get the feeling I want, such as reduced negative emotions or increased pleasure.	0	1

(Continued)

13. I have tried to cut down or stop eating certain kinds of food.	0	1
Total		

3. Brain imaging (PET scans) shows that obese people and drug addicts have lower numbers of dopamine receptors, making them more likely to crave things that boost dopamine. This is, in part, genetically determined.

4. Foods high in fat and sweets stimulate the release of the body's own opioids (chemicals like morphine) in the brain.

5. Drugs we use to block the brain's receptors for heroin and morphine (naltrexone) also reduce the consumption and preference for sweet and high-fat foods in both normal-weight and obese binge eaters.

6. People (and rats) develop a tolerance to sugar—they need more and more of the substance to satisfy themselves; this is true of drugs such as alcohol or heroin.

7. Obese individuals continue to eat large amounts of unhealthy foods despite severe social and personal negative consequences, just like addicts and alcoholics.

8. Animals and humans experience "withdrawal" when suddenly cut off from sugar, just like addicts detoxifying from drugs.
9. Just like drugs, after an initial period of "enjoyment" of the food, the user consumes it not to get high but to feel normal.

Remember the movie *Super Size Me,* in which Morgan Spurlock ate three meals from McDonald's every day? What struck me about that film was not that he gained 24.5 pounds, or that his cholesterol went up, or even that he got a fatty liver. What was surprising was the portrait it painted of the addictive quality of the food. At the beginning of the movie, after he ate his first supersized meal, he threw it up, just like a teenager who drinks too much alcohol at his first party. By the end of the movie, he only felt "well" when he ate that junk food. The rest of the time he felt depressed, exhausted, anxious, and irritable and lost his sex drive, just like an addict or smoker withdrawing from his drug. The food was clearly addictive.

The problem of food addiction is compounded by the fact that food manufacturers refuse to release any internal data on how they put ingredients together to maximize consumption of their products, despite requests from researchers. In his book *The End of Overeating,* David Kessler, MD, the former head of the Food and Drug Administration, describes the science of how food is made into drugs—through the creation of hyperpalatable foods that lead to neurochemical addiction.

THE SPECIAL CASE OF LIQUID CALORIES

Liquid sugar calories are the most addictive "food" in our diet. Sugar-sweetened beverages are a unique category of food. Aside from being the single biggest source of added sugar in the diet, sugary drinks drive diabetes and obesity in ways that solid food (even solid junk food) doesn't.[5] And many of these beverages are also loaded with caffeine, which compounds their addictive properties.

Why are sugar-sweetened drinks so bad for us?[6] Here are a few good reasons:

1. If you drink your calories in sweetened beverages, you don't reduce your solid calories to compensate. So not only are these empty calories, but they're extra calories you normally wouldn't eat.
2. From 1977 to 2002, consumption of calories in sugar-sweetened beverages doubled and is the main source of added sugar calories to our diet.
3. During that time period, obesity rates doubled in children ages two to eleven and tripled in adolescents from ages twelve to nineteen.[7]

4. More than 90 percent of American children and teenagers drink sodas every day. Liquid calories account for up to 10–15 percent of the total daily calorie consumption of the average teenager.

5. The average consumption of sugar-sweetened beverages is 175 calories a day. Since these calories are in addition to calories from solid food, this would add 18 pounds to the average person's weight each year.

6. Each can of soda consumed by children per day increases their risk of being overweight by 60 percent.[8] Soft drinks are the largest source of added sugar to children's diets. Researchers from Harvard's Children's Hospital showed in a randomized trial that, if provided with easy access to alternatives to sugar-sweetened beverages, kids would reduce their intake of sugar-sweetened drinks by 82 percent and have significant weight loss.[9]

7. In the Nurses' Health Study of 91,249 women, those who had one sugar-sweetened soft drink had an 82 percent higher risk of having diabetes over 4 years. Those who drank fruit punch doubled their risk of developing diabetes.[10]

8. Other studies also link sugar-sweetened drinks to pre-diabetes, diabetes (particularly in African-Americans),[11] and heart disease.[12]

9. A review of over 30 studies, published in the *American Journal of Clinical Nutrition,* found clear evidence that drinking sugar-sweetened beverages led to weight gain.[13]

Bottom line: When you drink your calories, you don't feel full, so you end up eating more overall.

A large study by Harvard scientists, funded by the Centers for Disease Control and the Robert Wood Johnson Foundation, found that if people drank water instead of sodas, they would consume 225 fewer calories a day (equivalent to about one soft drink).[14] In a year, that is 82,123 fewer calories. That amounts to a weight loss of 24 pounds a year just by switching to non-sugar-sweetened drinks.

What should we be drinking? Water. Tap water. Filter it, chill it, squeeze a little lemon juice in it, and enjoy it. We have been brainwashed to think we can't drink just water, but it is what we are made of and it will help you lose weight. In fact, researchers found that drinking water before meals increases weight loss by about 44 percent.[15]

There is ample proof that sugar-sweetened drinks are harmful to our health. But even if they weren't, shouldn't manufacturers of these products have to prove that they are safe rather than expect under-funded scientists to prove they are harmful?

There have been some studies that found little or

no association between weight gain and sugar-sweetened beverages.[16] However, many of these studies were funded by the food industry, including the American Beverage Association (formerly known as the American Soft Drink Association). In fact, a 2007 review of more than 206 scientific studies found that if the food industry funded the study, there was up to an eightfold likelihood of the study findings proving favorable to the food industry.[17]

A little-known fact is that many food industry goliaths banded together to form the Center for Consumer Freedom,[18] which has created a media campaign stating that the obesity epidemic is a hoax. They tell us, "Don't believe your eyes; believe us." Owing to "privacy concerns," the website won't reveal its funders. Investigators discovered that Coca-Cola, PepsiCo, Kellogg, Kraft, and others were behind this but wanted to remain anonymous because, as reported on the website, they are afraid of food fascists — those vegetable-eating, organic-gardening militia groups. Oh my!

Under the food stamp program (SNAP), the U.S. Department of Agriculture spends $4 billion a year on soda for the poor. That buys almost 30 million servings a day or over 10 billion servings a year of corn-sugar-sweetened drinks. The government (our taxes) pays now and pays later through ballooning Medicaid and Medicare costs for obesity- and

Diet Drinks: Helpful or Harmful?

If you are thinking that diet soft drinks are the answer, think again. Diet drink consumption has increased 400 percent since 1960. They may or may not cause cancer, but the evidence is mounting that they lead to weight gain rather than weight loss. Those who consume diet drinks regularly have a 200 percent increased risk of weight gain, a 36 percent increased risk of pre-diabetes or metabolic syndrome, and a 67 percent increased risk of diabetes. A study of over 400 people found that those who drank two diet sodas a day had five times the increase in waist circumference as those who did not drink soda.

Seems you can't outsmart Mother Nature. Fooling your brain into thinking you are getting something sweet plays dirty tricks on your metabolism. Artificial sweeteners disrupt the normal hormonal and neurological signals that control hunger and satiety (feeling full). A study of rats that were fed artificially sweetened food found that their metabolism slowed down and they were triggered to consume more calories and gain more weight than rats fed sugar-sweetened food.[19]

In another alarming study, rats offered the choice of cocaine or artificial sweeteners always picked the artificial sweetener, even if the rats were previously programmed to be cocaine addicts. The author of the study said that, "[t]he absolute preference for taste sweetness may lead to a re-ordering in the hierarchy of potentially addictive stimuli, with sweetened diets...taking precedence over cocaine and possibly other drugs of abuse."[20]

The use of artificial sweeteners, as well as "food porn," the sexy experience of sweet, fat, and salt in your mouth, alters your food preferences. Your palate shifts from being able to enjoy fruits and vegetables and whole foods to liking only the sexy stuff.[21]

My advice is to give up stevia, aspartame, sucralose, sugar alcohols such as xylitol and malitol, and all of the other heavily used and marketed sweeteners unless you want to slow down your metabolism, gain weight, and become an addict.

diabetes-driven disease. They won't revise their policy because they say it's discriminatory to prevent the purchase of soda. To whom: the poor or industrial food and agriculture?

THE "SODA TAX"

Thomas Frieden, director of the Centers for Disease Control, and Kelly Brownell of Yale University authored an article in the *New England Journal of Medicine* advocating for a penny-an-ounce tax on sugar-sweetened beverages, known around the country as the "soda tax." Just as taxing cigarettes has reduced smoking, it is estimated this tax would reduce soda consumption by 23 percent a year. The 10-year savings in health care costs would be $50 billion. The increased revenue to strapped state governments would be $150 billion a year.

Now, taxing sugar-sweetened beverages would not eradicate obesity, but liquid calories are proving to be a clear target for public health intervention. Doing this could generate revenue for obesity prevention and treatment programs and reduce soda consumption. Funds from this initiative could be earmarked for community programs to address obesity in adults and children, especially for the poor.

This would cost nothing and have immediate impact. It could "supersize" the efforts of Michelle Obama, who only has $400 million to fight childhood obesity. The American Beverage Association, led by Coca-Cola and Pepsi, spent $1 million in lobbying against this idea in 2000. In 2009, they spent $20 million. If they didn't think it would affect policy or consumption, they wouldn't fight it. Their own internal studies show that when Coke increased prices by 12 percent, their sales dropped 14.6 percent.

We *can* alter the default conditions in the environment that foster and promote diabesity and addictive behavior. It's simply a matter of public and political will. If we don't, we will face an ongoing epidemic of obesity and illness across the nation and the globe.

If pushed, Big Farming can start growing healthy food to feed the nation, and Big Food can come up with innovative solutions that satisfy consumers and supply healthful, economical, convenient, and delicious foods for our world. However, these industries will *not* police themselves. And if the foods they market are addictive, what are the ethical, legal, and moral implications of allowing these food pushers unrestricted access to our children?

5

How Big Food, Big Farming, and Big Pharma Are Killing Us

What is the driving force behind all the cheap, low-quality foods that are little more than combinations of fat, sugar, and salt and, as we saw in the last chapter, have proven to be as addictive as any drug?

Junk food produced from and made cheap by government subsidies such as the 2010 Farm Bill are heavily marketed (to the tune of $30 billion a year) by mega–food corporations such as Altria (formerly known as Philip Morris–Kraft), ConAgra, Cargill, Tyson, Sara Lee, Unilever, General Mills, Kellogg, Coca-Cola, and PepsiCo. Government subsidization is how a Twinkie with thirty-nine different ingredients and a hefty marketing budget can cost less than a head of broccoli.

These processed foods are heartily consumed by our ever-widening population, driving obesity rates up to nearly three out of four Americans. The more they eat, the fatter they become. The fatter they become, the more they develop heart disease, diabetes, cancer, and a myriad of other chronic ailments. The sicker our population, the more medications are sold by Big Pharma for high cholesterol, diabetes, high blood pressure, depression, and many other lifestyle-driven diseases. One of the leading products of the American food industry has become patients for the American health care industry. The toxic triad of Big Farming, Big Food, and Big Pharma profits from a nation of sick and fat citizens. The government essentially stands in line next to you in fast-food chains helping you buy cheeseburgers, fries, and cola.

But in the produce aisle of your supermarket, you are on your own. The 2010 Farm bill provided $42 billion in subsidies to Big Farming to encourage the production of cheap sugar (from corn) and fats (from soy beans). It did not offer support for farmers to grow fruits, vegetables, or healthy whole foods. Aside from subsidies for corn, sugar, and wheat, the Farm bill does almost nothing to support the production of whole, fresh, local, seasonal, or organic produce.

That's one reason why everywhere you look—in stores, schools, and government institutions and food programs—you find cheap, high-calorie, nutrient-poor processed foods (or "food-like substances"). It's becoming increasingly difficult to avoid making food choices that drive obesity, especially when the price of fruits and vegetables has increased five times as fast as sugar-sweetened beverages.

It's not a coincidence that the poorest states, such as Mississippi, in our country are also the fattest. Poverty makes it impossible to make the best food choices, and poverty rates are higher than they have been in a generation. Not only are healthier foods almost always more expensive, they are often not available in poorer neighborhoods. This combination of factors is a direct link to obesity and diabetes.

Our government has not been very helpful in these areas. Its focus has been on education (e.g., the food pyramid or the new "my plate" initiative) and on encouraging personal responsibility rather than on regulating Big Food. Government actions are at best anemic. In 2011, the Federal Trade Commission (FTC) and other government agencies announced new food marketing guidelines.[1] The agencies would like Big Food to refrain from marketing foods to children with trans fats or more than 15 percent saturated fat, 210 milligrams of sodium, or 13 grams of added sugar per serving. But this was only a suggestion of guidelines that the FTC encouraged the food industry to consider implementing in five years. That's like suggesting tobacco companies consider not marketing cigarettes to children in five years. We need tougher policies, not buckling to lobbying interests.

The food industry has decided to preempt any food-labeling regulations that would give consumers real, credible information about the disease-causing or health-promoting effects of their products. At the request of the Centers for Disease Control, the Institute of Medicine, an independent scientific body, came out with food-labeling recommendations in late 2011. That is why in early 2011, two major food-industry trade associations, the Grocery Manufacturers of America (GMA) and the Food Marketing Institute, announced a new and voluntary nutrition-labeling system. Major food and beverage companies will use it on the front of packages to "help busy consumers make informed choices." Or to confuse the heck out of them. Their system lists the percents of various nutrients at their discretion. Most nutrition experts would have a hard time figuring out if the food was healthy or not, and that is the intent. In Europe, the red, yellow, and green labeling system provides consumers with an easy way to quickly assess their food choices. But the mantra of the food industry is that there are no bad foods. Nonsense. The science is clear—trans fats and high-fructose corn syrup are bad. So are pharmacological doses of sugar.

The general public, too, seems to prefer that government not regulate what we eat. We accept that the government mandates auto safety regulations and that the FDA oversees drug safety, so why are we so resistant to oversight for the food and farming industries? After all, poor diet causes many more deaths than auto accidents. We certainly can't leave it to the Toxic Triad to police themselves. It didn't work for Big Tobacco; why would it work for them?

THE CAUSES OF AN OBESOGENIC ENVIRONMENT

There is an element of blaming the victim in all of this that misses the environmental conditions that drive obesity and disease and lead to what is now being called an "obesogenic" environment. There are five main factors:

1. **Industrial processed, fast food, and junk food are addictive.** As we've seen, these foods are biologically addictive and drive excess calorie consumption.
2. **Big Farming's influence increases obesity around the world.** Surplus crops from the United States are sold cheaply to poor countries, which in turn destroys local farming economies and displaces farmers, creating unemployment

and making developing nations dependent on imported processed food and corn syrup.

3. **Unethical, manipulative food marketing drives eating habits.** There is very little government control over Big Food's marketing practices, especially in marketing to children. The government licenses the airwaves but doesn't police them.

4. **Families are not eating home-cooked meals together.** Family mealtime has disappeared in much of America. There are many reasons for this, but it's been helped along largely by the proliferation of convenience or fast foods. This has led to a generation of Americans who have trouble recognizing vegetables and fruits in their original form and can't cook except in a microwave.

5. **Environmental toxins abound.** These contribute to weight gain, obesity, and diabetes. We have to worry about not only what we eat but also the burden of plastics, metals, and pollutants that have been shown to poison and slow our metabolism and lead to weight gain.

To really change our obesogenic environment, we need to create healthier choices for everyone. We must focus on specific actions we can take personally, politically, and in our communities to alter our food landscape.

FOOD MARKETING PRACTICES: ARE THEY ETHICAL, MORAL, OR LEGAL?

Big Food takes advantage of the glut of processed food in our country to drive up profits through the use of mass media technologies. Other than drinking sugar-sweetened beverages, the number of hours of screen time is the single biggest factor correlating with obesity. The average American spends nine and a half hours a day in front of a screen, mostly television. In addition to the metabolism-slowing, hypnotic effect of watching television, relentless food marketing targeted to children is one of the major factors driving this problem. The average two-year-old can identify, by name, junk food brands in supermarkets, but many elementary school children can't readily differentiate between a potato and a tomato (as Jamie Oliver demonstrated in his television program, *Food Revolution*).

Think about this: If processed and junk foods are addictive, and we are pushing our children to consume them, what are the moral, ethical, and legal implications?

The Robert Wood Johnson Foundation is the largest organization working to address the epidemic of childhood obesity. They spend $100 million a year on public education and programs. How long do you think it takes the food industry to spend that amount on marketing processed and junk food to children? Four days. By January fourth each year, the largest funder fighting the battle against obesity is out of cash, leaving the food industry the rest of the year to push their "drugs."

The average child sees 10,000 ads for junk food on television a year. The food industry spends $13 billion a year marketing their products to children. Adding to the television onslaught, there are now product placements in toys, games, education materials, songs, and movies; celebrity endorsements; and stealth campaigns using word of mouth, text messaging, and the Internet. The food industry proudly uses terms such as "stealth," "viral," and "guerrilla" marketing to describe their practices on Facebook, YouTube, and Twitter, and in product placements in popular television shows such as *American Idol,* during which all the judges are drinking Coke, thanks to a multimillion-dollar deal with the show. The worse the food, the more companies spend on marketing.

These activities do an end run around conventional marketing as well as societal and parental controls. If you spoke to your child before every meal about healthy eating, you couldn't compete with the onslaught of coercive messaging from industry. A Yale study found that kids who watched food ads ate 50 percent more of the snacks placed in front of them. The visual stimuli trigger the brain to eat more. Snacking (an American invention) is seen as fun, exciting, and ultimately the source of happiness.

Dr. Kelly Brownell and his group from Yale's Rudd Center for Food Policy and Obesity published data showing that the breakfast cereals with the worst nutritional value had the most advertising (www.cereal facts.org). We stopped Joe Camel. We also need to stop this type of marketing. It is unfair at best; drug dealing at worst.

However, the government is shy about regulating food advertising. In 1978, the Federal Trade Commission ruled that sugary drink commercials were unethical, because they promoted tooth decay. The beverage industry lobbied Congress, and Congress, in turn, chose not to give the FTC money that year. The FTC was stopped in its tracks since it didn't have the funds to push forward with this legislation. The result? In the United States, food advertising to children knows almost no bounds. Yet in many other countries, including Sweden, Norway, and the United Kingdom, food advertising to children is banned.

The Center for Science in the Public Interest brought a lawsuit against Coca-Cola for deceptive marketing practices of its "Vitamin Water" product. Coke hired celebrities like Kobe Bryant and Lebron James to tout its healthful effects. At 125 calories a bottle (drinking one bottle a day would make you gain about 10 pounds in a year), the minuscule amount of vitamins in the bottle is irrelevant compared to the sugar. The lawsuit is based on the Jelly Bean Rule, which prohibits companies from selling junk foods with minimal health benefits by marketing them as healthy foods. The lawyers for Coca-Cola are defending the lawsuit by asserting that "no consumer could reasonably be misled into thinking Vitamin Water was a healthy beverage." Astounding. They defend themselves by saying that no one could be stupid enough to believe their ads that this is actually a healthy drink. Just ask some average teenagers what they think.

In 2005, the Institute of Medicine (IOM) published its report on *Food Marketing to Children and Youth: Threat or Opportunity?*[2] They reviewed more than 123 peer-reviewed studies addressing the links between food marketing and children's preferences, requests, consumption, weight gain, and diabetes. IOM was not permitted to review any internal research done by the food industry. Instead the organization performed research focused on children, including preschoolers, to ferret out the psychological drivers of food choices. The resulting report from IOM documents the comprehensive and deliberate effort made by the food industry to find ways to exploit the suggestibility of children. Remember, they are selling not just Nintendos but substances that are proven to be addictive and cause obesity, diabetes, heart disease, and cancer.

The IOM concluded that we need to "turn food and beverage marketing forces toward better diets for American children and youth." Some food companies appear to promote health and exercise programs and limit access to sugary drinks in schools, but they "fall far short of their full potential." While the food industry agreed to remove sugary drinks from schools under pressure from the Clinton Foundation, they later modified the agreement to allow "vitamin waters" and "sports drinks," erasing whatever gains were made in making schools healthier.[3] A recent study found that replacing sodas in school vending machines with "sports drinks" had zero impact on weight or health. It was good public relations, but just led to bigger profits for big food companies and bigger waist sizes for kids. Big Food will not voluntarily sacrifice profits or change their foods or practices. Its primary method for increasing profits is to get people to eat more. The IOM advises that "Congress should enact legislation mandating the shift [in food marketing practices]."

Big Food and the government's response to studies like these is that "individual choice" drives decisions—that people can choose for themselves how much unhealthy food they can or should consume. However, there are significant problems with this stance. In the first place, processed food is addictive. And research in behavioral economics shows that even when people think they are making free and rational choices, they are not.[4] The addictive biology, pervasive advertising, cheap prices, and other social and environmental factors all work together to shape our food preferences.

Americans support change: 72 percent of New Yorkers support a tax on sugar-sweetened beverages if the money is used for obesity prevention and treatment programs; 69 percent support changes in school nutrition; and 51 percent support an outright ban on junk food advertising.[5]

WHAT WE CAN DO TO CREATE A HEALTHIER NATION AND WORLD

Our global health and economic crisis is blamed on the personal sins of sloth, gluttony, and a weak will. The scientific evidence and a deeper examination of political and corporate policies and behaviors does not support this indictment of the individual. This is all to say that while you may suffer from diabesity, it is *not* your fault. It's not that you are simply weak-willed. Resolving these problems will require community, social, and political changes that foster and encourage healthy choices.

This starts with personal action and community

organization. Creating a healthier world is a revolutionary act, one you can start right now. Remember the words of Margaret Mead: "Never doubt that a small group of thoughtful, committed citizens can change the world; indeed, it's the only thing that ever has."

In the next chapter you will learn how a new science-based model of health care called functional medicine can be the lever for a sea change in how we approach illness and take back our health by addressing the causes of imbalances in our interconnected biological and social systems.

6

Functional Medicine: A New Approach to Reverse This Epidemic

The way modern medicine operates is like trying to diagnose what's wrong with your car by listening to the noises it makes instead of looking under the hood. We often miss the problems right in front of us. Most doctors would guarantee 100 percent that you don't have pre-diabetes if you have a normal blood sugar (under 100 mg/dl) or a normal glucose tolerance test (when your blood sugar is measured 2 hours after a sugary drink). Unfortunately they are 100 percent wrong. That's because they don't look under the hood.

Many of my patients have perfectly normal blood sugars but sky-high insulin levels and every other metabolic breakdown that goes with pre-diabetes, yet when they come to see me, most have not been diagnosed with pre-diabetes. Even with the limited conventional approach of diagnosing pre-diabetes as a blood sugar over 100 mg/dl and a 2-hour glucose tolerance over 140 mg/dl, 90 percent of people who currently have the condition are not diagnosed. This is because doctors don't measure insulin.

Think about it for a minute — the most common chronic disease in America, the country with the "best" health care in the world, is *not* diagnosed in 90 percent of people who have it.

FUNCTIONAL MEDICINE: THE FUTURE

My goal in medicine is to help provide a way to navigate and sort through health information based on an entirely new way of thinking about health and disease. I want to find the right treatment for each person, regardless of what that treatment might be. If a medicine is the best treatment, I will choose that; if a change in diet, supplements, herbs, or lifestyle works best, then I will choose that. We must learn to treat the person, not the disease; *the system,* not just the symptoms. This is personalized medicine, the medicine of the future.

An understanding of the body's basic systems, how they get out of balance, and how to get them back in balance allows us to create an individualized program for each person. Ralph Snyderman, MD, of Duke University, calls this "P4 Medicine," or "Prospective Medicine"—personalized, preventive, predictive, and participatory (meaning that you have to actively participate in your own care).[1]

This is also known as patient-centered health care, rather than disease-focused medicine, and it is a fundamental underpinning of **functional medicine**—a revolutionary new way to understand the underlying causes of disease and how our genes, our environment, and our lifestyle interact to determine health or disease.

In functional medicine, we want to answer the question "Why?"—not just "What is the right drug for this disease?" The question isn't "What disease do you have?" but "Which system or systems in your body are out of balance?" The goal is to understand what disturbs the normal function of these systems, and how we can best create optimal function. I am not so much interested in helping patients get perfect lab tests, because, as we have seen, these don't tell the whole story. I'm interested in helping them identify how the particular systems in their bodies are working or not working, and then how we can get them into balance.

This must be done by treating the whole system,

not the symptom. It is like treating the soil, not the plant. Just as there is no need for fertilizer or pesticide if the soil is healthy, there is no need for medication if your body is healthy.

THE CONTINUUM OF DISEASE: A MORE HELPFUL WAY TO DIAGNOSE ILLNESS

Most medicine today is based on clear-cut, yes-or-no diagnoses that often miss the underlying causes and subtler manifestations of illness. Most conventional doctors are taught that you either have a disease or you don't; you have diabetes or you don't. There are no gray areas.

Practicing medicine this way is plainly misguided because it misses one of the most fundamental laws of physiology, biology, and disease: **the continuum concept.** There is a continuum from optimal health to hidden imbalance to serious dysfunction to disease. Anywhere along that continuum, we can intervene and reverse the process. The sooner we address it, the better.

For example, when it comes to diabesity, most doctors just follow blood sugar, which only rises very late in the disease process. If your blood sugar is 90 or 110, you don't have diabetes. If it is over 125, you do have diabetes. But these distinctions are completely arbitrary, and they do nothing to help treat impending problems. I remember one patient, Daren, who came to see me with mildly elevated blood sugar. I asked Daren if he had seen his doctor about this, and he said yes. I then asked, "What did your doctor say?" Daren's doctor had told him, "We are going to watch and wait until your blood sugar is more elevated, and then we are going to treat you with medication for diabetes."

This attitude is absurd and harmful in the face of what we know about the problems that occur even in the absence of full-blown diabetes. And it completely ignores subtler clues from symptoms and signs of disease, which may highlight underlying metabolic imbalances (especially when further testing is done). These imbalances may be remedied by the appropriate treatment—treatment that is not focused on some disease, but instead works to balance the system by removing those things that alter or damage our functioning and providing those things that enhance, optimize, and normalize our function.

That attitude is also why diabesity is so woefully and inadequately diagnosed and treated, leaving millions of Americans suffering needlessly from chronic symptoms.

THE IMPORTANCE OF EARLY DIAGNOSIS

The truth is that the road to diabetes can start in childhood.[2] In fact, we are now seeing an epidemic of type 2 diabetes in children as young as eight years old.[3] Pediatric diabetes specialists, who for years took care of only type 1 diabetes, an autoimmune disease, now have their offices overwhelmed with type 2 diabetes, a lifestyle and environmental disease. By the time you're diagnosed with diabetes, you have problems with insulin and blood sugar that could have been detected 20–30 years earlier. That is, if you knew where to look, which most doctors are not trained to do.

Insulin resistance and the diabesity associated with it are often accompanied by increasing belly fat, fatigue after meals, sugar cravings, blood sugar swings or hypoglycemia, high triglycerides, low HDL, high blood pressure, low sex drive, problems with blood clotting, and increased inflammation. These clues can often be picked up long before you ever get diabetes, and may help you prevent diabetes entirely. If you have a family history of obesity (especially around the belly), diabetes, early heart disease, or even dementia or cancer, you are even more prone to this problem.

Fortunately, many people with pre-diabetes

never get diabetes. Unfortunately, they are at severe risk of disease and death just the same.

The fact is that both the symptoms and the long-term complications of diabetes and insulin resistance overlap. The classic diabetic symptoms of excess thirst, urination, and weight loss are specific to diabetes, but *all* the other warning signs (blood sugar and insulin imbalances, for example) are there for many years before those telltale symptoms crop up. We could eliminate many of the long-term complications of diabesity if we simply addressed these warning signs and diagnosed the problem much earlier in the process.

All the phenomena that we see in diabesity are the results of the same thing: imbalances in the seven key systems in your body that form the web or network of your biology. Understanding this web is the basis of functional medicine,[4] a method of treatment grounded in a whole new scientific field called systems biology, which seeks to understand how systems in the body are interconnected rather than as simply discrete organs and body parts that have no relationship to one another. The perspective of medical specialization — organizing medicine by organs and diseases, by geography (location) and symptoms — is flawed and has placed modern medicine at a crisis point.

Our way of thinking about disease is outdated and does not take advantage of the latest scientific advances. Functional medicine, on the other hand, implements the best of current science and systems thinking.

THE SEVEN STEPS TO ULTRAWELLNESS

Over the last twenty years an emerging body of scientific knowledge that forms the foundation of the functional medicine approach has pointed to a number of factors that are the true drivers of diabesity and all chronic disease, but they are not the things we usually think of as causing these conditions.

There are seven fundamental systems in your body that can get out of balance. To heal from diabesity, or overcome any of the other chronic illnesses you suffer from, you must rebalance these seven key systems. In Part II, we will explore the imbalances in these systems and how to correct them:

- Step 1: Boost Your Nutrition
- Step 2: Regulate Your Hormones
- Step 3: Reduce Inflammation
- Step 4: Improve Your Digestion
- Step 5: Maximize Detoxification
- Step 6: Enhance Energy Metabolism
- Step 7: Soothe Your Mind

In Parts III and IV, I will provide you with a comprehensive program for rebalancing these systems. Along with my plan to Take Back Our Health (Part V), this personalized approach will allow you to leverage the latest science so you can heal from this modern plague.

PART II

THE SEVEN STEPS TO TREATING DIABESITY

Between the health care that we have now and the health care that we could have lies not just a gap, but a chasm.

— Committee on Quality of Health Care
in America,
Institute of Medicine, 2001

We can't solve problems by using the same kind of thinking we used when we created them.

— Albert Einstein

7

Understanding the Seven Steps

I often joke that I am a "wholistic" doctor because I take care of patients with a "whole list" of problems. Typically when someone has multiple complaints and they ask their doctor about them, they get told, "We can only deal with one problem at this visit." Or they get referred out to a half-dozen different specialists — one for the skin rash, one for joint pain, one for reflux, one for migraines, and so on. No one asks, "How is everything connected?" It's no wonder that the average Medicare patient has six doctors and is on five medications.

The trick is to see the connections. When the seven systems are out of balance, illness occurs, whether it's weight gain, diabetes, heart disease, cancer, or anything that may be on your "whole list." The key is not to treat each thing separately, but to look for and treat the fundamental underlying causes.

In pre-diabetes, diabetes, and all other diseases, imbalances, symptoms, and illness occur because of just a very few things that cause disease.

THE REAL CAUSES OF DISEASE

In addition to single-gene genetic disorders, there are just **five causes of all disease:** poor diet, chronic stress, microbes, toxins, and allergens, all of which wash over our DNA causing changes in our gene expression, and turning off or on different genes and messages that affect our metabolism. The five causes interact with the seven key systems in the body. When those systems are out of balance, symptoms occur and doctors diagnose diseases.

And there are just **a few "ingredients"** needed to make a healthy human — real, whole, fresh food, nutrients (vitamins and minerals), light, water, air, sleep, movement, rhythm, love, connection, meaning, and purpose.

When you take out the bad stuff and put in the good stuff, the body knows what to do and creates health. Disease goes away as a side effect of creating health.

The approach functional medicine takes to disease is not a new treatment or modality or specialty or technique. It is not integrative or alternative medicine. It is the future of medicine — applying new discoveries in biology about how we really get sick and how we can create health. It is about treating your whole system, not the symptom. It applies the most advanced science in a practical clinical method in the service of our health. It is a way of thinking that focuses on the question of "why," or the cause, and not just "what," or the name of the disease.

The names of your diseases become irrelevant when we understand the causes. In fact, one factor can cause dozens of "diseases." Take celiac disease—an allergic and autoimmune reaction to gluten. It can show up as rheumatoid arthritis, diabetes, heart disease, cancer, inflammatory bowel disease, depression, autism, osteoporosis, and more. On the other hand, one disease, such as dementia, can have many causes, including B12 deficiency, viruses, insulin resistance, and heavy metal toxicity.

Imagine that you go to the doctor and say you have no energy, you feel sad, helpless, hopeless, you can't sleep, and you have no interest in food or sex.

Your doctor will probably say, "Oh, I know what's wrong with you. You're depressed. You need an anti-depressant." But "depression" is just a label we give to that collection of symptoms. It tells you nothing about what caused the symptoms.

The symptoms of depression could result from an emotional trauma; an autoimmune reaction to gluten that causes low thyroid function; vitamin B12 deficiency because you are taking an acid blocker that prevents its absorption; vitamin D deficiency because you live in Seattle; inflammation in your gut from taking too many antibiotics that kill the normal flora; a high body burden of mercury because you love fish; an omega-3 deficiency because you hate fish; or insulin resistance because you eat too much sugar. The diagnosis and treatment of each of those causes is very different. The same is true for obesity and diabetes and any of the thousands of symptoms labeled as "diseases" in our medical books.

We now have a system of classifying disease based on the location or geography in your body (heart, joint, stomach) and by symptoms. There are over 12,000 diagnoses now, and in the new classification system we will have 155,000 different diseases. This is nonsense. Functional medicine recognizes that almost all disease arises out of imbalances in the few key systems of your body (the seven steps) that occur when you have too much of something (toxins, microbes, allergens, poor diet, stress) or not enough of something (real, whole food, nutrients (vitamins and minerals), light, water, air, sleep, movement, rhythm, love, connection, meaning, and purpose).

Seeing the connections and teasing apart the real causes of disease is how I helped Evelyn.

Evelyn's Story: Seeing Connections, Identifying Causes

Evelyn, a forty-eight-year-old woman, came all the way across the country from Northern Canada to get help, because after seeing twelve doctors over ten years and being diagnosed with twenty-nine different "diseases," she didn't get any answers or any better. She was over 237 pounds and had a BMI of 37 (35 is considered morbidly obese).

Evelyn had a "whole list" of problems that we found when we looked under the hood. Rather than organizing them by disease or medical specialty, by location or symptoms, we organized them based on understanding the body as a whole system.

All her symptoms were connected, but no one connected the dots. She had:
- Irritable bowel syndrome
- Reflux
- Hypertension
- Hypoglycemia
- Metabolic syndrome
- Obesity
- Hypothyroidism
- Polycystic ovarian syndrome (PCOS)

- Environmental allergies/postnasal drip
- Latex allergy
- Frequent yeast infections
- Osteoarthritis
- Migraines
- Fibromyalgia
- Chronic pain
- Chronic fatigue syndrome
- Headache
- Migraines
- Frequent weight fluctuations
- Bulimia and anorexia
- Binge eating disorder
- Kidney stones
- Gout
- ADD
- Asthma
- Chronic sinusitis
- Sleep apnea
- Psoriasis
- Depression/anxiety
- Infertility

What she really had were some basic imbalances caused by her diet. She was eating too much gluten (an allergen), she had too much yeast and toxic bacteria in her gut (microbes), and she had several nutritional deficiencies. This triggered systemic inflammation, leading to weight gain and pre-diabetes, as well as an autoimmune disease of her thyroid, which had not been diagnosed.

I organized her symptoms by the seven key systems, and then figured out what was causing the imbalances.

She had **Hormone/Metabolic/ Neurotransmitter Imbalances:**

- Insulin resistance (pre-diabetes) and obesity
- Hypoglycemia
- Hypertension
- Frequent weight fluctuations
- Bulimia and anorexia
- Binge eating disorder
- Polycystic ovarian syndrome (PCOS)
- Hypothyroidism
- Estrogen toxicity
- Irregular menstrual bleeding
- Premenstrual syndrome
- Uterine fibroids
- Depression and anxiety
- Migraines
- Gout
- ADD
- Sleep apnea
- Infertility

She had **Immune/Inflammatory Imbalances:**

- Food allergies
- Chronic sinusitis and postnasal drip
- Environmental allergies
- Asthma
- Rosacea
- Psoriasis
- Vaginal/yeast infections
- Mold exposure
- Edema or swelling of her legs
- Osteoarthritis

She had **Digestive Imbalances:**

- Irritable bowel syndrome
- Bloating after meals
- Small intestinal bacterial overgrowth
- Yeast overgrowth
- Reflux

She had **Detoxification Imbalances:**

- Fibromyalgia
- Chronic fatigue
- Multiple chemical sensitivities
- Edema
- High body burden of toxins and mercury
- Mercury amalgam fillings
- Kidney stones

She had **Energy Imbalances:**

- Chronic pain

And she had **Nutritional Imbalances:**
- Vitamin D deficiency
- Magnesium deficiency
- Zinc deficiency

I started by treating the five systems within which she was experiencing imbalance, not all of her twenty-nine separate diseases.

We began by simply cleaning up her diet—she started a whole foods low-glycemic-load diet without gluten or dairy. We cleared out the bad bugs in her gut with antibiotics and treated the yeast with antifungals. I gave her some digestive enzymes and probiotics to help normalize her gut.

I then helped her get her hormones back in balance. I suspected she had a low-functioning thyroid even though doctors had told her that her tests were normal (I learned in medical school to treat the patient and not the test), so I gave her a low dose of Armour® Thyroid, a type of natural hormone replacement therapy. Her symptoms of premenstrual syndrome, heavy bleeding, and fibroids told me she had too much estrogen and not enough progesterone. So I gave her magnesium, vitamin B6, and hormone-balancing herbs. I also gave her support for improving her blood sugar and insulin with PGX (a super fiber), a multivitamin with extra chromium, biotin, and alpha lipoic acid, and I prescribed a high dose of vitamin D3 (5,000 units a day because she lived in Northern Canada).

Six weeks later I got her lab results back. They confirmed what I had thought—she had very high antibodies to gluten, which triggered inflammation and an autoimmune reaction in her body, including in her thyroid gland. She had high uric acid, which causes gout and results from too much sugar and high-fructose corn syrup.[1] This is a classic sign of insulin resistance and pre-diabetes. Her blood tests showed very high insulin and blood sugar two hours after a sugar drink, and her sex hormones were out of balance. And she had very low vitamin D of 16 ng/dl.

At our six-week phone call, she told me she was doing great. I went down the list of symptoms expecting some ongoing issues, but after struggling for ten years, she had no more symptoms. *None.* No more fibromyalgia, chronic fatigue syndrome, brain fog, or depression; no more sinus problems or congestion; no more irritable bowel or reflux; no more migraines; no more PMS, heavy bleeding, or feeling tired and cold all the time. Even her psoriasis and rosacea had gone away. And as a nice side effect, she lost 21 pounds without even trying! The same things that make you sick make you fat, so when you address the underlying causes of disease, the weight loss is automatic.

___

Not all of my patients have a list as long as Evelyn's, but the approach is the same: Focus on identifying and treating the underlying causes of disease and helping the body's systems, and the disease (and weight loss) takes care of itself.

DISCOVERING YOUR IMBALANCES: PERSONALIZING THE BLOOD SUGAR SOLUTION

In each chapter in Part II, I provide quizzes to help you identify which systems in your body are out of balance. Is it your hormones, your gut, your immune system? Are you toxic? Which system is causing you the most problems? These quizzes are based on three factors:

1. Decades of clinical experience and testing of more than 10,000 patients
2. A review of thousands of scientific papers
3. Collaboration with many of the physicians at the forefront of functional medicine and science.

The quizzes will help you identify where you are out of balance and guide you to restoring balance in each of those systems.

Everyone who has diabesity will go on the basic foundational *Blood Sugar Solution* diet and lifestyle program as outlined in Part IV. However, depending on the answers you give in the quizzes in Part II, you may need to add a few extra "self-care" steps to personalize the program. You will do this in Week 6. If you do, follow the recommended personalization of your plan in Part IV. For the majority of you, *The Blood Sugar Solution* and a little self-care will solve your problems. You will be able to accomplish these steps on your own or with others through the online support program and guidelines for creating social support that is detailed in Part IV. You can learn more about our online community and access a set of free tools to help you through the program (including an online version of all the quizzes in Part II) at www.bloodsugarsolution.com.

A few of you may score in the "medical care" range on the quizzes. In this case, you should complete *The Blood Sugar Solution* basic and self-care program starting in week 6. Then retake the quizzes after another six weeks on the self-care plan. If your score still indicates "medical care" or you don't see the improvement you'd like, it may mean you have deeper problems that require more diagnostic testing and medical treatment. In this case, I have provided a detailed online companion guide called *How to Work with Your Doctor to Get What You Need.* This guide, which you will find at www.bloodsugarsolu tion.com, outlines information on how to get the special laboratory tests needed to confirm or investigate suspected imbalances and guidelines for correcting these imbalances. I have also provided resources for you to find a doctor who is aware of or experienced in functional medicine and can be your partner in health at www.bloodsugarsolution.com.

I strongly encourage you to visit the website now and take advantage of all the information, tools, and community support available as you start on your journey to healing.

Now let's explore the seven key biological systems at the root of diabesity, starting with nutrition.

8

Step 1: Boost Your Nutrition

Our current American diet is a problem both for what it contains — too much sugar, processed fats, salt, additives, hormones, pesticides, and genetically altered inflammatory proteins — and for what it doesn't contain — omega-3 fats, fiber, magnesium, zinc, B and D vitamins, antioxidants, and more. Except for most omega-3 fats, all these come from a plant-based diet. Plants contain nearly all the vitamins, minerals, antioxidants, phytonutrients, and fiber in our diet. These are essential for keeping our biology in balance and, in particular, for regulating our metabolism and weight.

The paradox today is that the most obese children and adults are also the most nutritionally deficient.[1] Rickets and scurvy are now being seen in obese children. Most of us don't realize that the more calories you eat, the more nutrients you need — vitamins and minerals are the grease that lubricate the wheels of our metabolism and help all the chemical reactions in our bodies run properly, including those involved in regulation of sugar and fat burning. Our current diet is energy dense (too many calories) but nutrient poor (not enough vitamins and minerals). All these "empty calories" we consume cause our metabolisms to break down and disease and obesity to flourish.

The leading cause of diabesity is our SAD (Standard American Diet). Whole, real, fresh food that you cook yourself is the most potent medicine you can use to prevent, treat, and reverse diabesity.

Overfed and Undernourished: A Patient's Story

Sarah, a nineteen-year-old girl, walked into my office with a "whole list" of complaints, including obesity, fatigue, and muscle pain. She had been sick and fat since she was eight years old. While many factors contributed to her poor health, her poor-quality diet (high in sugar, junk food, fast foods full of trans fats and high-fructose corn syrup) led to nutritional deficiencies that compounded her health and weight problems. The only colorful food she ate was Cheetos. The sugar and caffeine in sodas depleted her magnesium levels. And because she had hated fish her whole life, she had a severe omega-3 fat deficiency. She was so tired and sick that she never went outside; sitting on the couch watching television led to a serious vitamin D deficiency.

Slowly we got her off her junk food, sugar, and caffeine. We corrected her nutritional deficiencies with both diet and supplements of magnesium, fish oil, and vitamin D. Over the course of six months her muscle pain went away, she got her energy back, and she lost 54 pounds.

Our nutrient-poor, calorie-rich diet is the main factor driving the epidemic of diabesity. It has led to a nation of overfed but undernourished people. In this chapter we will look at some of the major dietary shifts that have led to the diabesity epidemic. Then I will explain the exciting new science of **nutrigenomics,** which promises to help us cure the problem by seeing food not just as calories or energy to burn but as **information** that provides instructions to our genes to gain or lose weight, get sick or get healthy.

But before we get to that, take the following quizzes to see where your nutritional imbalances lie. Take all the quizzes in Part II before you start the program and again after the six weeks are over to measure the "before and after" change in your health. You may need extra individualized support based on your scores; I explain this in Week 6 of the plan (see Chapter 24).

BOOST YOUR NUTRITION QUIZZES

There are several important nutritional deficiencies that can lead to diabesity. The following quizzes will help you determine which you suffer from.

Magnesium Quiz

Magnesium is the relaxation mineral and helps regulate blood sugar. The following quiz will help you learn if you are deficient. For any symptom you have experienced in the last month, place a check in the "Before" box. Then find out how severe your problem is by using the scoring key below. Place a check in the "After" box after you've completed the six-week program to see how much you've improved.

	Before	After
I have a low intake of dark green leafy vegetables, kelp, wheat bran or germ, almonds, cashews, and buckwheat.		
I am tired often.		
I have trouble falling asleep or have insomnia.		
I am sensitive to loud noises.		

(Continued)

	Before	After
I have fewer than two bowel movements a day.		
I have asthma.		
I experience muscle twitching.		
I experience leg or hand cramps.		
I frequently experience headaches or migraines.		
I have premenstrual syndrome most months.		
Swallowing is sometimes difficult for me.		
I have restless leg syndrome.		
I have acid reflux.		
I frequently feel irritable.		
I am depressed.		
I am anxious.		
I have attention deficit disorder		
I have a lot of stress in my life.		
I am autistic.		
I have kidney stones.		
I experience heart flutters, skipped beats, or palpitations.		
I have heart disease or heart failure.		

	Before	After
I have mitral valve prolapse.		
I have diabetes.		
TOTAL		

Score	Severity	Care Plan	Action to Take
0–3	You may have a slightly low level of magnesium.	*The Blood Sugar Solution*	No personalization needed. Simply complete *The Blood Sugar Solution.*
4–12	You may have a moderately low level of magnesium.	Self-Care	Complete *The Blood Sugar Solution* and optimize your magnesium levels by following the steps in Chapter 24.
13+	You may have a severely low level of magnesium.	Medical Care	Do both of the above steps and see a physician for additional assistance if you are not better after the first six weeks of the program.

Vitamin D Quiz

Over 80 percent of Americans are deficient in vitamin D. The quiz below will help you learn if you are low in vitamin D. For any symptom you have experienced in the last month, place a check in the "Before" box. Then find out how severe your problem is by using the scoring key below. Place a check in the "After" box after you've completed the six-week program to see how much you've improved.

	Before	After
I work indoors.		
I hardly ever go out in the sun.		
I wear sun block most of the time.		
I have seasonal affective disorder (SAD) or the winter blues.		
My home is north of Florida.		
I have dark skin (any race other than Caucasian).		
I am sixty years old or older.		
I don't eat small fatty fish such as mackerel, herring, sardines (the main sources of dietary vitamin D).		
My muscles are sore or weak.		

	Before	After
My bones are tender. (Press on your shin bone — if it hurts, you are vitamin D deficient.)		
I have osteoarthritis. (Vitamin D deficiency weakens bones and leads to deterioration.)		
I have osteoporosis.		
I have broken more than two bones or fractured a hip.		
My mental sharpness and/or memory are not what they used to be.		
I have an autoimmune disease (e.g., multiple sclerosis).		
I seem to have more infections than most people I know.		
I have prostate cancer.		
Total		

Score	Severity	Care Plan	Action to Take
0–3	You may have a low level of vitamin D.	*The Blood Sugar Solution*	No personalization needed. Simply complete *The Blood Sugar Solution.*

(Continued)

Score	Severity	Care Plan	Action to Take
4+	You may have a severely low level of vitamin D.	Medical Care	Do the above step and see a physician for additional assistance if you are not better after the first six weeks of the program.

Essential Omega-3 Fatty Acids Quiz

Over 90 percent of Americans are deficient in omega-3 fats, which are critical to control inflammation, blood sugar, and metabolism. The quiz below will help you find out if you need an oil change. For any symptom you have experienced in the last month, place a check in the "Before" box. Then find out how severe your problem is by using the scoring key below. Place a check in the "After" box after you've completed the six-week program to see how much you've improved.

	Before	After
My skin is dry, itchy, scaling, or flaking.		
My nails are soft, cracked, or brittle.		

	Before	After
I have dandruff.		
I have hard earwax.		
I have tiny bumps on the backs of my arms or on my trunk.		
I am thirsty most of the time.		
My joints feel achy or stiff.		
I have fewer than two bowel movements a day.		
My stool is light-colored, hard, or foul-smelling.		
I am depressed, have ADD/ADHD, and/or memory loss.		
My genetic background is Irish, Scottish, Welsh, Scandinavian, or coastal Native American.		
I have fibrocystic breasts.		
I suffer from premenstrual syndrome almost every month.		
My blood pressure is higher than it should be.		
My LDL cholesterol is too high, my HDL cholesterol is too low, and my triglycerides are high.		
TOTAL		

Score	Severity	Care Plan	Action to Take
0–4	You may have a mild fatty acid deficiency.	*The Blood Sugar Solution*	No personalization needed. Simply complete *The Blood Sugar Solution.*
5–7	You may have a moderate fatty acid deficiency.	Self-Care	Complete *The Blood Sugar Solution* and optimize your fatty acid levels by following the personalization steps in Chapter 24.
8+	You may have a severe fatty acid deficiency.	Medical Care	Do both of the above steps and see a physician for additional assistance if you are not better after the first six weeks of the program.

Now that you have identified three of the most common nutritional deficiencies of our modern life, and those particularly important to metabolism and blood sugar control, let's look at how we got into this terrible mess of being overfed and undernourished.

NUTRITIONAL CHANGE 1:
SUGAR IN ALL ITS FORMS

Our diet has changed dramatically within the last 100 years. It has changed even more dramatically in the last 30–50 years. The biggest change has been our increased sugar consumption. Our Paleolithic ancestors ate 22 teaspoons of sugar per year.[2] At the beginning of the 1800s, the average person consumed 10 pounds a year. And now the average American eats 150–180 pounds per year. That's almost half a pound of sugar per person per day![3] All sugar is harmful when consumed in those pharmacologic doses. When one 20-ounce HFCS-sweetened soda, sports drink, or tea has 17 teaspoons of sugar (and the average teenager often consumes more than 20 ounces a day), we are conducting a largely uncontrolled "drug" experiment on the human species.

In the last 30 years, the sugar calories we consume from high-fructose corn syrup (HFCS) have increased from 0 percent to 66 percent, mostly in the form of liquid calories from soft drinks and other sweetened beverages. And we know that liquid calories in the form of sugar pile on the pounds much more than solid calories do. Following are four reasons why we need to eliminate HFCS from our diet:

1. **HFCS and cane sugar are not biochemically identical or processed the same way by the body.**

High-fructose corn syrup is an industrial food product and far from "natural." It is extracted from corn stalks through a chemical process and is a biochemically novel compound that is sweeter and cheaper than cane sugar (sucrose).

There is no chemical bond between the glucose and the fructose that make up HFCS, so no digestion is required and it is more rapidly absorbed into your bloodstream. Fructose goes right to the liver and triggers *lipogenesis* (the production of fats like triglycerides and cholesterol), which leads to a major cause of liver damage—called fatty liver—in this country affecting 70 million people. The rapidly absorbed glucose triggers big spikes in insulin. Both these features of HFCS lead to increased metabolic disturbances that drive increases in appetite, weight gain, diabetes, heart disease, cancer, dementia, and more.

Research done at the Children's Hospital Oakland Research Institute found that every molecule of free fructose from HFCS* requires more energy to be absorbed by the gut and soaks up two phospho-

---

* Normally in regular table sugar, glucose and fructose molecules are joined together in a chemical bond and are not "free." In high-fructose corn syrup all the fructose is "free" and acts very differently in the body, causing more damage.

rous molecules from ATP (our body's energy source). This depletes the ATP required to maintain the integrity of our intestinal lining.

Little "tight junctions," or connections, between the intestinal cells in the gut cement each intestinal cell together, preventing food and bacteria from "leaking" across the intestinal membrane and triggering an immune reaction and body-wide inflammation. High doses of fructose have been proven to literally punch holes in the intestinal lining, allowing nasty by-products of toxic gut bacteria and partially digested food proteins to enter your bloodstream and trigger inflammation. Naturally occurring fructose in fruit is part of a complex web of nutrients and fiber and doesn't exhibit the same biological effects as the high fructose found in corn sugar.

Cane sugar and the industrially produced, euphemistically named corn sugar are not biochemically or physiologically the same, despite millions of dollars of television commercials by the corn industry claiming otherwise.

2. **HFCS contains contaminants such as mercury that are not regulated or measured by the FDA.**

An FDA researcher asked corn producers to ship a barrel of high-fructose corn syrup to her so that she could test for contaminants. Her repeated requests were denied until she claimed she represented a newly created soft drink company. She was then promptly shipped a big vat of HFCS, which was used in a study that showed that HFCS often contains toxic levels of mercury because of chlor-alkali products used in its manufacturing.[4] Poisoned sugar is certainly not natural.

When HFCS is run through a chemical analyzer or a chromatograph, strange chemical peaks show up that are not glucose or fructose. What are they? Who knows? But it calls into question the purity of this processed form of supersugar. The exact nature, effects, and toxicity of these compounds have not been fully explained, but shouldn't we be protected from the presence of untested chemical compounds in our food supply, especially when the contaminated food product provides up to 15–20 percent of the average American's daily calorie intake?

3. **Independent medical and nutrition experts do not support the use of HCFS in our diet, despite the assertions of the corn industry.**

The corn industry's happy-looking websites www .cornsugar.com and www.sweetsurprise.com bolster their position that cane sugar and corn sugar are the same by quoting, or should I say misquoting, experts.

Barry M. Popkin, PhD, Professor, Department of

Nutrition, University of North Carolina at Chapel Hill, has published widely on the dangers of sugar-sweetened drinks and their contribution to the obesity epidemic. In a review of HFCS in the *American Journal of Clinical Nutrition*,[5] he explains the mechanism by which free fructose may contribute to obesity. He states that:

> The digestion, absorption, and metabolism of fructose differ from those of glucose. Hepatic metabolism of fructose favors de novo lipogenesis. In addition, unlike glucose, fructose does not stimulate insulin secretion or enhance leptin production. Because insulin and leptin act as key afferent signals in the regulation of food intake and body weight [to control appetite], this suggests that dietary fructose may contribute to increased energy intake and weight gain. Furthermore, calorically sweetened beverages may enhance caloric overconsumption.

He concludes by saying that "the increase in consumption of HFCS has a temporal relation to the epidemic of obesity, and the overconsumption of HFCS in calorically sweetened beverages may play a role in the epidemic of obesity."

The corn industry takes his comments out of context to support its position, that "all sugar is the same."

True, large doses of sugar of any kind are harmful, and in the end it might be the pharmacologic doses of any type of sugar that kill you. But the biochemistry and the effects on absorption, appetite, and metabolism are different and Dr. Popkin knows that.

4. **HFCS is almost always a marker of poor-quality, nutrient-poor, disease-creating industrial food products or "food-like substances."**

The last and most important reason to avoid products that contain HFCS is that they are a marker for poor-quality food full of empty calories and artificial ingredients. If you find "high-fructose corn syrup" or the new term "corn sugar" on the label, you can be sure it is not whole, real, fresh food full of fiber, vitamins, minerals, phytonutrients, and antioxidants. Stay away if you want to stay healthy. We must reduce our overall consumption of sugar, but with this one simple dietary change (cutting out HFCS), you can radically reduce your health risks and improve your overall health.

NUTRITIONAL CHANGE 2: OUR LOW-FIBER DIET

Along with our increased sugar consumption, our fiber consumption has decreased tremendously. Our

Paleolithic ancestors ate 50–100 grams of fiber per day. We now eat fewer than 15 grams per day.[6]

Fiber is important because it slows the absorption of sugar into the bloodstream from our gut, makes us feel full, and reduces cholesterol. The fiber in our diet comes predominantly from plant foods such as fruits and vegetables, including nuts, seeds, whole grains, and beans. Those who eat a refined, processed diet out of boxes, packages, or cans typically get less fiber than those who eat whole, real foods.

The lack of fiber in our diet has enormous implications for our health. It contributes to heart disease, diabetes, obesity, cancers, and many other chronic diseases.[7] In fact, studies show that the addition of high levels of fiber to the diet is as effective as diabetes medication in lowering blood sugar, without any of the side effects.[8]

NUTRITIONAL CHANGE 3: AN EPIDEMIC OF NUTRITIONAL DEFICIENCIES

In America, we eat more than we ever have, yet we are nutritionally depleted. As a result, we now see the epidemic of diabesity and many other chronic diseases.

A number of nutrients are particularly important in the prevention and treatment of diabesity, including vitamin D,[9] chromium,[10, 11] magnesium,[12] zinc,[13] biotin,[14] omega-3 fats,[15] and antioxidants such as alpha lipoic acid.[16] These are necessary for proper control and balance of insulin and blood sugar. When these are deficient, our biochemical machinery slows down and can grind to a halt. We become more insulin resistant, our blood sugar swings out of balance, and we gain weight.

THE NUTRITIONAL SOLUTION: NUTRIGENOMICS

We generally think of food as a way to get energy, a means to feed our bodies the fuel they need to function. However, new science has shown that food literally speaks to our genes. The information your body receives from the foods you eat turns your genes on and off. This provides your body with instructions on how to control your metabolism from moment to moment and day to day, every time you take a bite of food. This is the science of **nutrigenomics,** or how food talks to your genes, and it is the nutritional approach that underlies *The Blood Sugar Solution*. In fact, Dr. Dean Ornish showed that after just three months on an intensive lifestyle program including a whole-foods plant-based diet, over 500 genes that regulate cancer were beneficially affected, either turning off the cancer-causing genes or turning on the cancer-protective genes.[17] There is no medication that can do that. Recently, scientists found the genetic material of plants in the blood of humans. Think about it for a minute — plant genes are telling our genes what to do — this is revolutionary.

To illustrate how powerful this approach is, let me share a remarkable study that shows how quickly and powerfully the quality of the food you eat affects your genes, independent of calories, carbs, protein, fat, or fiber. This study focused on people with pre-diabetes. They were divided into two groups. Each group was fed exactly the same amount of calories, with equivalent amounts of protein, fat, carbohydrates, and fiber, for 12 weeks.[18]

The only difference between the groups was this: One group was fed whole-kernel rye bread and rye pasta; the other group was fed oats, wheat, and potatoes as its sources of carbohydrates. After 12 weeks, the researchers performed a subcutaneous fat biopsy, looked at gene expression, and gave the participants in the study a glucose challenge to assess how their blood sugar and insulin were affected by these dietary changes.

The results were groundbreaking. Remarkably, people in the group that ate rye had smarter, smaller fat cells and were more insulin-sensitive. Diabesity-reversing genes were switched on because of the information contained in the rye (a phytonutrient called lignans) independent of calories or grams of carbs eaten. In other words, it didn't matter how many calories or grams of carbs this group ate—it was the *kind* of carbs that was important. The quality of our food matters as much as the quantity we eat.

Even more amazing was how much their genes had changed in such a short time. Dozens of genes that had made participants fat and diabetic were turned off, and dozens of genes that would help them become healthy and thin were turned on. Seventy-one genes that promoted insulin resistance and cell death were turned off in the rye group. The foods they ate beneficially affected their genes, turning off the very genes that predisposed them to diabesity.

On the other hand, 62 genes that promote diabesity were turned on in the group that ate oats, wheat, and potatoes, and that led to increased stress molecules, increased inflammation, and increased oxidative stress, or free radicals. All this, in turn, causes diabesity.

Remember, these two groups ate *exactly* the same number of calories and *exactly* the same percentage of fat, protein, carbohydrate, and fiber. The only difference was in the *type* of carbohydrates they consumed. This one study (among many others that point to the same conclusions) illustrates that food is not just calories. **Food is information.**

If you want to turn off the genes that lead to diabesity and turn on the genes that lead to health, the key is the **quality and type** of food you eat, not necessarily the number of calories you consume or the ratio of protein to fat to carbohydrate in your diet.

You need to put your genes on a diet. As David Ludwig, one of the leading obesity researchers at Harvard Medical School, said, "Molecular pathways involved in hormone action [like insulin resistance] have been the target of a multibillion-dollar pharmaceutical research effort. However, many of these pathways may normally be under dietary regulation. The results of the present study [on nutrigenomics] emphasize the age-old wisdom to 'use food as medicine'—in this case, for the targeted prevention and treatment of obesity, diabetes, and heart disease."[19]

Shifting from a nutrient-poor diet to a nutrient-rich diet that is abundant in plant foods such as fruits, vegetables, nuts, seeds, beans, and whole grains improves the expression of hundreds of genes that control insulin function and obesity. An optimal diet to prevent and treat diabesity also includes healthy fats such as olive oil, nuts, avocados, and omega-3 fats, along with modest amounts of lean animal protein. This is commonly known as a Mediterranean diet.[20] It is a diet of whole, real, fresh food that has been prepared in a kitchen, not a factory. This way of eating has been shown to prevent and even reverse diabesity. It has broad-ranging benefits for our health, and beneficially affects our entire physiology, reducing inflammation, boosting detoxification, balancing hormones, and providing powerful antioxidant protection—all things that fix the underlying causes of disease.

What you put on your fork is the most powerful medicine you can take to correct the root causes of chronic disease and diabesity.

In addition to these dietary changes, you also need a full complement of vitamins and minerals, and you may need to individually correct specific deficiencies, including deficiencies in chromium, biotin, vitamin D,[21] magnesium,[22] zinc, alpha lipoic acid,[23] and omega-3 fats.[24, 25] We need these additional nutrients because our soils, farming, food processing, and food distribution systems result in nutrient-depleted foods.

Sir Albert Howard, who started the organic agriculture movement, said in his landmark book, *The Soil and Health,* that we must "treat the whole problem of health in soil, plant, animal, and man as one great subject."

Even with a perfect diet, the combination of our depleted soils, the storage and transportation of our food, genetic alterations of traditional heirloom species, and the increased stress and nutritional demands resulting from a toxic environment make it impossible for us to get the vitamins and minerals we need solely from the foods we eat.[26] The evidence shows that we cannot get away from the need for nutritional supplements.[27]

In Part IV, you will learn precisely how you need to eat and what supplements you need to take to reverse diabesity. For now, just keep in mind that our common ideas about food being no more than a source of energy are very limited. Nutrigenomics is the future of medicine. It will help us both understand and successfully treat diabesity.

9

Step 2: Regulate Your Hormones

This book is mostly focused on the hormone insulin, but balancing *all* of your hormones, including sex hormones, adrenal or stress hormones, and thyroid hormones, is important if you want to heal. They are all interconnected; they interact with one another like a big musical symphony. When this symphony is playing out of tune, problems arise.

To overcome diabesity, you must identify and treat thyroid imbalances that control your metabolism; overactive stress hormones that worsen insulin resistance and blood sugar; and insulin imbalance and its harmful effects on your sex hormones. Let's look at how each of these major hormonal imbalances can be contributing factors in diabesity.

THYROID HORMONE: CONTROLLING YOUR METABOLISM

Your thyroid controls your metabolism. If it is working slowly, your metabolism slows and your risk of diabesity goes up. Thyroid disease affects 1 in 5 women and 1 in 10 men, yet 50 percent of people with thyroid disease are undiagnosed. Undiagnosed thyroid disease worsens insulin resistance,[1] and insulin resistance worsens thyroid function.[2] Many who are diagnosed are treated inadequately with medications such as Synthroid.

Hidden Thyroid Disease and Diabesity: A Patient's Story

Rene, a graduate student, was a serious and determined twenty-five-year-old woman who did everything she could to take care of herself. She ate a clean, whole foods diet rich in fruits and vegetables, nuts, seeds, beans, and whole grains, and she exercised an hour every day with a trainer. She got enough sleep and balanced work and play. But she had one problem. She was 20 pounds overweight and nothing she did seemed to matter. Digging into her story, I found some clues to the mysterious weight gain and insulin problems. Her periods were never regular, she had dry skin, she was constipated, her hair was coarse, and she was cold all the time. Despite seeing the best doctors in Los Angeles, no one had looked deeply into the obvious explanation for all those symptoms: low thyroid function. Of course, they did the standard thyroid test (TSH), but because the result of 3.5 was within the "normal" range, they didn't look further.

I always give the full spectrum of thyroid function tests, including TSH (normal is now considered less than 3.5 by the American College of Endocrinology; however, most labs' reference ranges have not been changed to reflect the new guidelines). I also check the thyroid hormone levels, T4 and T3, as well as the thyroid antibodies to see if there is an autoimmune reaction against the thyroid. Most physicians only check TSH, missing many people with subtler thyroid problems. Rene had a very low T3 and high thyroid antibodies, so even though her TSH was "normal," I treated her with a natural thyroid hormone containing T4 and T3. All her symptoms went away, her periods became regular, and she lost 20 pounds.

Do you suffer from a sluggish, low-functioning thyroid? Take the following quiz and find out. Remember to take this quiz before you start the program and again after the six weeks are over to measure the "before and after" change in your health. You may need extra individualized support or natural thyroid replacement based on your scores; I explain this in Week 6 of the plan.

Thyroid Quiz

The thyroid gland is very sensitive to the effects of environmental toxins, infections, nutritional deficiencies (iodine, selenium, and zinc), and stress. One in five women and one in ten men have low thyroid function, and more than half don't know it. The quiz below will help you self-diagnose hidden thyroid problems. For any symptom you have experienced in the last month, place a check in the "Before" box. Then find out how severe your problem is by using the scoring key below. Place a check in the "After" box after you've completed the six-week program to see how much you've improved.

	Before	After
The outer thirds of my eyebrows are thinning.		
I am sensitive to cold.		
My hands and feet are cold all the time.		

(Continued)

	Before	After
My hair is thinning, I lose hair, or I have coarse hair.		
I have thick skin and fingernails.		
My skin is dry.		
I experience muscle fatigue, pain, or weakness.		
I have heavy menstrual bleeding, serious PMS, other menstrual problems, or infertility.		
My sex drive has decreased.		
I am tired all the time, especially in the morning.		
My memory and concentration are not what they used to be.		
I retain fluid (swelling of hands and feet).		
I have difficulty losing weight or have recently gained weight.		
I am frequently constipated.		
I am depressed and apathetic.		
I have an autoimmune disease (e.g., rheumatoid arthritis, multiple sclerosis, lupus, allergies, or yeast overgrowth).		

	Before	After
I have low blood pressure and a low heart rate.		
I am gluten-sensitive or have celiac disease.		
I have been exposed to environmental toxins.		
I consume a lot of tuna and sushi, and/or I have multiple dental silver (mercury) fillings.		
I have been exposed to radiation treatments.		
I drink chlorinated or fluoridated water.		
Thyroid problems run in my family.		
TOTAL		

Score	Severity	Care Plan	Action to Take
0–3	You may have slightly low thyroid function.	*The Blood Sugar Solution*	No personalization needed. Simply complete *The Blood Sugar Solution.*

(Continued)

Score	Severity	Care Plan	Action to Take
4–7	You may have moderately low thyroid function.	Self-Care	Complete *The Blood Sugar Solution* and optimize your thyroid levels by following the personalization steps in Chapter 24.
8+	You may have severely low thyroid function.	Medical Care	Do both of the above steps and see a physician for additional assistance if you are not better after the first six weeks of the program.

If you scored over 3, I encourage you to follow the personalization steps for the thyroid in Week 6 of Part IV and to read my e-book, *The UltraThyroid Solution* (www.bloodsugarsolution.com/ultrathyroid), for more information on how to identify and treat thyroid disease.

STRESS HORMONES: THE DANGERS OF CHRONIC STRESS

Stress hormones also play a critical role in diabesity. Chronic stress increases the production of *cortisol,* the main stress hormone. Chronically elevated cortisol causes increased blood sugar and cholesterol, depression, and even dementia,[3] and promotes the accumulation of belly fat that we so commonly see in patients with insulin resistance or diabetes. Too much cortisol also causes muscle loss, interferes with thyroid and growth hormones, and negatively impacts sleep, all of which promote weight gain. Sleep deprivation increases appetite and sugar cravings. In a study of healthy young men deprived of just 2 hours of sleep, their blood levels of ghrelin (the hunger hormone) increased and PYY (the brake on appetite) decreased.[4] This made them crave and eat more refined carbohydrates and sugar. Getting enough quality sleep is important in the treatment of diabesity and can prevent weight gain, diabetes, and heart disease.

But even more important is decreasing our stress levels.

Stress is defined as a real or imagined threat to our body or ego. We will always have intermittent acute stressors. That can't be avoided. But it is not the acute stress that comes and goes that causes problems with your health. What has such a dramatic impact on diabesity as well as on so many other chronic illnesses is the unremitting stress that is created, in part, by your attitude toward that stress: Do you believe that things will work out in the end? Do you see the glass as half empty or half full? Do you think the world a safe place or a dangerous place?

The effects of stress are shaped by our thoughts, attitudes, and beliefs. We *can* change what we think and believe, and we can reduce the impact of daily stress on our lives as a result. You shouldn't believe every stupid thought you have!

In Chapter 14, "Step 7: Soothe Your Mind," we further explore the links between stress and diabesity. You can also follow the additional personalization steps for calming the mind in Part IV as well as use my audio CD program *UltraCalm* (www.blood sugarsolution.com/ultracalm), to help you relieve chronic stress with a few simple tools.

SEX HORMONES: MEN BECOMING WOMEN AND WOMEN BECOMING MEN?

Too much insulin has a negative effect on your sex hormones. If you are a man, it makes you more like a woman, and if you are a woman, it makes you more like a man. Insulin resistance leads to hair growth on the face and body and loss of hair on the head in women. Many women also get acne and irregular menstrual cycles. It makes women grow a mustache or beard, go bald, and get pimples.

Insulin resistance can also be an unrecognized cause of polycystic ovarian syndrome,[5] which causes infertility in women. This is a nutritional problem caused by our toxic diet and environment.

Infertility: A Patient's Story

Lisa desperately wanted children. After failing treatment with the best infertility specialists in the New Jersey–New York area, she came to see me. Her doctors told her she had polycystic ovarian syndrome (PCOS), which is really a nutritional and metabolic problem that affects hormones. It is primarily caused by pre-diabetes. Symptoms include irregular or heavy periods, acne, facial hair, loss of scalp hair, and increased belly fat.

After pills and shots and hormone cocktails that pushed and prodded her ovaries to work properly, after multiple in vitro fertilization (IVF) attempts at $15,000 a pop, there was still no baby for Lisa. But the problem wasn't her ovaries—it was her diet.

Three months after she transformed her diet from processed to whole, fresh, real foods and started exercising daily and taking nutritional supplements that support normal blood sugar metabolism, Lisa got pregnant naturally. And a year later I got a cute baby picture with a little note attached that said, "Thanks Dr. Hyman for getting me pregnant." I wasn't sure how to explain that to my wife! In fact, using the principles in this book, I have gotten many women pregnant, and my office wall is full of baby pictures.

Dr. Walter Willett of Harvard wrote about his research on infertility caused by pre-diabetes in *The Fertility Diet*. Researchers studied fertility in 19,000 women from the Harvard Nurses' Health Study.[6] They found that a majority of infertility, which affects one in seven couples, might be treated effectively through diet, lifestyle, and supplements. Fixing nutritional deficiencies by taking a multivitamin,[7] and eating a whole-foods, low-glycemic-load, nutrient-rich, plant-based diet can have an enormous impact on fertility.

In addition, Dr. David Ludwig found that a low-glycemic-load diet prevented preterm labor in overweight women.[8] So eating according to the plan in this book can help you not only get pregnant but stay pregnant.

Sugar Makes You Less of a Man:
A Patient's Story

Steve, a fifty-four-year-old author, is another patient who couldn't seem to lose weight. Despite working aggressively with a trainer three to five days a week doing strength training and aerobics, he couldn't get his appetite under control, build muscle, or lose any of the considerable belly fat that hung around his 285-pound body. His sex drive was low and erections were weak. We found that he had sky-high insulin levels but rock-bottom testosterone levels.

By improving his diet and applying some topical bioidentical testosterone gel, he was able to build muscle, lose weight, control his appetite, and resume having sex with his beautiful wife.

In men, insulin resistance drives down testosterone levels.[9] Sex drive and sexual function are significantly impaired as a result. Low testosterone also leads to other problems, such as decreased muscle mass and more fat deposition in the belly, seen in all those big guts in men over forty years old. Over time, diabetic men become more like women because insulin and excess body fat result in a higher estrogen level, leading to soft skin; increased breast size; loss of hair on the legs, arms, and chest; loss of muscle mass; low sex drive; and trouble getting erections.

Are your sex hormones out of balance? Take the quiz below to find out. Remember to take this quiz before you start the program and again after the six weeks are over to measure the "before and after" change in your health. You may need extra individualized support based on your scores; I explain this in Week 6 of the plan.

Sex Hormone Imbalance Quiz

Many symptoms people suffer from are related to imbalances in their sex hormones. Men and women each respond differently to those imbalances. Take the appropriate quiz to find out if hormonal imbalances are making you miserable. For any symptom you have experienced in the last month, place a check in the "Before" box. Then find out how severe your problem is by using the scoring key below. Place a check in the "After" box after you've completed the six-week program to see how much you've improved.

For Women	Before	After
I have irregular cycles, heavy bleeding, or light bleeding.		
Prior to my period, I often get headaches and/or migraines.		
My breasts are tender and enlarged.		
I frequently have PMS.		
I am experiencing peri- or menopausal symptoms.		
I have hot flashes.		
I no longer have any interest in sex.		
I have dry skin, hair, and/or vagina.		
I experience monthly weight fluctuation.		
I have gained weight around the middle.		
I feel bloated most of the time.		
I experience edema, swelling, puffiness, or water retention.		
I get premenstrual cravings (especially for sweet or salty foods).		
I have frequent mood swings.		
I feel anxious.		

(Continued)

For Women	Before	After
I am depressed.		
I feel unable to cope with ordinary demands.		
I have back, joint, or muscle pain.		
I suffer from infertility.		
I use birth control pills or other hormones.		
I have breast cysts or lumps, or fibrocystic breasts.		
Breast, ovarian, or uterine cancer runs in my family.		
I have uterine fibroids.		
I have night sweats.		
I have trouble sleeping.		
I sometimes have heart palpitations.		
My memory and concentration are not what they used to be.		
I have facial hair.		
I have been exposed to pesticides or heavy metals (in food, water, and/or the air).		
TOTAL		

Score	Severity	Care Plan	Action to Take
0–9	You may have a mild sex hormone imbalance.	*The Blood Sugar Solution*	No personalization needed. Simply complete *The Blood Sugar Solution*.
10–14	You may have a moderate sexual hormone imbalance.	Self-Care	Complete *The Blood Sugar Solution* and optimize your sex hormone levels by following the personalization steps in Chapter 24.
15+	You may have a severe sexual hormone imbalance.	Medical Care	Do both of the above steps and see a physician for additional assistance if you are not better after the first six weeks of the program.

For Men	Before	After
I have "man boobs" or have lost hair on my arms, legs, and chest.		
I am often tired or have low energy.		
I feel a sense of apathy toward my life and future.		
I have lost my vitality and sex drive.		
I have trouble achieving or maintaining an erection.		
I am infertile or have low sperm counts.		
I have loss of muscle.		
I have increased abdominal fat.		
I feel weak.		
I have bone loss or bone fractures.		
My cholesterol levels have increased.		
My insulin and blood sugar levels have increased.		
I am suffering from depression.		
I have been exposed to pesticides or heavy metals (in food, water, and/or the air).		
TOTAL		

Score	Severity	Care Plan	Action to Take
0–4	You may have a mild sex hormone imbalance.	*The Blood Sugar Solution*	No personalization needed. Simply complete *The Blood Sugar Solution*.
5–6	You may have a moderate sexual hormone imbalance.	Self-Care	Complete *The Blood Sugar Solution* and optimize your sex hormone levels by following the personalization steps in Chapter 24.
7+	You may have a severe sex hormone imbalance.	Medical Care	Do both of the above steps and see a physician for additional assistance if you are not better after the first six weeks of the program.

If your sex hormones are out of balance, the problem is likely related to increased insulin resistance. These imbalances are completely reversible through *The Blood Sugar Solution.*

10

Step 3: Reduce Inflammation

Anything that causes inflammation will, in turn, cause insulin resistance. And anything that causes insulin resistance will cause inflammation. This dangerous spiral is at the root of so many of our twenty-first-century chronic maladies.

Inflammation is something we are all familiar with — from a sore throat, an allergic reaction with hives, or a cut that gets infected and swollen, red, hot, and tender. But the inflammation that drives obesity and chronic disease is invisible and doesn't hurt. It is a hidden, smoldering fire created by your immune system as it tries to fight off bad food (sugar, processed foods, inflammatory fats), stress, toxins, food allergens, an overgrowth of bad bugs in your gut, and even low-grade infections.

These triggers all cause an increase in the inflammatory molecules of your immune system called *cytokines*. They are important in fighting off infection and cancer, helping your body distinguish between friend and foe. But when inflammatory cytokines get out of control, chronic diseases of every stripe result.

INFLAMMATION, INSULIN RESISTANCE, AND CHRONIC DISEASE: THE MISSING LINK

One of the most significant medical discoveries of the twenty-first century is that inflammation is the common thread connecting not just the obvious autoimmune and allergic diseases but most chronic disease, including heart disease, obesity, diabetes, cancer, dementia, and depression. In fact, out-of-control inflammation causes insulin resistance, which, as we now know, is the main factor in all these diseases apart from autoimmunity and allergy. The insulin resistance then creates even more inflammation, and the whole biological house burns down.

Anything that triggers cytokines will make your cells more insulin-resistant, which will in turn make your pancreas pump out more insulin in order to get glucose inside your cells to burn for energy. But since your cells are resistant to the insulin, you require even more of it. Insulin resistance is a state of starving in the midst of plenty.

As we said earlier, insulin is a fat storage hormone that makes you eat more and gain more weight. We now know that fat cells (or adipocytes) also produce their very own highly inflammatory cytokines called *adipocytokines* (or *adipokines* for short).[1] These adipokines (IL-1, IL-6, and tumor necrosis factor alpha) worsen insulin resistance, obesity, and diabetes, and inflame many other chronic diseases.

What triggers this inflammation? A number of recent studies have pointed to a few basic causes that we can identify and treat directly.

Sugar, refined carbohydrates, trans fats, too many inflammatory omega-6 fats from processed plant oils (such as soybean or corn oil), artificial sweeteners, hidden food allergies and sensitivities, chronic infections, imbalances in gut bacteria, environmental toxins, stress, and a sedentary lifestyle all promote inflammation. Of course, which of these factors is the source of inflammation for you is a key question, and the answer is different for everyone. You must locate all the sources of inflammation in your life and eliminate them if you want to overcome diabesity. *The Blood Sugar Solution* will help you do that.

Diabesity, Depression, and Inflammation: A Patient's Story

Depression and obesity are two problems that often go together. That was true for J.P., an eighteen-year-old who came for help with fatigue, depression, anxiety, and a 27-pound weight gain. When he first saw me, he weighed 201 pounds. He had severe pre-diabetes and didn't know it.

We found many clues in his story and on his tests that all pointed to inflammation driving his obesity and depression. He had canker sores (gluten problem[2]); cracking at the corners of his mouth (B vitamin deficiencies); acne on his face, chest, back, and shoulders (dairy or sugar intake and gut inflammation); and seasonal allergies. He also was cold and tired (thyroid problems), especially in the mornings. He had trouble falling asleep, and had been on Paxil for four years to treat his anxiety and depression. He had other telltale symptoms of inflammation and immune dysfunction, including itchy ears (allergies or fungus) and white spots on his nails (zinc deficiency).

He had horrible eating habits: no breakfast, fast food for lunch and dinner, and diet and regular sodas throughout the day. He hated seafood (omega-3 fat deficiency). He did, at least, exercise for 25 minutes a day on the treadmill and 1–2 times a week with a trainer. And he slept 10 hours a night.

His lab tests showed omega-3 fat,[3] vitamin D,[4, 5, 6] B6,[7] and B12[8] deficiencies, all associated with pre-diabetes and depression. He had autoimmune thyroid antibodies with otherwise "normal" thyroid function.[9] He also had high cholesterol, low HDL, and high triglycerides, all of which are classic for pre-diabetes. He had a normal blood sugar but a sky-high insulin level after a sugar drink (linked to acne,[10] depression,[11] weight gain, and carbohydrate cravings).

We also found antibodies to gluten (linked to fatigue, depression,[12] hypothyroidism,[13] and acne) and many other foods,[14] indicating a "leaky gut" (see Chapter 11), which also causes diabesity.

By removing the food allergens from his diet, getting him on a whole-foods, low-sugar, and unprocessed diet, cleaning up his gut with antifungals and giving him a probiotic, supporting his thyroid function, and fixing his nutritional deficiencies, all his symptoms cleared up. We didn't need to treat all his individual "diseases." We helped his system get back in balance and his symptoms went away as a side effect of getting healthy. In the first two months he lost 20 pounds and his cravings stopped. He had many causes of inflammation and we had to address them all.

Mounting evidence underscores the critical role that inflammation plays in the development and continuation of diabesity. In fact, those who have a high C-reactive protein (a marker of systemic inflammation) blood level have a 1,700 percent increased probability of developing diabetes.[15] In medicine, 20 or 30 percent increases are considered significant; a seventeenfold increase should be headline news.

The increased rate of chronic illness we see in our society is a direct outcome of increased rates of inflammation. There is no longer any debate about this in the world of medicine. The important questions are, "What's causing the inflammation, and how do we treat it most effectively?"

I can assure you the answer is *not* simply to take more aspirin or Advil. That's like taking painkillers while a horse is standing on your foot. The treatment is getting the horse off your foot—and that means finding the underlying causes of inflammation and eliminating them. I will explain the primary causes in a moment, but first take the quiz below to find out how inflamed you are. Remember to take this quiz before you start the program and again after the six weeks are over to measure the "before and after" change in your health. You may need extra individualized support based on your scores; I explain this in Week 6 of the plan.

Inflammation Quiz

Hidden inflammation makes you fat and diabetic and causes many other chronic diseases including heart disease, cancer, and dementia. For any symptom you have experienced in the last month, place a check in the "Before" box. Then find out how severe your problem is by using the scoring key below. Place a check in the "After" box after you've completed the six-week program to see how much you've improved.

	Before	After
I frequently get colds and infections.		
I have recurring sinusitis.		
I have seasonal or environmental allergies.		
I have a history of chronic infections, such as hepatitis, skin infections, canker sores, cold sores.		
I have food allergies or sensitivities, or I don't feel well after eating (sluggishness, headaches, confusion, etc.).		
My work environment includes poor lighting, chemicals, and/or poor ventilation.		

	Before	After
I have had a heart attack or have heart disease.		
I have diabetes or am overweight (BMI greater than 25).		
I have bronchitis or asthma.		
I have eczema, acne, and/or rashes.		
I have arthritis (osteoarthritis/ degenerative).		
I have an autoimmune disease (rheumatoid arthritis, lupus, hypothyroidism, etc.).		
I suffer from colitis or inflammatory bowel disease.		
I have irritable bowel syndrome (spastic colon).		
I have neuritis (ADHD, autism, mood, and behavior problems).		
Parkinson's or Alzheimer's disease runs in my family.		
My life is very stressful.		
I drink more than three alcoholic beverages a week.		
I don't exercise more than 30 minutes three times a week.		

(Continued)

	Before	After
At work, I am exposed to pesticides, toxic chemicals, loud noise, heavy metals, and/or toxic bosses and coworkers.		
TOTAL		

Score	Severity	Care Plan	Action to Take
0–6	You may have a low level of inflammation.	*The Blood Sugar Solution*	No personalization needed. Simply complete *The Blood Sugar Solution.*
7–9	You may have a moderate level of inflammation.	Self-Care	Complete *The Blood Sugar Solution* and optimize your results by following the personalization steps in Chapter 24.
10+	You may have a severe level of inflammation.	Medical Care	Do both of the above steps and see a physician for additional assistance if you are not better after the first six weeks of the program.

My guess is that most of you found you are inflamed. Let's review the top seven causes of inflammation in our society. In Part IV, I will show you how to correct these problems.

CAUSE OF INFLAMMATION 1: DIETARY SUGARS, REFINED FLOURS, AND ARTIFICIAL SWEETENERS

Dietary sugars and refined flours are the biggest triggers of inflammation. They cause insulin levels to spike and start a cascade of biochemical reactions that turn on genes and lead to chronic and persistent inflammation. This begins a downward spiral into more inflammation, more insulin resistance, poorer blood sugar control, and more disease.

However, it is not just sugar, but also artificial sweeteners that drive inflammation, as we learned in Chapter 4. Diet drinks and artificial sweeteners of all stripes likely increase insulin resistance.

Lack of fiber, too many inflammatory omega-6 fats (soybean and corn oil), and not enough anti-inflammatory omega-3 fats (fish oil, flaxseeds) also contribute to the development of systemic inflammation, and that leads to worsening insulin resistance.

CAUSE OF INFLAMMATION 2: FOOD SENSITIVITIES AND ALLERGIES

Food sensitivities and allergens also may play a role in the development of insulin resistance and diabesity. The allergies I am talking about here are not the typical hypersensitivity or acute allergies we are most familiar with, such as peanut or bee sting allergies. These are known as immediate-acting "IgE-mediated responses," and while they can be deadly, they are not a major contributor to insulin resistance.

Delayed, or hidden, allergies (known as "IgG-mediated responses") do, however, play a significant role. Some people suffer from allergic responses to inputs—like certain foods—which cause a broad array of subtle symptoms. These sensitivities don't cause your throat to swell shut like IgE-mediated allergies do, but they do create systemic low-grade inflammation in the body that can manifest itself in any number of ways. Recent research indicates that these sensitivities may contribute to insulin resistance.

In fact, in a study that compared obese children to normal-weight children, the obese children had threefold higher levels of C-reactive protein and a two-and-a-half-fold higher level of IgG antibodies for the 277 different foods tested.[16] In addition, these obese children had thicker carotid arteries, an indication of cholesterol-laden plaque lining the arteries and a strong predictor of heart disease and stroke. Plaque results from inflammation that starts in the gut but spreads throughout the body as food particles "leak" across a damaged gut barrier and trigger the production of cytokines such as IL-1, IL-6, and TNF (tumor necrosis factor) alpha.

This highly significant study points to the previously unrecognized connection between food allergies, weight gain, and insulin resistance. Diets eliminating common food sensitivities can help treat diabesity. For patients who have trouble losing weight, I often recommend a six-week elimination of dairy and gluten, the most common culprits, as a critical part of *The Blood Sugar Solution*. In fact, this is the single most important part of the program for many people, resulting in the greatest weight loss and reversal of diabesity.

In my practice, using IgG food sensitivities as a guide to treatment has been one of the most powerful interventions to treat and reverse a whole host of chronic ailments. In my book *The UltraSimple Diet* (www.bloodsugarsolution.com/ultrasimple-diet), I provide a comprehensive elimination diet to test for these hidden sensitivities. I have seen dramatic effects in weight loss, inflammatory conditions like autoimmune disease, and even mood and behavioral disorders (which I explain in my book *The UltraMind*

Solution — www.bloodsugarsolution.com/ultra mind-solution). But most physicians, especially allergists, do not accept or believe in these food reactions. That is unfortunate because there is solid evidence for the benefits of an elimination diet, including a remarkable study, published in one of the world's most prestigious journals, the *Lancet,* showing that attention deficit hyperactivity disorder (ADHD) improved dramatically through an elimination diet based on IgG food-sensitivity testing.[17] Interestingly, ADHD and childhood obesity often show up together and may be caused by similar factors.[18]

Gluten Makes You Fat: A Patient's Story

In medical school, we were trained to think that people with celiac disease were skinny kids with diarrhea, bloated bellies, and abdominal pain. Today we know differently; you can be fat, old, and constipated (or have no digestive symptoms) and still have celiac disease.

That was the case for Ron, who was a hefty 350 pounds when he came to see me. He was a weight loss expert, having tried every program from very low-calorie diets to no-carb diets to liquid diets. He could never maintain the weight loss.

He had many symptoms, including joint pain, a chronic cough, postnasal drip, and asthma, all of which were clues that inflammation might be driving his weight. He went from 180 pounds in high school to over 300 during graduate school. Cravings were his constant companion. He was a self-proclaimed carb addict. Exhausted all the time, he propped himself up with diet sodas and fast food. Since he was so big, he couldn't sleep lying down and spent every night sleeping in a chair. He was a heavy snorer and likely had sleep apnea. His doctor put him on a statin and aspirin, but that didn't make him feel better or address the underlying causes of his symptoms.

When we tested him, we found he had very high levels of inflammation with a C-reactive protein of 8.5 (normal is less than 1.0); his insulin was 183 after a sugar drink (normal is less than 25); and he had high uric acid and lots of dangerous small LDL particles (statins lower the total amount of LDL but don't affect particle size or the quality of your cholesterol). All these indicated severe pre-diabetes. But most important, we found very high levels of anti-gliadin (AGA) and tissue transglutaminase (TTG) antibodies, which indicate an autoimmune reaction to gluten. He had celiac disease, which explained all his health problems, including obesity, pre-diabetes, asthma, joint pain, and fatigue.

Six weeks after being on a gluten-free diet, not only did he lose three notches on his belt, but his knees didn't hurt, his asthma was gone, he wasn't hungry, his energy was back, and he didn't need a nap every day. And he could finally sleep in his bed. Anytime I see anyone with serious health problems, I always check for gluten sensitivity.

How Gluten Triggers Weight Gain, Pre-Diabetes, Diabetes, and More

Gluten-free is hot these days. There are books and websites, restaurants with gluten-free menus, and grocery stores with hundreds of new gluten-free products on the shelves. Is this a fad, or a reflection of response to a real problem?

Sadly, chronic illness is increasingly caused by eating our beloved diet staple, bread, the staff of life, and all the wheat products hidden in everything from soups to vodka to salad dressing to lipstick to envelope adhesive. In a moment I will explain why gluten sensitivity and celiac disease have been increasing and now affect at least 20 million Americans. Unfortunately, 99 percent of the people who

There is also some striking new research showing that adverse immune reactions to gluten may result from problems in very different parts of the immune system than those implicated in celiac disease. Most doctors dismiss gluten sensitivity if you don't have a diagnosis of celiac disease, but this new research proves them wrong. Celiac disease results when the body creates antibodies against the wheat (adaptive immunity), but another kind of gluten sensitivity results from a generalized activated immune system (innate immunity). This means that people can be gluten-sensitive without having celiac disease or gluten antibodies and still have inflammation and many other symptoms.[21]

Too Many Gluten-Free Products: Another Cause of Weight Gain

Too many people, trying to eat healthy, are eating too much gluten-free junk food like cookies, cakes, and processed food. Just because a food is gluten-free doesn't mean it's healthy. Gluten-free cookies and cake are still cookies and cake! Vegetables, fruits, beans, nuts and seeds, and lean animal protein are all gluten-free—stick with those.

How Can Gluten Sensitivity Be Diagnosed?

In the past, doctors would only diagnose celiac disease based on positive intestinal biopsy. But Dr. Alessio

Fasano of the University of Maryland School of Medicine suggests a more inclusive way to diagnose celiac disease and gluten intolerance or sensitivity. He suggests that any four out of the five factors below are diagnostic.[22] I would agree for full-blown celiac, but except for only a positive gene test, I think any of these factors warrants a trial of a strict 100 percent gluten elimination diet for six weeks.

And I believe if you have just three out of five criteria, you should be gluten-free for life.

1. You have symptoms of celiac (any digestive, allergic, autoimmune, or inflammatory disease including diabesity).
2. You get better on a gluten-free diet.
3. You have elevated antibodies to gluten (anti-gliadin [AGA] or tissue transglutaminase [TTG] antibodies).
4. You have a positive small intestinal biopsy.
5. You have the genes that predispose you to gluten sensitivity (HLA DQ2/8).

CAUSE OF INFLAMMATION 3: CHRONIC HIDDEN INFECTIONS

Chronic infections can also trigger inflammation. New studies show that infections such as adenovirus (the kind of virus that causes upper respiratory infections or infectious pinkeye) may be linked to obesity and insulin resistance.[23] These can be identified and treated by experienced practitioners in functional medicine. You can also boost your immune system in order to suppress and control these latent infections.

To learn more about what tests to get in order to check for latent infections, see *How to Work with Your Doctor to Get What You Need* at www.blood sugarsolution.com.

CAUSE OF INFLAMMATION 4: TOXINS

Toxins also play a large role in inflammation and can lead to diabesity. The increasing load of persistent organic pollutants (such as PCBs and pesticides) and heavy metals (such as arsenic, mercury, and lead) has been linked to both diabetes and insulin resistance.[24] The link between toxins, inflammation, and diabesity[25] will be discussed further in Chapter 12, "Step 5: Maximize Detoxification."

CAUSE OF INFLAMMATION 5: CHRONIC STRESS

Chronic stress is yet another cause of inflammation in the body.[26] That's one more reason for you to relax and learn how to calm your mind. I discussed this in the last chapter and we will go into greater detail about the impacts of stress in Chapter 14, "Step 7: Soothe Your Mind," where I explain how chronic stress and the resultant high levels of cortisol increase insulin and weight gain around the middle.

CAUSE OF INFLAMMATION 6: SEDENTARY LIFESTYLE

It's hard to imagine that doing nothing can make you inflamed, but that is exactly what happens. Lack of regular exercise creates low-grade inflammation in the body. And regular exercise dramatically reduces inflammation,[27] which is why exercise is so critical to the reversal and treatment of diabesity.

CAUSE OF INFLAMMATION 7: NUTRITIONAL DEFICIENCIES

Studies show that deficiencies in basic nutrients such as vitamin D, omega-3 fats, and antioxidants promote inflammation, and that simply taking a multivitamin and mineral supplement is as effective for lowering inflammation as taking a statin medication, with a lot less expense and fewer side effects.[28] In Part IV, I will guide you in how to choose and take the best nutrients to correct inflammation and diabesity.

Locating and addressing each of the causes of inflammation in your life is essential not only for overcoming diabesity but also for addressing virtually every other health-related issue. There is no doubt about it: Inflammation is one of the common pathways to illness. Cooling off the fires is essential if you want to heal.

11

Step 4: Improve Your Digestion

New evidence points to an unexpected source of metabolic problems and diabesity—a toxic digestive system. As I've mentioned, our diet has changed dramatically in the last 10,000 years, and even more so in the last 100 years, with the industrialization of our food supply. This highly processed, high-sugar, high-fat, low-fiber diet has substantially altered the bacteria that historically grew in our digestive tracts, and the change has been linked to weight gain and diabetes.[1] Many other modern inventions—including antibiotics, acid blockers, anti-inflammatory medication, aspirin, steroids, antibiotics in our food supply, chronic stress, and even cesarean section births—all injure the gut, alter our gut flora, and lead to systemic inflammation.

Bad Bugs Caused a Big Belly: A Patient's Story

Jennifer was a forty-one-year-old flight attendant who had struggled with her health for years—weight problems, bloating after every meal, diarrhea, heartburn, depression, fatigue, premenstrual syndrome, and irregular periods. She was skinny in high school at 120 pounds and then ballooned up to 215 pounds, most of which she carried around her middle. She tried many diets but could never stick with them. She had given up and was eating pizza, ice cream, and lots of Splenda.

When we did her tests, we found not only inflammation with a high C-reactive protein of 7.2 (normal is less than 1), but abnormal digestive function. She had an overgrowth of bacteria in her small intestine (which normally has very few bacteria) that caused fermentation of all the carbs and sugars she was eating. She was bloated because of all the gas produced by the bad bugs as they munched on the starches. In her stool, we found almost no healthy bacteria. We also found many food sensitivities, including dairy, gluten, and eggs. These often occur because the bad bugs in the small intestine cause a leaky gut, and the partially digested food particles leak across the intestinal lining, triggering antibodies. The bad bugs and the food allergens led to inflammation and weight gain.

We treated her obesity and pre-diabetes with nonabsorbed antibiotics that killed the bad bugs in her gut. To help her heal her leaky gut, we got her off the foods she was sensitive to and her acid blockers, and put her on enzymes, probiotics, fish oil, and zinc. Not only did her reflux, bloating, cravings, and PMS go away, but her C-reactive protein went back to normal. She lost 65 pounds as a side effect of fixing her gut and cooling off the inflammation.

Is your gut contributing to your diabesity? Take the quiz below to find out. Remember to take this quiz before you start the program and again after the six weeks are over to measure the "before and after" change in your health. You may need extra individualized support based on your scores; I explain this in Week 6 of the plan.

Digestion Quiz

The health of your digestion mirrors your overall health, and increasingly gut problems are linked to weight gain and obesity. Take this quiz to assess your gut issues. For any symptom you have experienced in the last month, place a check in the "Before" box. Then find out how severe your problem is by using the scoring key below. Place a check in the "After" box after you've completed the six-week program to see how much you've improved.

	Before	After
I get heartburn.		
I regularly use antacids (Tums, Maalox, acid-blocking drugs, etc.).		
I feel bloated or full, and/or have belching, burning, or flatulence, right after meals.		
Eating bread or other sugars causes bloating.		
I have chronic yeast or fungal infections (jock itch, vaginal yeast infection, athlete's foot, toenail fungus).		
I have chronic abdominal pain.		
I feel fatigued after eating.		
I often experience diarrhea.		
I have a bowel movement less than once or twice a day.		
My stools are greasy, large, poorly formed, or foul-smelling.		

(Continued)

	Before	After
I sometimes notice food that is not fully digested in my stool.		
I have food allergies, intolerance, or reactions.		
I have thrush (whitish tongue).		
I have bleeding gums or gingivitis.		
I have a map-like rash on my tongue indicating food allergy or yeast overgrowth.		
I have sores on my tongue.		
I frequently get canker sores.		
I drink more than three alcoholic beverages a week.		
I crave sweets and bread.		
My life is excessively stressful.		
I have a history of NSAID (ibuprofen, naproxen, etc.) or other anti-inflammatory use.		
I frequently use antibiotics or have frequently used them in the past (more than 1–2 times in three years).		
I have taken prednisone or other steroid drugs.		
I have taken birth control pills or hormone replacement.		

	Before	After
When I take supplements, I feel nauseous.		
I experience anal itching.		
I have or have had the following diseases or conditions (score 1 point for each): ■ Acne after adolescence ■ Chronic hives ■ Eczema ■ Rosacea ■ Psoriasis ■ Chronic fatigue syndrome ■ Chronic autoimmune disease(s) ■ Autism ■ ADHD ■ Fibromyalgia ■ Inflammatory bowel disease ■ Irritable bowel syndrome ■ Celiac disease (gluten allergy)		
TOTAL		

Score	Severity	Care Plan	Action to Take
0–8	You may have a low-level problem with your gut.	*The Blood Sugar Solution*	No personalization needed. Simply complete *The Blood Sugar Solution*.

(Continued)

Score	Severity	Care Plan	Action to Take
9–12	You may have a moderate problem with your gut.	Self-Care	Complete *The Blood Sugar Solution* and optimize your results by following the personalization steps in Chapter 24.
13+	You may have a severe problem with your gut.	Medical Care	Do both of the above steps and see a physician for additional assistance if you are not better after the first six weeks of the program.

If you have found out you have digestive imbalances, you are not alone. They are among the most common reasons people see their doctor. Some of the top-selling drugs of all time are acid blockers such as Prilosec, Prevacid, and Nexium used for reflux, which affects up to 44 percent of the population. Irritable bowel syndrome affects 15 percent of the population and there is no effective drug treatment. Inflammatory bowel diseases such as colitis or

Crohn's are on the rise. Clearly there is something amiss with our digestive systems. Getting your system back in balance will not only relieve your digestive symptoms, but will also help you reverse diabesity. In Part IV, you will learn how to set your tummy right.

THE MICROBIOME: HOW GUT BACTERIA MAKE YOU FAT

Think of your gut as one big ecosystem. It contains 500 species of bacteria that amount to three pounds of your total weight. There are more than 100 trillion microbial cells. There is 100 times more bacterial DNA than human DNA in your body. You are outnumbered! These bugs control digestion, metabolism, inflammation, and your risk of colon and other cancers. They produce vitamins and beneficial nutrients, as well as molecules that sustain your body and your ecosystem through symbiosis.

A whole new field of research has emerged on the human "microbiome" (the community of microbes and their genes within the human gut) and how it affects weight and health.[2] In fact, your weight may be controlled more by what your bacteria eat than what you eat. A remarkable study found that mice with sterilized digestive tracts, or *no* bacteria in their guts, had 42 percent less body fat, despite the fact that they ate 29 percent *more* calories than the control mice.[3] Even more remarkable, when normal bacteria were reintroduced into the guts of those mice, there was a 57 percent increase in body fat and insulin resistance *without* any increase in food consumption or decrease in exercise. This explodes the myth that weight loss is just a matter of calories in and calories out.

Gut bacteria thrive on what you feed them. If you feed them whole, fresh, real foods, good bugs will grow. If you feed them junk, bad bugs will grow. And bad bugs produce nasty toxins. Instead of symbiosis—a mutually beneficial relationship between you and your bugs—you create *dysbiosis*—a harmful interaction between bugs and host that damages your gut lining, creating a leaky gut. Partially digested food particles and microbial toxins then "leak" across your gut, triggering an immune response to these "foreign" proteins.

That inflammation, in turn, damages your metabolism, affects how your brain controls appetite, and creates insulin resistance and weight gain. Supplements of probiotics (the good bacteria) can help improve the quality of your gut ecosystem and are potential partners in weight loss.

The process by which bad bugs in your gut produce toxins was described in a paper published in 2007 in *Diabetes Journal*.[4] The study showed how *metabolic endotoxemia* (the production of toxins from bad bugs in your gut) initiates and promotes obesity and insulin resistance. The findings were striking.

In rats fed a high-fat, low-fiber diet, bad bugs took over. The bad bugs released bacterial toxins called *lipopolysaccharides (LPS)* into the bloodstream through the gut. These toxins bound to immune cells (white blood cells, or lymphocytes). The white blood cells, aggravated by the bacterial toxins, produced an inflammatory molecule called *tumor necrosis factor alpha (TNF-α)*. This molecule then sets into motion a well-described cascade of inflammation, causing insulin resistance. You know what happens from there. The bottom line is this: The toxic bugs in your gut may make you fat and inflamed.

Improving the quality of your diet with whole, fresh, high-fiber foods can significantly reduce inflammation and the resulting weight gain simply by supporting healthy flora in your intestine. Putting good bugs such as *Lactobacillus, Bifidobacterium,* and the healthy type of *E. coli* back into your gut will help cool the inflammation and help you shed pounds. You may need a special stool test if you are not getting better, but for most people what we in functional medicine call the 4R program works very well: **Remove** the bad bugs, drugs, and food allergens; **replace** needed enzymes, fiber, and prebiotics;

reinoculate your gut with good bacteria or probiotics; and finally **repair** the gut lining with omega-3 fats, zinc, glutamine, quercitin, and other healing nutrients. I will explain exactly how to do this in Part IV.

12

Step 5: Maximize Detoxification

Over the last few years, scientists have uncovered an unexpected fact: Environmental toxins make you fat and cause diabetes. This should be headline news, but it isn't because there are no drugs to treat it. Everyone is focused on lifestyle, calories in–calories out, and medication for diabetes. But the scientific data tells us something else is contributing to the epidemic. We have found that environmental toxins interfere with blood sugar and cholesterol metabolism, and cause insulin resistance.[1]

Toxic and Fat: A Patient's Story

Vicky was a health nut, but she had 40 extra pounds she couldn't lose. She ate an organic, whole-foods, low-sugar, high-fiber diet, but she loved tuna fish (full of mercury). She was a fitness trainer and coach and exercised 90 minutes a day.

In addition to not being able to lose weight, she had severe premenstrual syndrome, stomach bloating, fatigue, and mild depression. Clearly her lifestyle wasn't the problem.

When I can't solve a patient's problem, or when they have tried everything else, I often think about the role of environmental toxins on metabolism, obesity, and insulin resistance. Toxins also act as hormone disruptors and are linked to many female complaints.

We looked at Vicky's heavy metal levels and found she had very high levels of mercury— 76 mcg/gram/cr (normal < 3).* Metabolic and health effects are being identified at lower and lower levels of mercury. Once we identified the problem, we carefully and slowly helped her detoxify, by supporting her own detoxification pathways with sulfur molecules like n-acetyl-cysteine (which boosts glutathione, the body's main detoxifier); methylating B vitamins (B6,

---

* The tests for measuring metals are controversial. Most doctors just look at blood levels, but that only indicates recent exposure, usually from eating fish like tuna with high levels of mercury. Hair analysis tells you only about mercury exposure from eating fish and goes back a few months. A random urine test will only show if you have current ongoing exposures from something in your environment or workplace. That is why we do a challenge test with a chelating agent that binds to mercury in the blood and tissues and pulls it out and dumps it in the urine. That gives a better idea of total body burden of metals.

folate, B12); the broccoli family of vegetables, which boosts detoxification; and detoxifying minerals, including zinc and selenium. Saunas also helped her body get rid of metals and other toxins, and they can be a great aid in weight loss. We also used oral doses of DMSA, a chelating agent. Slowly her mercury came down from 76 to 5, and she lost 35 pounds. All the rest of her symptoms—PMS, fatigue, depression, and bloating—went away, too.

If you have struggled with weight loss and diabetes despite eating a perfect diet and exercising your butt off, it may be the effect of the load of toxins in your body interfering with your metabolism.

Take the quiz below to find out if you are toxic. Remember to take this quiz before you start the program and again after the six weeks are over to measure the "before and after" change in your health. You may need extra individualized support based on your scores; I explain this in Week 6 of the plan.

Toxicity Quiz

We often don't connect our ill health or symptoms directly with the effects of environmental toxins. This quiz will help you make that link. For any symptom you have experienced in the last month, place a check in the "Before" box. Then find out how severe your problem is by using the scoring key below. Place a check in the "After" box after you've completed the six-week program to see how much you've improved.

	Before	After
I produce small amounts of urine only a few times a day, and it is dark and strong-smelling.		
I have bowel movements only every other day or less often.		
I have hard, difficult-to-pass bowel movements every day or every other day.		
I almost never break a real sweat.		
I have one or more of the following symptoms (score 1 point for each): ■ Concentration and memory problems ■ Headaches ■ Fatigue ■ Muscle aches		
Most of my clothes are dry-cleaned.		
I drink bottled water from plastic containers, unfiltered tap water, or well water.		
I get my house or apartment treated for bugs by an exterminator and/or use household or lawn garden chemicals.		

	Before	**After**
I work or live in a "tight" building with poor ventilation or windows that don't open.		
I live in a large urban or industrial area.		
My diet includes swordfish, tile fish, tuna, shark, or other large fish more than once a week.		
I have more than two mercury fillings in my teeth.		
I am bothered by one or more of the following (score 1 point if you are bothered by any of these, not 1 point for each): ■ Perfumes ■ Soaps ■ Gasoline or diesel fumes ■ New car smells ■ Tobacco smoke ■ Chlorinated water ■ Detergents ■ Dry cleaning ■ Fabric stores ■ Hair spray ■ Other strong odors		

(Continued)

	Before	After
When I drink caffeine, I experience anxiety, palpitations, sweating, or dizziness. I feel wired up, and experience an increase in joint and muscle aches.		
I have a negative reaction when I consume foods containing MSG, sulfites (found in wine, dried fruit, salad bars), sodium benzoate (preservative), red wine, cheese, banana, chocolate, or even a small amount of alcohol, garlic, or onions.		
I regularly consume the following substances or medications (score 1 point if you take any of these, not 1 point for each): ■ Acetaminophen ■ Ibuprofen or naproxen ■ Acid-blocking drugs (Tagamet, Zantac, Pepcid, Prilosec, Prevacid) ■ Medications for colitis, Crohn's disease, recurrent headaches, allergy symptoms, nausea, diarrhea, or indigestion ■ Hormone-modulating medications in pills, patches, or creams (birth control pills, estrogen, progesterone, prostate medication)		

	Before	After
I have had jaundice (turning yellow) or I have Gilbert's syndrome (an elevation of bilirubin).		
I have a history of any of the following conditions (score 1 point if you have a history of any of these, not 1 point for each): ■ Breast cancer ■ Smoking-induced lung cancer ■ Other type of cancer ■ Food allergies, sensitivities, or intolerances ■ Prostate problems		
I have a family history of Parkinson's, Alzheimer's, ALS (amyotrophic lateral sclerosis), multiple sclerosis, or other neurodegenerative diseases.		
I get regular flu vaccines (which contain mercury or thimerosal).		
I have fibromyalgia or chronic fatigue syndrome.		
TOTAL		

(Continued)

Score	Severity	Care Plan	Action to Take
0–6	You may have a low level of toxicity.	*The Blood Sugar Solution*	No personalization needed. Simply complete *The Blood Sugar Solution.*
7–9	You may have a moderate level of toxicity.	Self-Care	Complete *The Blood Sugar Solution* and optimize your results by following the personalization steps in Chapter 24.
10+	You may have a severe level of toxicity.	Medical Care	Do both of the above steps and see a physician for additional assistance if you are not better after the first six weeks of the program.

NEW EVIDENCE LINKING TOXINS TO DIABESITY: FAT BABIES AND FAT RATS

The most recent example of how toxins make us fat can be seen in the dramatic increase in obesity in babies. In 2006, scientists at the Harvard School of Public Health found that the rate of obesity in infants less than six months old has risen 73 percent since 1980. This is not related to lack of exercise or diet—after all, babies that age are only drinking breast milk or formula. They don't say, "Hey, Mom, take me out for a twelve-hundred-calorie McDonald's breakfast or a giant tub of buttered popcorn." And you can't point to watching too much television or video games as a risk factor. So what's the cause? It appears it may be the load of environmental toxins in their little bodies. The toxins make them fat.

The average newborn has 287 chemicals in her umbilical cord blood, 217 of which are neurotoxic (poisonous to nerves or nerve cells). The chemicals these infants are exposed to include pesticides, phthalates, bisphenol A, flame retardants, and heavy metals such as mercury, lead, and arsenic.[2] These chemicals have a broad range of negative effects on human biology; they damage the nervous system and increase the risk of cancer, and now they have been shown to contribute to obesity.

A study published in the *Journal of the American Medical Association* found that bisphenol A, a petrochemical that lines water bottles and canned food containers, increases a person's risk of diabetes, heart disease, and abnormal liver function or fatty liver caused by insulin resistance.[3]

Data from the government's National Health and Nutrition Examination Survey 1999–2002 found a striking correlation between diabetes and blood levels of six common persistent organic pollutants (POPs): polychlorinated dibenzo-*p*-dioxins (PCDDs), polychlorinated dibenzofurans (PCDFs), polychlorinated biphenyls (PCBs), hexachlorobenzene (HCB), and two organochlorines used as pesticides.[4] Those people who had the highest levels of pollutants in their blood had a dramatically higher risk of diabetes. This isn't just a coincidence. Experimental studies prove you can induce obesity through direct exposure to toxins, independent of calorie intake or exercise.

A recent paper in the *Journal of the American Medical Association* documented that arsenic exposure increases the risk of diabetes.[5]

Studies of Air Force veterans of the Vietnam War found that those who had been exposed to Agent Orange (dioxin) had a much higher risk of diabetes.[6]

The National Institutes of Health, the Food and Drug Administration, the Environmental Protection Agency, and the National Academy of Sciences recently convened a conference to examine this new phenomenon of *obesogens*—toxins that cause obesity.

The old idea that weight gain is simply a matter of calories in–calories out is falling apart. New evidence shows that it can occur in the absence of excess calorie intake. For example, in a recent study, rats given toxic chemicals gained weight and increased their fat storage *without* increased caloric intake or decreased exercise. In six months, these rats were 20 percent heavier and had 36 percent more body fat than rats not exposed to those chemicals.[7]

Here is the take-home message: If you are toxic, you can gain weight without eating any more calories or doing any less exercise.

Toxins interfere with and slow down metabolism and contribute to weight gain and diabetes. In 2007, I published a paper called "Systems Biology, Toxins, Obesity, and Functional Medicine," which provides a detailed description of many of the mechanisms by which toxins cause obesity[8] (available at http://drhyman.com/downloads/Diabetes-and-Toxins.pdf). One of the key mechanisms that leads to insulin resistance and diabesity is that toxins block the function of very important receptors on the nuclei of your cells. These receptors, called peroxisome proliferator-activated receptors (PPARs), are needed for optimal insulin function and blood sugar control.[9] Using new techniques of genetic and metabolic analysis, scientists have shown that toxins cause increases in glucose, cholesterol, and fatty liver, and slow down your thyroid function.[10] They also may cause an increase in appetite and problems with brain signals that control hunger.

This is no longer something that can be ignored. Toxins make you fat and cause diabesity, and they must be addressed in any treatment program for diabesity.

You will learn how to enhance your body's own detoxification systems and remove toxins from your environment and your body in Part IV.

13

Step 6: Enhance Energy Metabolism

Among the most exciting and important findings in recent science is the discovery of how differences in our metabolism affect our risk for diabesity. Our metabolism turns calories and oxygen into the energy that fuels every cell in our body. This energy is made in little factories in our cells called *mitochondria*.

So what are mitochondria and what do they have to do with having more energy, losing weight, reversing diabesity, and living disease-free to 120?

Everything.

In each cell there are hundreds to thousands of these little energy factories. They exist in greater amounts in active organs and tissues, like the muscles, heart, and brain. The role of your metabolism is to take the oxygen you breathe and the food you eat and process it to make energy, the fuel for life.

When your mitochondria are not working properly, you suffer all the symptoms of low energy: fatigue, slow metabolism, weight gain, memory loss, pain, rapid aging, and more. Many things can go wrong and impede your metabolism, make it run less efficiently, or shut it down.

We have more than 100,000 trillion of these powerhouses in our body, and each one contains 17,000 little assembly lines for making ATP, our major fuel. They use over 90 percent of the oxygen we breathe. They take up 40 percent of the space inside the heart cells. Unfortunately for us, they are sensitive to damage from eating too much sugar and processed foods, environmental toxins, and anything that causes inflammation.

People with diabesity don't produce energy in their mitochondria as well as healthy people do.[1] And surprisingly, thin and otherwise healthy first-degree relatives of diabetics have mitochondria that are 50 percent less active than those of people without a family history of diabetes, making them much more likely to develop diabetes at some point in their lives.[2] Often the cause of damage to our mitochondria is something we call *oxidative stress*. We are familiar with the process — it is seen as rust on a car, wrinkles on your face, an apple that turns brown in the air. But you can wrinkle on the inside, too.

The good news is that there are ways to enhance

and optimize mitochondrial function, boost energy production, and reduce oxidative stress. The even better news is that doing these things can reverse diabesity and insulin resistance.

Slow-Burning Mitochondria: A Patient's Story

Jane, a fifty-eight-year-old patient of mine with pre-diabetes, had difficulty getting her weight and blood sugar under control. She ate well and exercised regularly, but just couldn't get things to fall into place. We looked at a special urine test called "organic acids" that measures mitochondrial function in a different way from V02 max, or oxygen consumption.

We measured all the various steps in Jane's metabolism that turn fat and carbohydrates into energy and we found a number of roadblocks. She needed more carnitine, alpha lipoic acid, and coenzyme Q10. After a few months on mitochondrial-boosting, energy-burning amino acids and nutrients, we tested her again and found her metabolism significantly improved. As a side effect, she lost 23 pounds, her energy increased, and her blood sugar normalized.

In my medical practice I often test all the steps in metabolism to see if there are any that are blocked or slow. Each step requires different helpers or cofactors. These are usually vitamins and minerals or amino acids. Your mitochondria need help transporting and burning calories. Specific nutrients, including carnitine, alpha lipoic acid, coenzyme Q10, the B vitamins (especially riboflavin [B2] and niacin [B3]), and branched-chain essential amino acids (BCAA) are critical in these steps.

You may be wondering how your metabolic engine is working and if you are rusting on the inside. Take the two quizzes below to see if your mitochondria are damaged and if you have too much oxidative stress. Remember to take this quiz before you start the program and again after the six weeks are over to measure the "before and after" change in your health. You may need extra individualized support based on your scores; I explain this in Week 6 of the plan.

Energy Metabolism Quiz

Some people do indeed have a slow metabolism and reduced capacity to burn calories from food. Use this quiz to assess the severity of your damaged or slow metabolism. For any symptom you have experienced in the last month, place a check in the "Before" box. Place a check in the "After" box after you've completed the six-week program to see how much you've improved.

	Before	After
I am experiencing chronic or prolonged fatigue.		
I'm too tired to do many of the things I would like to do.		
Fatigue interferes with my work, family, or social life.		
I am not refreshed when I wake up.		
I have trouble falling or staying asleep, or I wake up too early.		
I have aching muscle pain or discomfort.		
I have muscle weakness.		
I have a poor tolerance for exercise and I'm incredibly tired afterward.		
My concentration and memory are not what they used to be.		
I am irritable and moody.		
I gained weight and developed diabetes after an acute stressor, infection, or trauma.		

(Continued)

	Before	After
I frequently overeat.		
I have been exposed to pesticides, unfiltered water, nonorganic food, or other environmental chemicals.		
I have chronic fatigue syndrome or fibromyalgia.		
I have a history of chronic infections.		
I have been under prolonged stress.		
I have Gulf War syndrome.		
I have a neurologic disease (Alzheimer's, Parkinson's, ALS, etc.).		
I have autism or ADHD.		
I suffer from depression, bipolar disease, or schizophrenia.		
TOTAL		

Score	Severity	Care Plan	Action to Take
0–6	You may have a mild loss of energy.	*The Blood Sugar Solution*	No personalization needed. Simply complete *The Blood Sugar Solution.*

Score	Severity	Care Plan	Action to Take
7–9	You may have a moderate loss of energy.	Self-Care	Complete *The Blood Sugar Solution* and optimize your results by following the personalization steps in Chapter 24.
10+	You may have a severe loss of energy.	Medical Care	Do both of the above steps and see a physician for additional assistance if you are not better after the first six weeks of the program.

Oxidative Stress or Rusting Quiz

Free radicals or oxidative stress slow our metabolism and cause weight gain, diabetes, and aging.

Take the quiz below to find out if you are at risk for high levels of oxidative stress. For any symptom you have experienced in the last month, place a check in the "Before" box. Then find out how severe your problem is by using the scoring key below. Place a check in the "After" box after you've completed the six-week program to see how much you've improved.

	Before	After
Exercise is not a part of my regular routine, or is too much a part of my regular routine (more than 15 hours a week).		
I am overweight (BMI more than 25).		
I am fatigued on a regular basis.		
I sleep less than eight hours a night.		
I regularly experience deep muscle or joint pain.		
I am sensitive to perfume, smoke, or other chemicals or fumes.		
I am exposed to a significant level of environmental toxins (pollutants, chemicals, etc.) at home and/or at work.		
I drink more than three alcoholic beverages a week.		
I smoke cigarettes or cigars (or anything else).		
There is a significant amount of secondhand smoke where I work or live.		

	Before	After
I don't use sun block, I like to bake in the sun, or I go to tanning booths.		
I would rate my life as very stressful.		
I eat fewer than five servings of deeply colored vegetables and fruits a day.		
My diet includes a fair amount of fried foods, margarine, or a lot of animal fat (meat, cheese, etc.).		
I eat white flour and sugar more than twice a week.		
I suffer from chronic colds and infections (cold sores, canker sores, etc.).		
I don't take antioxidants or a multivitamin.		
I take prescription, over-the-counter, and/or recreational drugs.		
I have arthritis or allergies.		
I have diabetes or heart disease.		
TOTAL		

Score	Severity	Care Plan	Action to Take
0–9	You may have a low level of oxidative stress.	*The Blood Sugar Solution*	No personalization needed. Simply complete *The Blood Sugar Solution.*
10+	You may have a severe level of oxidative stress.	Medical Care	Do the above step and see a physician for additional assistance if you are not better after the first six weeks of the program.

WHAT DAMAGES YOUR MITOCHONDRIA

Your mitochondria are sensitive to a variety of insults, particularly calorie-rich, high-sugar, nutrient- and antioxidant-poor foods. Toxins, infections, and anything causing inflammation can further damage our mitochondria. This leads to oxidative stress, or free radical production, which damages our mitochondria, cells, and tissues. When unchecked, oxidative stress turns on genes that increase insulin resistance and inflammation and reduce mitochondrial function and energy production in the body.[3]

You can reduce free radical activity and oxidative stress, and improve energy production in your cells, by combining a whole-food, nutrient-, phytonutrient-, and antioxidant-rich diet with supplemental antioxidants such as alpha lipoic acid and other mitochondrial-boosting supplements, as well as with special types of exercise. These are essential components of *The Blood Sugar Solution* program (see Part IV).

If you have diabetes, or a family history of diabetes, exercise is especially important. In fact, your genetic predisposition toward reduced mitochondrial function can be overcome by exercise. I recommend including strength training and a special type of aerobic conditioning called *high-intensity interval training (HIT)* in your regular routine. This combination has been shown to dramatically improve mitochondrial function, and leads to weight loss and improved cellular metabolism.[4] In Part IV, I will explain how you can incorporate both forms of exercise into your daily life.

THE HOLY GRAIL OF HEALTHY AGING: KEEPING THE MITOCHONDRIA HEALTHY

The single most important biological phenomenon that causes aging is diminished energy production in the mitochondria, which results in the development of insulin resistance. In fact, the "disease" of aging is really a disease of accelerated insulin resistance. If we fix that, we can reverse the aging process. Treatments are being developed to address mitochondrial dysfunction, including one based on *resveratrol,* the antioxidant compound in red grapes. Resveratrol acts on a master class of genes called *sirtuins,* which regulate insulin function and mitochondrial energy production. When these genes are turned on, they basically reverse the mitochondrial aging process and insulin resistance.

You might have heard of the rats fed high doses of resveratrol. They lived thirty percent longer and became fitter, even while eating the equivalent of the standard American poor-quality diet. They did it by having the equivalent of about 1,500 bottles of red wine, so don't try this at home.

Calorie restriction also helps improve mitochondrial function, although it is hard to do. Excellent animal studies have shown that if you eat 30 percent fewer calories per day, you will live 30 percent longer.[5] In an effort to extend their lifespan, a group of brave souls in the Calorie Restriction Society eats food high in nutrients but very low in calories. One man I met ate 5 pounds of celery for breakfast and a few pounds of tomatoes and cucumbers for lunch!

However, exciting new research points to a novel way to prevent the ravages of aging without having to eat 5 pounds of celery a day. In his medically dense book, *Avoiding the First Cause of Death,* Wulf Dröge explains how to extend your lifespan to 120 years old. All you have to do is carefully balance, repair, and rebuild your mitochondria. You can do that by reducing insulin production and optimizing amino acid and protein intake, as well as by exercising. Bottom line: Consume small amounts of low-glycemic-load carbs, along with easily used and absorbed amino acids and protein throughout the day. That's *The Blood Sugar Solution* program. Studies show that taking the basic amino acid protein building blocks as supplements for repair and healing actually helps slow aging and reverses insulin resistance and diabetes.[6] In Part IV, I recommend exactly what to take and how to get the nutrients and amino acids you need to reverse diabesity and promote healthy aging.

Remember, by modifying your lifestyle, doing interval training and exercising, eating a nutrient-dense diet, and taking certain supplements, such as carnitine, alpha lipoic acid, coenzyme Q10, the B vitamins, and branched-chain amino acids (BCAA), you can boost your mitochondrial function.[7]

14

Step 7: Soothe Your Mind

Stress makes you fat and contributes to the development of diabesity. When I worked in the emergency room, I frequently saw patients with high blood sugar. These people were not diabetic. Acute stress had caused their blood sugar to skyrocket. Doctors have long known there is a relationship between stress and blood sugar. What we now understand is that, in the face of chronic stress, our levels of insulin, cortisol, and inflammatory compounds called *cytokines* all increase. This drives the relentless metabolic dysfunction that leads to weight gain, insulin resistance, and ultimately diabetes.

Bad Relationships Cause Weight Gain: A Patient's Story

Rebecca was fifty-two, single, and still lived with and cared for her eighty-four-year-old mother.

Despite a highly successful professional career as a social worker, she lived under the cloud of her mother's daily criticism. The chronic stress affected her ability to care for herself and to make healthy choices about her food, exercise, and social life. Her body secreted high levels of cortisol, which helps protect us from danger in times of acute stress but causes weight gain, increases hunger, causes pre-diabetes and diabetes, and contributes to or exacerbates every known chronic disease. Rebecca developed severe pre-diabetes, but what she most needed wasn't a healthier diet or more exercise. She needed to get a "mother-ectomy" and move out. With support and encouragement, she reclaimed her life and her health.

Are your stress levels contributing to your diabesity? Take the quiz below to find out. Remember to take this quiz before you start the program and again after the six weeks are over to measure the "before and after" change in your health. You may need extra individualized support based on your scores; I explain this in Week 6 of the plan.

Stress and Adrenal Fatigue Quiz

Chronic stress contributes to many diseases including diabesity. For any symptom you have experienced in the last month, place a check in the "Before" box. Then find out how severe your problem is by using the scoring key below. Place a check in the "After" box after you've completed the six-week program to see how much you've improved.

	Before	After
My life is very stressful.		
I am easily startled and suffer from panic attacks.		
I feel tired but wired.		
When I'm nervous, my palms and feet get sweaty.		
I feel fatigued.		
I often feel weak and shaky.		
When I stand up, I feel dizzy.		
I have dark circles under my eyes.		
I crave sweets.		
I crave salt.		
I don't feel refreshed after a night's sleep.		
I have difficulty either falling or staying asleep.		
I have trouble concentrating or suffer from mental fogginess.		

	Before	After
I frequently experience headaches.		
I catch colds easily and suffer from frequent infections.		
I can't start my day without caffeine.		
I retain water.		
I experience heart palpitations.		
I have poor tolerance for alcohol, caffeine, and other drugs.		
I don't tolerate exercise well and I'm incredibly tired afterward.		
I have hypoglycemia (low blood sugar).		
My muscles are weak.		
My blood pressure is low.		
TOTAL		

Score	Severity	Care Plan	Action to Take
0–7	You may have low adrenal dysfunction.	*The Blood Sugar Solution*	No personalization needed. Simply complete *The Blood Sugar Solution.*

(Continued)

Score	Severity	Care Plan	Action to Take
8–10	You may have moderate adrenal dysfunction.	Self-Care	Complete *The Blood Sugar Solution* and optimize your fatty acid levels by following the personalization steps in Chapter 24.
11+	You may have severe adrenal dysfunction.	Medical Care	Do both of the above steps and see a physician for additional assistance if you are not better after the first six weeks of the program.

An increased stress response and the resultant high levels of cortisol worsen diabesity, damage your brain, and impair appetite control, making you hungrier and increasing your craving for sugar.

Diabetics have a much higher risk of getting depression.[1] And depressed people have a higher risk of getting diabetes. In a major study published in the *Archives of Internal Medicine*,[2] scientists found that women who were depressed were 17 percent more likely to develop diabetes even after the researchers adjusted for other risk factors such as weight and lack of regular exercise. Those women who were taking antidepressants were 25 percent more likely to develop diabetes than their counterparts who were not depressed. Women who already had diabetes were 29 percent more likely to develop depression after taking into account other depression risk factors, and those women who took insulin for their diabetes were 53 percent more likely to develop depression during the 10-year study. More insulin triggered more depression.

While certain factors such as inflammation, toxins, lack of physical activity, and obesity may partially explain the link between depression and diabetes, they do not completely explain it. They may also be linked by stress. People who are depressed have elevated levels of cortisol, which can lead to problems with glucose or blood sugar metabolism, increased insulin resistance, and the accumulation of belly fat.

As important as this mind-body connection is, it's still only one part of the puzzle. What most people don't realize is that what you do to your body affects your brain as well. As your metabolism, insulin resistance, and diabetes improve, you may find that your mood improves dramatically without the help of antidepressants or other drugs. Healing your body is an essential step for healing your brain. My book

The UltraMind Solution (www.bloodsugarsolution
.com/ultramind-solution) explains how the body
affects the brain and how diabesity is linked to mood
disorders, cognitive disorders, and brain aging.

The links between stress, weight gain, mental disorders, and blood sugar imbalances show that managing stress is a critical component of obesity and
diabetes treatment.

There are many ways to effectively reduce your
stress response. You can try relaxation therapies,
meditation, breathing exercises, yoga, group support,
massage, exercise, saunas, dancing, praying, laugh-
ing, and much more. Getting together to get healthy
is another powerful way to reduce stress.

Actively engaging your relaxation response is a
critical part of the process of healing diabesity. Find
a few things you enjoy and do them every day. Relaxing is as important as breathing, sleeping, or eating.
Not doing it will kill you. In Part IV, I share a number of extremely effective tools to help you engage
your relaxation response. You can try those or my
UltraCalm audio program (www.bloodsugarsolution
.com/ultracalm).

PART III

THE BLOOD SUGAR SOLUTION: PREPARATION

A journey of a thousand miles begins with a single step.

— Lao Tzu, Tao Te Ching

15

Start the Journey

Now that you understand the causes of diabesity and the extent of this problem, the next step is creating a solution—for ourselves, our families, our communities, and our society.

Eat better and exercise more. This is what we are told by doctors, nutritionists, and government agencies. How has that advice worked for you so far?

The Blood Sugar Solution is based on an entirely different approach—a systems approach—that connects the dots among all your symptoms and health problems. By applying this science, we can correct imbalances in the body and create health.

The secret is that you don't have to treat diabesity.

CREATING HEALTH

You simply have to create health.

We have been going about things backward. As you learn which obstacles stand in your way and the ingredients you need to generate health, you can simply remove the obstacles (toxins, allergens, microbes, stress, poor diet, and others) and add the ingredients (whole, fresh food, nutrients, hormones, sleep, movement, rhythm, relaxation, love, connection, meaning, and purpose). When you do this, your symptoms and diseases will take care of themselves.

Part IV of this book outlines a six-week action plan to get healthy and happy. In Part III, you will find a two-week preparation phase that will provide the foundation for vibrant and sustainable health. It is about celebration, not deprivation, about finding all the delicious benefits that come from eating real food and caring for our bodies and souls.

Over the course of this program, you will slowly and systematically integrate changes in your diet and lifestyle. Along the way I will teach you the information and skills you need to safely reinvent your kitchen, negotiate your supermarket, optimize your nutrition, add supplements, eliminate toxins, exercise, find your pause button, and more. You will learn how to use medication intelligently, discover natural alternatives for medications, and get started with a meal plan that includes menus, recipes, and shopping lists. Learn more about the online support program I developed at www.bloodsugarsolution .com. It will guide you through the entire program.

We will also explore how, together, as a community, we can create a movement for changing this horrible life-robbing, economy-busting epidemic. Through collective actions, we can *Take Back Our Health.*

Changing a lifetime of bad habits, learning new skills, and correcting misinformation take time. Two weeks to be exact. So don't skip this critical preparation phase.

GETTING HEALTHY TOGETHER

As you move forward on your journey to healing, remember that it is easier to get healthy together than to do it alone. In Chapter 16, you will learn how to harness the power of community, create your own group (even a group of two), and understand why having support is so important to long-term success, health, and happiness.

Social connection, support, and community are critical for long-term success and very powerful in the short term for making and sustaining lifestyle and behavior changes. Friends and community have a powerful influence over us. You are more likely to be overweight if your friends are overweight than if your family members are obese. It is not the genetic threads but the social threads that connect us and that ultimately have the most power to change the obesity, diabetes, and chronic disease epidemic.

Being connected to others is a necessary ingredient for health, just like food, water, air, sleep, or movement. We are hardwired for community and connection. It doesn't matter what group you belong to, what church, temple, or mosque you attend, what community you connect to — it is no accident that if Facebook were a country, its users would comprise the third largest country after China and India. Create or join a group. It is the most effective way to achieve lasting change.

GETTING TESTED

In Chapter 17, you will learn about getting tested. You will need to collect information about yourself, your story, and your symptoms to get a complete picture of the imbalances you suffer from and the changes you need to make on the program. The quizzes, body measurements, and basic baseline blood and urine tests outlined in this step will help you see where you are out of balance and become a yardstick by which you measure your progress and success.

GETTING STARTED

Let's get started.

There are five important steps you need to take to prepare your mind, your body, and your kitchen for *The Blood Sugar Solution* program:

1. **Prepare your mind.** Connect to your motivation so you can successfully get on and stay on the program.
2. **Prepare yourself.** Commit to the program and plan a start date.
3. **Prepare your kitchen.** Clean toxic substances out of your kitchen and stock it with the foods that create health, not disease.
4. **Prepare your inner shopper and inner chef.** Learn how to navigate the toxic food terrain in the modern supermarket and develop simple cooking skills that will support your health.
5. **Prepare your body.** Get your body ready to heal by taking a "drug holiday" from sugar, stimulants, and sedatives.

Please do not shortcut this process. Setting the stage for success is essential if you are going to make the most of the program.

PREPARE YOUR MIND: FIND YOUR MOTIVATION

Are you ready?

Your life is about to change.

You have made a decision to get healthy. But that is only the first step.

The second step is preparing for action.

The third step is acting on what you have decided.

The final step is sustaining healthy changes for life.

When you make a decision to create health, you will face many obstacles. In our fast-paced, media-saturated, overworked, overstressed, underactive, over-fed lives, choosing health is a revolutionary act. And it will take a revolution to change all the conditions that lead to illness, obesity, and diabetes. But revolutions start with small changes that are specific, measurable, attainable, realistic, and timely.

Identifying Obstacles and Connecting to Your Motivation

First you must identify the obstacles in front of you and get clear about your motivation to change. Overcoming your inertia will require focused intention and a repeated reinforcing of that intention. Journaling, creating a group support system, and my online

support curriculum and tools at www.bloodsugar
solution.com can help you overcome these obstacles.

What are your obstacles? They might include:

- Beliefs about what is possible, or not ("I can't cure
  diabetes or lose weight")
- A negative relationship to your body and to
  food ("Eating makes me fat and sick, but I *love*
  to eat.")
- Self-defeating thoughts and behaviors
- Biological addiction to sugar
- A toxic food landscape of fast, processed, depleted,
  calorie-rich foods
- Aggressive food marketing practices ("Buy this; it
  will make you healthy and feel good")
- Lack of available high-quality foods, high in
  nutrients and low in calories
- Saboteurs at home and at work (food pushers)
- Too many responsibilities (trouble saying no to
  others and yes to yourself)
- History of failed attempts to change

The biggest belief that obstructs our path to success is the idea that we really can't change our health
that much. We may lose a few pounds, feel a little
better, but our health destiny is preprogrammed. Just
look at my diabetic father or my obese grandmother

or my sister who had that heart attack at fifty-two. What can I really do to change that?

Everything.

There may be many beliefs and attitudes, negative thought patterns and behaviors that prevent you from starting a process of self-care and self-nourishment. Focus on what is important to you. Feeling well? Living a long vibrant life? Contributing to your community? Spending more time with your family? Working through your bucket list? Taking a trip to the zoo with your grandchild? Having sex until you are ninety? Starting a business? Walking in the woods with your loved one? Riding your bike across America at eighty-five years old?

For me, the definition of health is being able to get up in the morning and do what nourishes me— being present with my family, doing a good job at work, climbing a mountain in the winter on snowshoes, playing basketball with my son, learning something new, having the energy and strength to make a contribution to my community and friends. That is what helps guide my choices every day. What is important for you?

Start a Journal Now

Journaling is an excellent way to get in touch with your inner motivations, to break the cycle of mindless eating and activity, to be honest and accountable and present to yourself. We often overeat because something is eating us. We stuff ourselves with food in order to stuff our feelings away. We use food to block feelings, but you can use words to block food. You can write in order to better metabolize your feelings so they don't end up driving unconscious choices or overeating. A diet of words and self-exploration often results in weight loss. You metabolize your life and calories better.

You will also use the journal to track your food intake every day, your exercise, sleep, symptoms, and your "numbers," including weight, waist size, and lab tests. Recognizing how you feel and what you experience as you alter your food intake, begin taking supplements, and start to exercise more is like "innercise," building the self-awareness needed to strengthen your ability to create high-level wellness and wholeness.

Be honest about your food intake; record everything you eat and the amount. This simple act will bring insight into how you care for your body and well-being. In her book *The Writing Diet*, Julia Cameron suggests you ask yourself four simple questions right before you choose to eat something:

1. Am I hungry?
2. Is this what I feel like eating?
3. Is this what I feel like eating now?
4. Is there something else I could eat instead?

Get The Blood Sugar Solution
Online Support Tools Now

I recommend you use my online companion course tools to record your journey. To start your journal, please go to www.bloodsugarsolution .com. The online companion course tools are a great place to track your progress (your story, your numbers, and your blood work), and to track your food intake and exercise, your inner journey, obstacles, and successes.

I also have my patients ask two related questions:

1. What am I feeling?
2. What do I need?

You may be hungry and need food, or lonely and need a friend, or tired and need a nap, or angry and need to sort out why. Not all of these feelings need food, although for many of us, that is our default action when we don't feel right.

As you journal, remember: This is for you. So be completely honest and transparent. This means not only recording what you are eating and how much you exercise, but what you *really* are feeling at the moment—there are no right or wrong answers.

Do not underestimate the power of this program. Research has shown that keeping track of your feelings, habits, and numbers creates a system of feedback and accountability that by itself is healing and will help you change your behavior. You don't have to believe it. Just do it.

Getting Rid of Mental Obstacles

Take out your journal (or use the course tools online) and respond to the questions below. Think about what depletes your energy and what gives you energy as you record responses:

- What are the top three things you do that hold you back from your health and weight loss goals? These may include things like smoking, not getting enough sleep, not relaxing enough, excess sugar consumption, unconscious or emotional eating, choosing poor-quality foods, eating late, skipping breakfast, and more.
- What are the top three emotions or mental habits that keep you from your health and weight loss goals? Is it putting things off, depression, low self-esteem, fear, anger, resentment, or something else?

- Do you have any "toxic relationships" in your life right now? Do they serve a purpose for you? Is there a way you could give them up or change them? If so, how could you do that?
- How would your life be different without these behavioral habits, mental and emotional constructs, and relationships?
- Are you really too busy to change your habits and life? Do you spend hours in front of the television or on the computer? How much time would you have to connect with friends, and to find and prepare healthy food, exercise, and relax if you took a "media fast"?
- What are some behaviors, habits, and relationships you could choose to engage in that would give you energy and mental, spiritual, and physical health?
- What motivates you in life? What makes you want to wake up each morning? What is your life's purpose?
- How does being overweight or ill diminish or detract from your life's purpose?
- How would following this program and getting well allow you to fulfill your life's purpose more effectively?

Each of us has unique reasons for wanting to create change in our health or life. There is no right or wrong reason, just what's most important to you.

Define Your Specific Goals for Creating Health and Happiness

Start by writing a list of your personal goals. Identify what you want and how you will get there. These questions are meant to get you started, but feel free to write whatever you like. Set aside a few hours. Be specific.

My Health Goals

- **Physical:** What physical or health problems do I want to heal from and how will I achieve that?
- **Food:** What is my relationship to food and how do I want to nourish myself?
- **Exercise:** What is my relationship with my body and exercise? How will I change that?
- **Sleep:** Do I prioritize quality sleep? What will I do to get enough sleep and recharge my body daily?
- **Weight:** How do I feel about my weight? What changes will I make to love my body rather than fight with it? What are my goals?

My Psychological and Social Goals

- **Emotional health:** Am I anxious, depressed, or angry? Am I a glass half-full or half-empty person? What thoughts and beliefs keep me stuck? Are there physical causes of my emotional state (food, stress, nutritional deficiencies, etc.)? What will I do to find out the source of my feelings and be the person I want to be?

- **Relationships:** What healing do I have to do in my relationships? What do I have to do to be a better child, partner, parent, friend, coworker, etc.?
- **Work:** What is my relationship to my work? How do I want to spend my time, energy, focus, skills, and talents? If I am not happy, what I can do to change how I am in my work or change what I am doing?

Meaning and Purpose

- **Spiritual goals:** What is important to me? What would I like to be my epitaph? What do I have to do to live up to that?
- **Getting to what's important now:** What are the "someday I hope to" thoughts I have that I can make happen now?

PREPARE YOURSELF

If you were going on vacation, you would organize your life to be sure everything was taken care of— the house, work, the kids, the bills, and the dog. You would arrange your travel, buy your tickets, pack your bags, and decide on a date and place to go. You would make a decision and pick a date to begin your journey.

Do the same thing for the most important trip you will ever take—the journey to wellness. Put a date on the calendar by which you will start your journey. Record it in your journal. The date you select will be the day you start the elimination phase of the program outlined in the section titled "Prepare Your Body" in this chapter. This phase will last for one week. When that week is over, you will start the six-week program described in Part IV. At the end of the six weeks, you will learn how to stay healthy for life. Choose the date on which you want to begin this process now.

PREPARE YOUR HEALTHY KITCHEN

Your kitchen is one of the most important rooms in your home. It has been hijacked by the food industry. It is time for you to reclaim it, to bring real food in and throw fake food out, to build on traditions of cooking and sharing meals with family and friends. Make mealtime a time of connection and celebration and nourishment for body and soul. It doesn't have to be hard or complicated. You simply have to get organized.

If you don't have a nourishing home full of

delicious, easy-to-prepare foods, snacks, and emergency meals, you will have a hard time succeeding. Don't put obstacles in your path by leaving disease-creating foods in your kitchen. Our fat storage hormones such as insulin and stress hormones such as cortisol control our appetite and behavior. If they surge and you have a big chocolate cake in the fridge, there is no way you can overcome the reptilian part of your brain that controls feeding behavior. We have hundreds of genes that protect us from starvation, but very few that protect us from overeating.

Here is how to get your kitchen ready for your journey.

Rid the Kitchen of Disease- and Obesity-Producing Frankenfoods

Take an afternoon to hunt and gather in your kitchen. Be merciless. If it is not real food, throw it out. You will restock your pantry and fridge with real food in Week 1 of the program.

I've outlined below my top 10 rules for eating safely for life. If you read these rules and think there will be nothing left to eat, then you have been eating in exactly the way that will make you sick and will keep you that way. The good news is that if your diet is all sugar, flour, and processed foods, you have the biggest gains to achieve.

These rules are mostly about what not to eat. You should follow them forever. We will get to all the wonderful foods you can eat later in Chapter 19.

10 Rules for Eating Safely for Life (and What to Remove from Your Kitchen)

1. Ideally have **only food without labels** in your kitchen or foods that don't come in a box, a package, or a can. There are labeled foods that are great, such as sardines, artichoke hearts, or roasted red peppers, but you have to be very smart in reading the labels. There are two things to look for: **the ingredient list and the nutrition facts.** Watch my video on how to buy food with labels that is safe and review how to interpret nutrition facts at www.bloodsugarsolution .com. Where is the primary ingredient on the list? If the real food is at the end of the list and sugar or salt is at the beginning, beware. The most abundant ingredient is listed first and the others are listed in descending order by weight. Be conscious, too, of ingredients that may not be on the list; some ingredients may be exempt from labels. This is often true if the food is in a very small package, if it has been prepared in the store, or if it has been made by a small manufacturer. Beware of these foods.

2. If a food has a label, it should have **fewer than five ingredients.** If it has more than five ingredients, throw it out. Also beware of foods with health claims on the label. They are usually bad for you — think "sports beverages." I recently saw a bag of deep-fried potato chips with the health claims "gluten-free, organic, no artificial ingredients, no sugar" and with fewer than five ingredients listed. Sounds great, right? But remember, cola is 100 percent fat-free and that doesn't make it a health food.

3. If **sugar** (by any name, including organic cane juice, honey, agave, maple syrup, cane syrup, or molasses) is on the label, throw it out. There are 39 teaspoons of sugar in the average bottle of ketchup. The same goes for **white rice and white flour,** which act just like sugar in the body. If you have diabesity, you can't easily handle any flour, even whole-grain. Throw it out.

4. Throw out any food with **high-fructose corn syrup** on the label. It is a supersweet, super cheap, subsidized liquid sugar that is in nearly every processed food. Some high-fructose corn syrup also contains mercury as a by-product of the manufacturing process.[1] Many liquid calories, such as sodas, juices, and "sports" drinks, contain this metabolic poison. It always signals low-quality or processed food.

5. Throw out any food with the word **hydroge-nated** on the label. This is an indicator of trans fats, vegetable oils converted through a chemical process into margarine or shortening. They are good for keeping cookies on the shelf for long periods of time without going stale, but these fats have been proven to cause heart disease, diabetes, and cancer. New York City and most European countries have banned trans fats, and you should, too.

6. Throw out any **highly refined cooking oils** such as corn, soy, etc. (I will explain which oils to buy in Week 1 of the program.) Also avoid toxic fats and fried foods.

7. Throw out any food with **ingredients you can't recognize or pronounce,** or are in Latin.

8. Throw out any **foods with preservatives, additives, coloring, or dyes,** "natural flavorings," or flavor enhancers such as MSG (monosodium glutamate).

9. Throw out food with **artificial sweeteners** of any kind (aspartame, Splenda, sucralose, and sugar alcohols—any word that ends with "ol," such as xylitol or sorbitol). They make you hungrier, slow your metabolism, give you bad gas, and make you store fat.

10. If it came from the earth or a farmer's field, not a food chemist's lab, it's safe to eat. As Michael

Pollan says, **If it was grown on a plant, not made in a plant, then you can keep it in your kitchen.** If it is something your great-grandmother wouldn't recognize as food (such as a "Lunch-able" or "Go-Gurt"), throw it out. Stay away from "food-like substances."

You will find a complete list of foods to avoid and more tips for cleaning out your pantry on my website—www.bloodsugarsolution.com. Also check out the Center for Science in the Public Interest's website for further information and updates at www .bloodsugarsolution.com/center-for-science-in-the-public-interest (click on Chemical Cuisine). And you can also watch my video on how to clean out your kitchen at www.bloodsugarsolution.com.

Get Your Essential Kitchen Tools

Before you start changing your diet, you need the right tools to support your journey to optimal health.

Kitchens are often bereft of even the most basic tools for preparing and cooking food. I've listed below the basic tools I feel are needed for the care and feeding of a human being. Invest in the highest-quality tools you can. Good kitchen equipment will last a lifetime.

Before you start the program, make sure you have most of the following:

- A set of good-quality knives
- Wooden cutting boards — one for animal prod-ucts, another for fruits and vegetables
- An 8-inch nonstick sauté pan
- A 12-inch nonstick sauté pan (Nonstick pans can vary in quality. Buy the highest quality, such as Calphalon or All-Clad, because of the health risks of poorer-quality nonstick pans using Teflon.)
- An 8-quart stockpot
- A 2-quart saucepan with lid
- A 4-quart saucepan with lid
- An 11-inch-square nonstick (non-Teflon) stovetop griddle
- Dutch oven
- Grill pan
- Three or four cookie or baking sheets
- A food processor
- A blender
- An immersion blender
- An instant-read chef's thermometer
- A can opener
- A coffee grinder for flaxseed or spices
- Wire whisks
- Spring tongs
- A fish spatula
- Rubber spatulas
- Assorted measuring cups (1 quart, 1 pint, and 1 cup), dry and liquid style

- A lemon/citrus reamer
- Microplane graters in assorted sizes

You will find further resources and product recommendations at www.bloodsugarsolution.com.

PREPARE YOUR INNER SHOPPER

Let's face it. You are a hunter and gatherer. You may carry a credit card instead of a spear, but make no mistake—you are on a mission for survival. Unfortunately our food landscape is a nutritional wasteland, consisting of supermarkets, convenience stores, fast-food outlets, restaurant chains, train stations, airports, highway rest stops, and your own kitchen.

We have no wisdom keepers who pass down the gathered knowledge of the ages of what to eat and what to avoid. Will this mushroom kill you or fill you? Will this fish heal you or paralyze you with a nasty fugu toxin? It's time to learn how to hunt and gather in the modern food desert. Buried in the mountains of sugar, fat, and salt in the average supermarket are nourishing foods. The American supermarket is a drug store—containing dangerous disease-promoting addictive drugs disguised as food as well as healing medicinal foods made by nature. The worst offenders are on the end caps of the aisles and in the middle of the shelves. The beans, salsa, and whole grains are hidden way down on the shelves or so up so high you can't see them. Yet once you become a skilled hunter-gatherer, you can emerge with real, whole, healing foods for your family.

While you won't be shopping for the foods in the meal plan until just before you begin the program, it's important to learn how to become an effective shopper during the preparation phase so you can be ready for that experience. I have created two short videos to give you a guided tour of the American supermarket. These will help you to safely navigate what can be a dangerous place. See *Supermarket Savvy: The Bad Stuff and The Good Stuff* at www .bloodsugarsolution.com.

I encourage you to make a shopping list every time you go to the supermarket and stick to it. You will save your money and your life.

PREPARE YOUR INNER CHEF

Not everyone likes cooking. That's okay. Not everyone likes school, or exercise. But it is an important life skill unless you have a personal chef or a spouse or partner who is happy to cook for you. When I was a boy, my mother told me, "If you can read, you can cook." You don't have to be Julia Child or Mario

Batali, but you can learn how to create nourishing, delicious, and healthy meals quickly and inexpensively without enrolling in cooking school.

I know this may seem like a lot to do when you already have a busy schedule. But the average American spends more time watching cooking on television than actually cooking. Learning to cook is worth it. So many people say they don't have the time or energy to cook, and I get it. I am very driven and have many "careers" — doctor, author, chairman of a nonprofit, volunteer, and educator as well as father, husband, son, brother, uncle, and friend. I have the energy to do all these things because I take care of my body and mind. I sleep 8 hours a night, exercise 4–6 times a week, and cook and eat good food. I have become an expert in instant (meaning quickly prepared) food. I can go into a fridge and pantry and prepare a delicious hot, fresh, whole-food meal in less time than it would take to bake a frozen pizza or order takeout.

Give me 15 minutes and I can feed my family and myself. You can do it, too. You just need to plan ahead a bit and get your kitchen ready for the week.

If you are resistant to cooking or think you don't have the time, the following journaling exercise may help.

Journaling Exercise: Why Don't I Cook?

Take out your journal and answer the following questions:

- What are the top three reasons you don't cook at present? Is it a lack of time? Do you cook poorly? Do you simply dislike cooking?
- How could you create more time to cook for yourself? Think of this in terms of priorities— are the "responsibilities" in your life really more important than your health, the health of your children, and the health of our world? How could you carve out 15–20 minutes to cook 2–3 times a day?
- What could you do that would make cooking more enjoyable? You might listen to music or get your family involved in cutting, chopping, peeling, and cleaning. Cooking is a wonderful family activity, giving you time together without distraction, a chance to catch up and nourish one another. Or you could chat with a friend on a headset while chopping and dicing.

You do have to learn how to put a meal together if you want to be healthy. Here are some easy ways to create simple, delicious meals.

Dr. Hyman's Favorite 3 Meals in 30 Minutes

I have provided a complete two-week set of menus, recipes, and shopping lists at the end of this book, and I will give you my Nutrition 101 course in Week 1 of the plan. But as long as you understand some basic nutritional principles and learn a few simple cooking techniques, you don't need to follow the meal plan. You can make a protein shake or have a couple of poached omega-3 eggs for breakfast or a bowl of brown rice, veggies, and protein for dinner. And you can learn to make some quick, easy, delicious, nourishing meals.

Here's what a very busy day's meals might look like for me and how much time it takes me to make great food. I sometimes *do* use things with cans and labels. But only real food with one or two ingredients I can recognize like "navy beans" or "artichoke hearts" or "wild salmon." I can make 3 meals in 30 minutes total. I work fast so it might take you a little longer. It won't be fancy, but it will be delicious and satisfying.

Breakfast shake: Protein powder (rice, soy, hemp, pea, or chia), frozen berries, unsweetened hemp milk, 1 tablespoon omega-3 oil, and a small handful of walnuts or almonds. Toss in a blender, blend, and drink. Time to make and consume: 5 minutes.

Lunch: Prewashed arugula or mixed greens, a can of rinsed white beans, a jar or can of artichoke hearts. Extra virgin olive oil, balsamic vinegar, a little salt and pepper. Combine, and eat. Time to make: less than 5 minutes.

Snacks: Raw almonds or cashews. Time to make: 0 minutes.

Dinner: Prepare a pot of short-grain brown rice ahead of time (it lasts 3–4 days in the fridge). Simply add 2 cups of water to 1 cup of rinsed brown rice, bring to a boil, cover, and then simmer for 45 minutes. I then take the rice, put some in a bowl, and heat it in the microwave (not ideal, but you do what you gotta do!) or sauté it in a nonstick pan with a little olive oil and salt (it tastes better this way). If I've sautéed it, I put the rice in a bowl and use the same pan to cook some prewashed spinach or other dark chopped green leafy veggies like kale, collards, chard, or some broccolini or asparagus. I add a little olive oil, some precrushed or prepeeled garlic (I told you I am very busy!) to the greens, and quickly sauté at medium heat in the pan. I add a little wheat-free tamari or salt and a few tablespoons of water to prevent it from sticking. I then put some canned wild salmon in the bowl with the rice. I put the greens (a *large* amount because they are filling, full of nutrients, and contain very few calories) on top of the fish and rice. And I have a delicious meal. Time to cook: 15 minutes at most—I do it in under 10. Imagine what you could do in an hour!

For more variety, you can use the same basic set of steps above and simply change the ingredients or the order. Use frozen blackberries and nut butter in your shake one day, blueberries and walnuts the next. Add canned salmon or sardines to the mixed greens for lunch. Try the navy beans at dinner or sauté a chicken breast to go with the brown rice and veggies (or dice it for chicken veggie stir-fry). Don't care for rice? Try quinoa or buckwheat instead—all are wonderful whole grains that can be cooked in advance.

You need to learn basic cooking skills in order to heal your body. The kitchen is where it all begins. Medical clinics of the future will include teaching kitchens where patients will learn basic cooking skills and food selection and preparation. Wouldn't you rather learn how to make food your medicine, than take a bunch of medications that don't work half as well and have only bad side effects?

Experiment with food, seek out local cooking classes, have a friend teach you how to cook. It's well worth the effort. You can also watch some cooking videos I have created at www.bloodsugarsolution .com.

PREPARE THE BODY

One week before you begin the program, you will start your "drug" holiday. The four top-selling items at supermarkets are all drugs: sugar, caffeine, alcohol, and nicotine. These drugs boost our energy or mood, or "relax" or calm us. But in the end they are false aids that deplete our energy and our health. A quick fix of sugar or caffeine gives you a brief boost, then you crash and crave. Not a good cycle. Alcohol is just sugar in another form, and it impairs your impulse control, so you will consume more. Once you get off these drugs, you will realize just how much they were robbing you of your energy and health.

Smoking is hard to quit. Seek help from your doctor or try hypnosis, acupuncture, or medication. I can get you off the other drugs without too much suffering.

One week before the program, cut out *all* of these addictive substances from your diet and your life:

- All sugar, including all flour products, breads, pastas, and other highly processed carbs that act like sugar

- All of the toxic, processed foods mentioned in my 10 Rules for Eating Safely for Life, on pages 233–236
- Alcohol (for seven weeks—one-week preparation and six-week program)
- Caffeine (for seven weeks—one-week preparation and six-week program)

Do not underestimate the power of eliminating these addictive substances that drive cravings and imbalances in your blood sugar. If you do nothing else in this book, these steps can change your life, boost your metabolism, balance your blood sugar, and help you lose weight.

Take Action! Cut Cravings for Sugar and End Food Addiction

Take the following steps to minimize your withdrawal symptoms as you eliminate addictive substances from your diet.

10 Tips for Cutting Your Cravings

1. **Balance your blood sugar.** Swings in blood sugar are the major driver of cravings, so keep your blood sugar stable. Eliminate sugar and artificial sweeteners 100 percent and your cravings will go away. Go cold turkey. Eliminate refined sugars, sodas, fruit juices, and artificial sweeteners from your diet, as these can trigger cravings.

Combine good protein (fish, organic eggs, small amounts of lean poultry, nuts, whole soy foods, and legumes), good fats (fish, extra virgin olive oil, unrefined coconut oil, olives, nuts other than peanuts, seeds, and avocados), and good carbs (beans, vegetables, whole grains, and fruit) at each meal to balance your blood sugar.

2. **Don't drink your calories.** Liquid calories drive up your appetite and your waist size more than anything else. You will pour on the pounds!

3. **Eat a nutritious protein breakfast.** Studies repeatedly show that eating a healthy **protein-containing** breakfast helps people lose weight, reduce cravings, and burn calories. Good proteins are eggs, nuts, seeds, nut butters, or a protein shake (see my UltraShake recipes on pages 494–496).

4. **Have small, frequent, fiber-rich meals throughout the day.** Eat every 3–4 hours and have some protein with each snack or meal (lean animal protein, nuts, seeds, or beans).

5. **Avoid eating within 3 hours of bedtime.** It drives up insulin before you sleep, which makes you store more belly fat. Belly fat drives cravings through inflammatory and hormonal triggers.

6. **Manage your stress.** Anything stressful can trigger hormones that activate cravings. If you

have the urge to eat, ask yourself two questions: "What am I feeling, and what do I need?" Is there something else besides food that will help you get what you need? Adopt a daily stress management program that includes deep-breathing exercises, meditation, and other relaxation techniques. (See Week 3 on pages 361–365 for specifics on how to do this.)

7. **Find out if hidden food allergies are triggering your cravings.** We often crave the very foods we are allergic to (which is why I recommend stopping gluten and dairy for the first six weeks of the program). Getting off them is not easy, but after two to three days without them, you will have renewed energy and relief from cravings and symptoms.

8. **Get moving.** Exercise helps control and regulate your appetite. (See Week 4 on pages 375–378 for tips on how to exercise.)

9. **Get 7–8 hours of sleep.** Not getting enough sleep drives sugar and carb cravings by affecting your appetite hormones. (See pages 369–371 for tips on how to sleep better.)

10. **Optimize your nutrient levels:**
    - **Optimize omega-3 fat.** Omega-3 fatty acids are important for controlling insulin function.
    - **Optimize your vitamin D level.** Your appetite control is impaired by low vitamin D levels.

- **Consider taking natural supplements for cravings control.** L-glutamine, PGX (a super fiber), chromium, alpha lipoic acid, dl-phenylalanine, N-acetyl-cysteine, and other natural dietary supplements can help reduce cravings.

Take Action! Eliminate Caffeine in Seven Days

When I was in medical school, everybody drank coffee, so I started drinking my daily cup of joe. I noticed I got very sleepy in the afternoon and needed some more caffeine or sugar to perk me up. I realized that coffee was the cause, so I stopped drinking it and my energy came back. I see many of my patients getting trapped in this cycle. Most also get too little sleep. But caffeine cannot compensate for lack of sleep.

When you eliminate caffeine, you will be more tired for the first few days. You may even get a headache. These withdrawal symptoms are a sure sign of addiction. But when you finally do get off caffeine, you will have more energy than you did when you were on it.

Here's how to end your addiction as painlessly as possible.

1. Start on a weekend, when you can catch up on sleep.
2. Cut your dose in half every day till you are down to one-half cup of coffee a day. Then stop.

3. Drink plenty of water.
4. Take 1,000 mg of vitamin C a day.
5. If you get a headache, go to bed, or if you have to, take a couple of Advil.

Take Action! Take a Break from Alcohol (Another Form of Liquid Calories)

A nice glass of red wine with a meal, a cold beer on a hot day, or a shot of tequila at a party are some of the sweet pleasures of life. But as a daily habit, alcohol can do more harm than you realize, especially if you have diabesity. It may raise triglycerides, elevate blood pressure, impair gut function, interrupt sleep, increase cancer risk, impair liver function, act as an additional calorie source, and prevent you from achieving a healthy weight. It is best that you avoid all alcoholic beverages while you are on the program.

Consider this: If you drink two glasses of wine a day, you will consume about 72,000 extra calories a year. If you don't reduce your food intake (which you won't because alcohol reduces your inhibitions around food), you could gain an extra 20 pounds a year. And these liquid calories go right to your belly.

Stop for six weeks. See how you feel. Then, if you want, enjoy one to three glasses of wine or alcohol a week (a "glass" is 5 ounces of wine, 1.5 ounces of distilled spirits, or 12 ounces of beer).

Remember, if you do nothing else recommended in this book, eliminating sugar, refined carbohydrates, processed food, trans fats, caffeine, and alcohol will have profound effects on your weight, energy, mood, and health in just a few weeks. So take that drug holiday. It will be the best vacation of your life.

16

Harness the Power
of Community

In the fall of 2010, I had dinner with Rick Warren, the pastor of the 30,000-strong Saddleback Church in Southern California. Over a healthy dinner of beet and cabbage autumn soup and a salad, he described his extraordinarily successful experiment for sustained personal growth and change. Rick had encouraged his congregation to form 5,000 small groups that met every week to study, learn, and grow together in their community.

In that moment, I envisioned using those same small groups as a means of creating healthy lifestyle change. With the help of Drs. Mehmet Oz and Daniel Amen, we created **The Daniel Plan,** a 52-week curriculum for physical and spiritual health and renewal that would be delivered through the small groups. Rick named it "The Daniel Plan" after the book of Daniel, which tells the story of King Nebuchadnezzar and the Israelites he imprisoned.

THE FIRST SUPPORT GROUP: DANIEL AND HIS FRIENDS

In the first chapter of the book of Daniel (Daniel 1:3–16), Daniel and his three enslaved friends, Shadrach, Meshach, and Abednego, were commanded to eat from the king's kitchen of rich foods and wine. Daniel and his friends were determined not to defile themselves by eating the food and drinking the wine. Daniel asked the chief of staff, Melzar, for permission to refuse the king's command. But Melzar implored Daniel to do as he was told, so that he, Melzar, would not be beheaded for going against the king's orders. He said that the king would know if Daniel and his friends hadn't eaten his food because they would look malnourished.

Daniel then gave him this challenge:

Please test us for 10 days on a diet of vegetables and water. At the end of 10 days, see how we look compared to the other young men who are eating from the king's food. Then make your decision in the light of what you see.

Melzar agreed to Daniel's challenge and tested them for 10 days. At the end of 10 days, Daniel and his three friends looked healthier and better nourished than the young men who were eating the food assigned by the king.

So after that Melzar fed them only vegetables instead of the food and wine provided for the others. God gave these four men an unusual aptitude for understanding every aspect of literature and wisdom.

On January 15, 2011, the day we launched The Daniel Plan at Saddleback Church, more than 8,000 people signed up to participate in small groups, track their progress, and be part of a research study. Within two months, 15,000 people had signed up. The plan includes a weekly curriculum, learning objectives, videos, webinars, seminars, and online support. From a survey taken after the first six weeks, we found that the congregation had lost an estimated 160,000 pounds total (or about 8 percent of their body weight). After 10 months, the average weight loss for those who did the program was 18.6 pounds, and many lost 50 to 100 pounds. But those who did the program **together** lost twice as much weight as those who did it alone. Many experienced relief from chronic symptoms, including migraines, asthma, reflux, irritable bowel, autoimmune diseases, depression, insomnia, cravings, joint pain, gout, acne, skin problems, and more. The Daniel Plan changed the entire culture of the church almost overnight. Local supermarkets and restaurants were offering Daniel Plan–friendly options. It worked as a treatment for disease. Diseases went away as a side effect of creating health. And one of the most important ingredients of the treatment is the healing power of the group itself. I realized that the group *is* the medicine, the community is the cure.

COMMUNITY: THE SOCIAL CURE FOR OUR SOCIAL DISEASE

The seed of this idea started in my mind when I went to Haiti with Paul Farmer after the earthquake in January 2010. His nonprofit organization, Partners in Health, has created a powerful and successful model for treating drug-resistant tuberculosis and AIDS in the most impoverished nations in the world. The brilliance of the vision wasn't in coming up with a new drug regimen or building big medical centers, but in a very simple idea: The missing ingredient in curing these patients was making sure they had the medication they needed, and making sure they took it. They needed someone to "accompany" them back to health. By recruiting and training more than 11,000 community health workers across the world, Farmer proved that the sickest, poorest patients with the most difficult-to-treat diseases could be successfully treated. The community was the treatment.

The same vision can be applied to the diabesity epidemic. A community-based support system is an effective way to guide people toward sustainable behavior and lifestyle change.

WHAT THE RESEARCH SHOWS: COMMUNITY SUPPORT WORKS BETTER THAN MEDICATION

Though the data from The Daniel Plan initiative is far from complete, we already know quite a bit about the impact community has on lifestyle change. The existing research proves that community and the use of small groups are more effective than any medication to treat obesity and diabetes. More studies are coming in every day showing that small groups of all kinds—led by trained laypeople, "peers," community health workers, nurses, health coaches, and health professionals in community health centers, churches, schools, and even people's homes—all work better than conventional care for diabesity and chronic disease.[1]

A landmark 2002 study based on the Diabetes Prevention Program[2] and a 10-year follow-up study[3] sponsored by the National Institutes of Health showed that group lifestyle intervention is much more powerful than any other treatment (including medication) to prevent diabetes in those with pre-diabetes. With regular lifestyle support and education, participants lost 5 percent of their body weight and reduced their risk of diabetes by 58 percent. This lifestyle-based group approach was also proven effective in a large Finnish Diabetes Prevention Study.[4]

I recently met one of the original participants in the Diabetes Prevention Program study. Her story astounded me. The lifestyle program was anemic and based on outdated nutrition advice. They met every few weeks in a group to share their progress and their difficulties. They had very basic nutrition counseling, which was mostly wrong (how to eat a low-fat diet for diabetes—the worst nutrition prescription we now know of for the illness). They had a journal to track their food intake, exercise, and weight, and they met for exercise only once a week. And still, this program worked better than any medication on the market. In fact, the study of the control group treated only with medication was stopped early. The ethics review board found it was unethical to continue to treat with medication and to withhold the lifestyle treatment.

The woman I met said the most powerful aspects

of the program were the group sessions and tracking her progress in a journal. Once the program stopped and she no longer had to track her progress or had the social support, her health declined.

The Look AHEAD Study, a 13-year study of 5,000 people funded by the National Institutes of Health, compared an intensive group lifestyle change program for diabetes prevention to regular medical care with individual visits to the diabetic educator, nutritionist, and doctor. To date, the group lifestyle program has proven remarkably more effective in lowering weight, cholesterol, blood sugar, and blood pressure than conventional medical care.[5] Once this study is completed, it will completely change our way of thinking about how to treat disease.

Group lifestyle intervention is not just effective with diabetes. Dr. Dean Ornish developed highly successful group treatment programs for heart disease and prostate cancer. These kinds of programs are more effective and will save more lives and money than medication and surgery for diseases caused by lifestyle and environmental factors.

Journaling Exercise: Why Won't I Join a Community?

Many of us don't consider ourselves "joiners." We find it difficult to get involved with a community of people. Ask yourself why you feel that way, and write about it. Remember that you can certainly start your own community, even if it's a community of two. Write down a list of friends, coworkers, or family members and invite them to start a small group.

Let me reiterate that almost all of the programs that have been studied were based on outdated or less than optimal lifestyle interventions, yet they *still* worked better than any medication. That is the power of the social group, the power of the social cure, the power of the group *as* medicine. The right information delivered in a fun curriculum through a social group has the power to turn our obesity and diabetes epidemic around.

Imagine the power of a more intensive program based on weekly group meetings or experiences, current nutrition science, and better exercise recommendations, supported by an improved journal and tracking system and interactive expert education and coaching to help participants optimize and personalize their diet, supplement regimen, and treatment recommendations. That is what I have created for you in *The Blood Sugar Solution* and its companion website. Go to www.bloodsugarsolution .com now to learn more about our online course community, create a group, and start using the tools today.

THE GROWING MOVEMENT TOWARD COMMUNITY SUPPORT

Two Portland doctors approached me after a lecture I gave and told me about their program for poor undocumented Hispanic women with chronic symptoms, obesity, and diabetes. For very little money (about $15 per person per session), they successfully guided these women to health in a program they called *Reclamado Su Salud* (Reclaim Your Health). They used a program based on *The Blood Sugar Solution* (which I have taught at many medical conferences). Their group of 20 women met weekly for 5 classes, then every two weeks for a total of eight 3-hour classes. The weight loss ranged from 5 to 20 pounds, blood pressures dropped an average of 10–20 points, and depression and inflammation scores dropped significantly.

Much can be done with a little help from your friends.

These examples represent just the beginning of what is possible when we work together. We are social beings and thrive on connection. I met with human resource and benefits executives at Google to advise them on creating a healthy workforce. A survey of their "Googlers" discovered that most of them wanted more ways to connect with one another.

Social networks and groups are spontaneously

sprouting up as support systems for lifestyle change. Not only can Facebook and Twitter help facilitate democratic revolution in countries such as Egypt, but they can link communities together in a common purpose to reclaim their health.

Smartphone applications including FitDay, DailyBurn, Gain Fitness, LoseIt, MyFitnessPal, and SocialWorkout all encourage tracking your progress and sharing it with your friends and community. These tools are early in development but speak to the need to build connection and community in support of health.

With the shift in health care policy prohibiting insurers from excluding sick patients or canceling insurance, and the mandate for universal coverage, insurers can no longer shift responsibility for prevention and health promotion. Large insurers such as UnitedHealthcare[6] and CIGNA are scrambling to create innovative community-based programs to address the tsunami of disease and costs they can no longer avoid.

This community-based group approach solves many enormous obstacles faced by the health care system. Today conventional doctors are the primary method by which people with diabesity receive health care. Unfortunately, most of these doctors have no training in lifestyle medicine or behavior change; lack the time, resources, and support team to facilitate such change; and do not get paid for helping patients create a sustainable lifestyle. Currently physicians and health care organizations have nowhere to refer patients and no clear, well-documented, proven solution to provide their patients. Telling their patients to eat better and exercise more is just not enough.

We can be part of a larger movement to create a healthy nation— *Take Back Our Health* (learn how to join in Chapter 27)—but it starts at home, with our families, our friends, our social network, our communities, our schools, our workplaces, and our churches, temples, and mosques.

You need to build yourself a support system to succeed long term. You need a team working together toward the same goals. It might be just one person— a health coach, a wellness champion, a community health worker, or a health professional—or an online community that can support, encourage, and guide you.

Start by finding people who will do the program with you. Create a small group, even if it is just one friend, who can support you through the process. Ask your friends, family, coworkers, and spiritual community members to join you. Use the guided online course and support program to help you along each week at www.bloodsugarsolution.com and find others who can be your support group. You can still be successful following this program by yourself, but it will be more fun, effective, and sustainable when done with others in community.

Take Action! Join or Create a Group

Learn more about our online support community at www.bloodsugarsolution.com, where you will find both personalized individual support tools and a way to create a support group on your own. At the website I have also provided a way for community health workers, health professionals, workplaces, and faith-based organizations to start their own groups. Using these tools, you can create a self-guided support group with friends (or even just one friend), other members online, family members, coworkers, neighbors, or members of your faith-based community. Here is what is available to support your journey back to health:

- A complete twelve-week course—two weeks of preparation, a six-week program, and a four-week transition to the Healthy for Life maintenance program. You can also access an optional ongoing program for those who want long-term education, coaching for themselves, and support for the group.
- Weekly education, including specific objectives, action items, educational videos, exercise instruction,

relaxation exercises, strategies for overcoming road-blocks and obstacles, and more.

- Tools to track your progress—measurements of weight, blood pressure, lab tests, symptoms, dietary and exercise tracking tools and many others, and an online journal with all the exercises and questions in the book and more.
- Online health and nutrition coaching with trained nutritionists and lifestyle educators to answer your questions and guide you.
- Webinars and workshops to support your journey.

Take Action! Ask for Support from Everyone Else

Ask for support from friends, family, and coworkers who are not in your "group."

Set clear boundaries with family, friends, and coworkers. Don't let them sabotage your efforts to reclaim your health. Learn how to cope with "food pushers" in your life. These are the people who say, "Don't worry about it. What can one little soda really do?" For some of us, that one little soda can set us on a downward spiral to overeating and all of the negative health consequences that come with it. Make a clear stand and explain to people why you are making these changes and why they are important to you. If they are true friends, they will see why it's essential that you take back your health.

Take Action! Support a Grass Roots Movement to Take Back Our Health

Use the online tools (www.takebackourhealth.org) and Chapter 27 in Part V to take action individually— at your workplace, your local schools, your faith-based communities, and your community centers—and to support the political changes needed to create health at home and in the world. Become part of the movement, become part of the conversation.

17

Take a Measure of Yourself

The Blood Sugar Solution translates scientific research into practical recommendations for anyone who wants to get and stay healthy. Soon you will start on this path toward balancing your insulin and your blood sugar. First you need to take some baseline measurements, take a quiz, and take some tests to determine which version of the program you should be following.

THE BASIC AND ADVANCED PLANS

There are two versions of the program. The basic program can be followed by anyone. It balances your blood sugar, reduces insulin spikes, balances hormones, cools off inflammation, helps improve digestion, boosts your metabolism, enhances detoxification, and calms your mind and nervous system. Eighty percent of you following the basic plan will have all the tools you need to heal from diabesity and take control of your health.

The advanced program is designed for people with more severe cases of diabesity, including all those who have been diagnosed with diabetes. The genomic revolution and our understanding of the various factors that create imbalances in our metabolism force us to move beyond the one-size-fits-all prescriptions of the past into personalized medicine and health. Some of us are genetically more susceptible to becoming insulin resistant and pump out much more insulin in response to a given sugar load, even if we are thin. Some of us are more likely to accumulate toxins or have inflammation from eating gluten or have sluggish mitochondria or odd populations of gut bacteria, or to have hormonal problems.

The advanced program will help those of you who have more serious biochemical and metabolic imbalances. If you qualify for the advanced program, you will take an additional set of supplements and make a few extra dietary changes.

To determine which plan is best for you and effectively track your progress, you will need to complete three action steps—get measured, take a quiz, and get tested.

Take Action! Gather and Record Your Body Measurements

You can quickly gather and track critical information about your health with four simple, easy-to-obtain measurements. They tell you volumes about your health and metabolism. Here is what to measure and how to measure it. (You can find special health trackers and online versions of these tools at www.bloodsugarsolution.com.)

1. Your Weight

- Weigh yourself first thing in the morning without clothes and after going to the bathroom. Track your weight once a week in your journal.

2. Your Height

- Measure it in feet and inches. Write it in your journal.

3. Your Waist Size

- Measure the widest point around your belly button. Track this weekly in your journal.

4. Your Blood Pressure

- Buy a home blood pressure cuff (see Resources), go to a drugstore that measures blood pressure for free, or get your doctor to measure it.
- Track it weekly in your journal.

- Measure it first thing in the morning before you start your daily activities. Ideal blood pressure is less than 115/75. Over 140/90 is significantly elevated.

I highly recommend getting the Wi-Fi Body Scale and Blood Pressure Monitor. They upload your weight, BMI, body composition, and blood pressure privately into your smartphone and our online tools and trackers. We can provide support and feedback as you go through *The Blood Sugar Solution*. Research shows that tracking your progress and being accountable doubles your results. You can share your progress with your friends and social network, which also doubles your results. To learn more, go to www.bloodsugarso lution.com/withings.

Once you have these critical measurements, you can determine other key numbers.

1. *Your Body Mass Index (BMI)*

- This is your weight in kilograms divided by your height in meters squared. For ease of calculation, use our online calculator at www.bloodsugarsolu tion.com/tracking-tools. Or use this calculation: BMI = weight in pounds × 703 divided by height in inches squared. For example, I am 185 pounds and 75 inches so my BMI = $185 \times 703/75^2 = 23$.
- This gives you a way of tracking if you are normal weight, overweight, or obese. Normal is less

than 25, overweight is 26 to 29, and obese is over 30. However, you should take into account your waist size as well. If you are a muscular body-builder with a small waist, you could be healthy. If you have skinny arms and legs and a skinny butt but a pot belly, you might have a normal BMI but be at big risk for diabesity. Also, certain ethnic groups, such as Asians, Hispanics, Native Americans, Pacific Islanders, Inuit, Indians, and Middle Easterners have diabesity at much lower BMIs.

■ Track your BMI weekly in your journal along with your other measurements.

2. *Your Waist-to-Height Ratio*

■ To calculate this, take your waist measurement and divide it by your height in inches. Move the decimal point two places to the right. See the chart below to interpret your waist-to-height ratio or go to www.bloodsugarsolution.com and enter your height and weight online. It will then be automatically calculated for you.

■ This number is very important. It tells you if you are fat around the middle. (If you stand sideways while looking in the mirror and have a big belly, or if you can't see your toes when standing up, then you have a problem.)

■ This number is a better predictor of diabesity, heart disease, and risk of death than almost any other number, including waist-to-hip measurement.[1] It is also easier to calculate.

- Measure this once a week while on the program and record it in your journal. Once you have gone off the program, you can measure it once a month.

Waist-to-Height Table

WOMEN

- Ratio less than 35: abnormally slim to underweight
- Ratio 35 to 42: extremely slim
- Ratio 42 to 46: slender and healthy
- Ratio 46 to 49: healthy
- Ratio 49 to 54: overweight
- Ratio 54 to 58: extremely overweight/obese
- Ratio over 58: highly obese

MEN

- Ratio less than 35: abnormally slim to underweight
- Ratio 35 to 43: extremely slim
- Ratio 43 to 46: slender and healthy
- Ratio 46 to 53: healthy, normal weight
- Ratio 53 to 58: overweight
- Ratio 58 to 63: extremely overweight/obese
- Ratio over 63: highly obese

After each week of the program has been completed, I recommend you come back to this section to reassess your measurements and see how much your body has changed. Getting feedback about your results is essential and motivating.

Record Your Numbers

Go to www.bloodsugarsolution.com to learn more about our online tools for tracking all your quiz scores, body measurements, blood tests, daily experiences, thoughts, and feelings so you can easily measure your progress over time. At the website you can also anonymously participate in our online research program to help demonstrate the benefits of this approach. More research should be taken out of large institutions and pharmaceutically driven agendas and put in the hands of the people. The collective sharing of data can transform health care from the bottom up. Tracking your progress will help you, but if you share your progress, you can also transform health care and improve the health of others. Please be part of *The Blood Sugar Solution* patient-driven research program by going to www.bloodsugarsolution.com to enter your data and numbers over time.

Take Action! Take the Comprehensive Diabesity Quiz

Now that you have recorded your BMI and waist-to-height ratio, you are ready to find out whether you should go on the basic or advanced plan. At the beginning of the book, you took a simple screening quiz to see if you may have diabesity. Now you can take a deeper look at the severity of your problem. To do that simply take the quiz below. Score **1 point** for each of the following questions you answer "yes" to. Note you can access an online version of this quiz at www.bloodsugarsolution.com.

Questions	Yes	No
Do you get an urge for something sweet, give in to it, experience a brief "sugar high," and later crash into the "sugar blues"?		
Did your doctor ever tell you your blood sugar was "a little high"?		
Would you describe yourself as an inactive person?		
If you go more than a few hours between meals, do you get irritable, anxious, tired, jittery, or have headaches intermittently throughout the day — and then feel better after you've eaten?		
Do you feel shaky 2–3 hours after a meal?		

(Continued)

273

Questions	Yes	No
Do you have trouble losing weight on a low-fat diet?		
If you miss a meal, do you feel cranky, irritable, weak, or tired?		
If you have a muffin, a bagel, cereal, pancakes, or other carbs for breakfast, is your eating out of control all day?		
Do you feel as though you can't stop eating once you start eating sweets or carbohydrates?		
Does a bowl of pasta or potatoes put you right to sleep, but a meal of fish or meat and vegetables make you feel good?		
Do you go for the breadbasket at the restaurant?		
Do you get heart palpitations after eating sweets?		
Do you tend to retain water after eating salty foods?		
If you skip breakfast, are you likely to have a panic attack in the afternoon?		

Questions	Yes	No
Do you absolutely positively have to have your cup of coffee in the morning in order to get yourself going?		
Do you often get moody, impatient, or anxious?		
Have you been having any problems lately with your memory and concentration?		
Do you feel calmer after you eat?		
Do you get tired a few hours after eating?		
Do you get night sweats (even if you are a man)?		
Do you feel the need to drink a lot of liquids?		
Do you feel that you get colds or infections more frequently than most people you know?		
Are you tired most of the time?		
Do you suffer from infertility or have symptoms of polycystic ovarian syndrome (irregular cycles, facial hair, and acne)?		

(Continued)

Questions	Yes	No
Do you suffer from impotence or erectile dysfunction?		
Do you have jock itch, vaginal yeast infections, anal itching, toenail fungus, dry scaly patches on your skin, or other symptoms of chronic fungal infections?		
Subtotal		

Next, score **3 points** for each of the following questions you answer "yes" to.

Questions	Yes	No
Is your BMI higher than 30?		
Is your waist-to-height ratio greater than 48 if you are a woman or 52 if you are a man?		
Have you been diagnosed with type 2 diabetes, pre-diabetes, or gestational diabetes?		
Has anyone in your family had diabetes, hypoglycemia, or alcoholism?		
Are you of nonwhite ancestry (African, Asian, Native American, Hispanic, Pacific Islander, Indian, Middle Eastern)?		

Questions	Yes	No
Do you have high blood pressure?		
Have you had a heart attack, angina, a transient ischemic attack, or a stroke?		
Do you have cataracts or have you ever had retinopathy (eye damage from diabetes)?		
Do you have levels of triglycerides over 100 mg/dl or HDL (good) cholesterol levels of less than 50 mg/dl, or a blood glucose over 110 mg/dl?		
Do you have kidney damage or protein in your urine?		
Do you have a loss of sensation in your feet or legs?		
Subtotal		
GRAND TOTAL (add subtotals together)		

Scoring Key

Once you have completed the quiz, determine how severe your condition is and whether you should go on the basic or advanced plan by using this scoring key:

Score	Severity	Basic or Advanced Plan
1–7	Mild Diabesity	The Basic Plan
8+	Moderate to Severe Diabesity	The Advanced Plan

Take Action! Get Your Blood and Urine Tested

While the quiz above will give you a good overall sense of how severe your condition is and an accurate assessment of whether to do the basic or the advanced plan, there are a set of laboratory tests I strongly encourage you to take. There are two levels of testing to properly assess diabesity, its complications, and its causes. No matter what your quiz score indicates, if the basic tests show you have advanced diabesity (see below for interpretation), then you should still do the advanced plan.

Basic Diabesity Testing: To Diagnose the Presence of Diabesity

I recommend testing for everyone who is considering following this program or who is overweight, has diabetes, or has a family history of type 2 diabetes. The tests listed below should be performed during the preparation phase of the program (more information on how and where to get these tests done will follow shortly).

I have created a special online guide called *How to Work with Your Doctor to Get What You Need,* where I provide detailed explanations for each of these tests and how to interpret the results. You can download the guide at www.bloodsugarsolution .com. I believe that people can become empowered to learn about their bodies, track their own test results, and use that information to track their disease risks and their progress. I encourage you to become an active partner in your health, and that includes knowing your numbers and following them over time.

NOTE: The abnormal levels noted are based on people who are *not* taking cholesterol or diabetes medications. If you are on medication, the numbers may look better but you may still have severe untreated diabesity.

- **Insulin response test.** This test measures fasting, 1-hour, and 2-hour glucose and insulin levels after a 75-gram glucose load. It's like a glucose tolerance test but measures both glucose and insulin. Your blood sugar can be normal but your insulin can be sky high. Fasting insulin should be < 5 IU/dl and 1- and 2-hour levels less than 30 IU/dl. Fasting blood sugar should be < 90 mg/dl and 1- and 2-hour less than 120 mg/dl. **Demand this test.** It is the most important indicator of the presence and severity of diabesity, but it is rarely done in medical practices today. That is why diabesity is not diagnosed in 90 percent of the people who have it. An alternative is to measure just fasting and 30 minutes post-glucose-load glucose and insulin levels. If you have already been diagnosed with diabetes, you don't need to do the 2-hour glucose-load test.

- **Hemoglobin A1c.** This test measures the average of the last six weeks of blood sugar. Abnormal is > 5.5% of total hemoglobin.

- **NMR lipid profile.** This test determines the particle size and number of LDL, HDL, and triglycerides. Small, dense particles are dangerous and an indicator of diabesity, even if your overall cholesterol is normal with or without medication. You should have fewer than 1,000 total LDL particles and fewer than 500 small LDL particles (the dense, dangerous type). This test is performed by Liposcience, but can be ordered through LabCorp, a laboratory testing company.

- **Lipid panel.** This panel shows total cholesterol (ideal < 180 mg/dl), LDL (ideal < 70 mg/dl), HDL cholesterol (ideal > 60 mg/dl), and triglycerides (ideal < 100 mg/dl).

- **Triglyceride/HDL ratio.** Abnormal is greater than 4.

- **Total cholesterol/HDL ratio.** Abnormal is greater than 3.

If your tests match those listed below, you should be on the advanced plan. If you are on cholesterol-lowering medication, you will have to rely on the insulin response test and the hemoglobin A1c to help you decide if you should be on the basic or the advanced plan.

Go on the advanced plan if:

- Fasting glucose > 110 mg/dl
- Fasting insulin > 12 IU/dl
- 1- or 2-hour glucose > 150 mg/dl
- ½ hour, 1- or 2-hour insulin > 80 IU/dl
- Hemoglobin A1c > 6.0 IU/dl
- Triglycerides > 200 mg/dl
- HDL < 40 mg/dl
- Triglyceride/HDL ratio greater than 5
- Total cholesterol/HDL ratio greater than 6

Additional Tests for Diabesity: To Assess Severity or Complications of Diabesity

These tests should be part of a normal screening and evaluation if you are at risk for or think you may have diabesity. If you have been diagnosed with type 2 diabetes or you qualify for the advanced program based on the quiz or the basic tests, it's important to make sure you get these additional tests done. I also believe they are important for everyone as part of an annual physical and checkup. I explain all these tests in greater detail in the online guide *How to Work with Your Doctor to Get What You Need* (download it at www.bloodsugarsolution.drhyman.com).

- High-sensitivity C-reactive protein (abnormal > 1.0 mg/liter) — to assess inflammation.
- Fibrinogen (abnormal > 350 mg/deciliter) — to assess clotting risk and thick blood.
- Lipoprotein (a) (abnormal > 30 nmol/L) — to assess treatable genetic cholesterol marker.
- Uric acid (abnormal > 7.0 mg/dl) — to assess gout risk caused by diabesity.
- Liver function tests (elevated AST, ALT, GGT are abnormal) — to assess fatty liver.
- Kidney function tests (BUN abnormal > 20 mg/dl, creatinine abnormal > 1.2 mg/dl) — to assess kidney function.
- Microalbumin (abnormal > 20 mg/dl) — to assess protein in urine, an early marker for damage to kidneys.
- 25 OH vitamin D (abnormal < 45–60 ng/dl) — for vitamin D status.
- Homocysteine (abnormal > 8.0 micromoles/liter): a sensitive marker for folate deficiency.
- Ferritin (abnormal > 200 ng/ml) — to assess inflammation and iron status.

- Thyroid hormones (abnormal TSH, free T3, free T4, TPO antibodies)—to assess thyroid function.
- Sex hormones (male—total and free testosterone; and female—FSH, LH, DHEA-S, estradiol, progesterone, free testosterone, and sex hormone binding globulin)—to assess sex hormones.

These tests can be done through your doctor, at most hospitals or laboratories, and even ordered yourself through personal testing companies such as SaveOn Labs (www.bloodsugarsolution.com/saveonlabs) and Direct Labs (www.bloodsugarsolution.com/directlabs). They have "Blood Sugar Solution Basic and Advanced Test Panels" that allow you to order the tests yourself.

While many of the problems you suffer from may be healed by going on *The Blood Sugar Solution,* some of you may need additional medical assistance. Others may already be seeing a doctor for treatment of diabesity. In either case, *How to Work with Your Doctor to Get What You Need* will give you important information that will help you interface with your medical practitioner in the most effective way possible. Download it at the website.

You should also get follow-up testing done at three-month, six-month, and one-year intervals. This will allow you and your doctor to accurately monitor your progress. Be sure to enter your results online at www.bloodsugarsolution.com to securely and privately track your progress and help revolutionize health care by participating in patient-driven research.

THE PREPARATION PHASE CHECKLIST

Preparation Phase Week 1—Lay the Groundwork	✓
Start Your Journal	☐
Visit *The Blood Sugar Solution* website at www.bloodsugarsolution.com to access our special set of support tools and online course.	☐
Connect to your motivation—review the journaling exercise on pages 222–224 for this	☐
Identify and overcome obstacles—review the journaling exercise on pages 227–228 for this.	☐
Identify your health and weight loss goals—review the journaling exercise on pages 229–230 for this.	☐
Set a date to officially start the six-week program.	☐
Prepare Your Healthy Kitchen	☐
Rid your kitchen of disease- and obesity-producing Frankenfoods—refer to the list on pages 233–236.	☐
Watch my video *Supermarket Savvy* at www .bloodsugarsolution.com.	☐
Get your essential kitchen tools—use the list on pages 236–238.	☐

Preparation Phase Week 1 — Lay the Groundwork (Continued)	✓

Prepare Your Inner Shopper   ☐

Watch my video *How to Read Labels* at www.bloodsugarsolution.com.   ☐

Watch my video *How to Understand Basic Nutrition Facts* at www.bloodsugarsolution.com   ☐

Prepare Your Inner Chef

Learn a few basic cooking skills — use the ideas I provide on pages 242–245, review the quick menus in Part VI, or consider taking a cooking class.   ☐

If you don't like to cook or feel you can't find the time, complete the journaling exercise on page 241 to identify why this is a problem for you and how to change that.   ☐

Prepare Your Community

Go To www.bloodsugarsolution.com to learn how to create a group in your community or join an online support group to double your success with the program.   ☐

Create a small support group in your community. Ask family, friends, and coworkers to do the program with you.   ☐

Preparation Phase Week 1 — Lay the Groundwork (Continued)	✓
Ask friends and family not involved in your group to support you on your journey toward health.	☐
Set clear boundaries with the people in your life who are "food pushers." Make sure they know you are doing this program and you are serious about it.	☐
Get involved! See Chapter 27 and the online tools at www.takebackourhealth.org to learn how you can become part of a social and political movement designed to help heal our nation and world.	☐
Take Measure of Yourself — Track Your Numbers	☐
Weigh yourself — use the tracking tools at www.bloodsugarsolution.com to help you.	☐
Record your height — use the tracking tools at www.bloodsugarsolution.com to help you.	☐
Record your waist size — use the tracking tools at www.bloodsugarsolution.com to help you.	☐
Record your blood pressure — use the tracking tools at www.bloodsugarsolution.com to help you.	☐

Preparation Phase Week 1 — Lay the Groundwork (Continued)	✓
Record your BMI — use the tracking tools at www.bloodsugarsolution.com to help you.	☐
Record your waist-to-height ratio — use the tracking tools at www.bloodsugarsolution .com to help you.	☐
Complete your diabesity quiz and determine whether you are on the basic or the advanced plan. Fill out the quiz and get your score online at www.bloodsugarsolution.com.	☐
Get the basic set of diabesity tests I recommend on pages 278–280.	☐
If you are at risk for or think you have diabesity, also complete the advanced testing I recommend on pages 281–283.	☐
Preparation Phase Week 2 — Prepare the Soil	✓
Starting on the first day of Week 2 of the program, stop all of the following:	☐
Flour and sugar products	☐
Toxic processed foods including HFCS, trans fats, additives, and preservatives (basically all processed food)	☐

Preparation Phase Week 2 — Prepare the Soil (Continued) ✓

Alcohol	☐
Caffeine — see my step-by-step program for eliminating caffeine on pages 249–250 to make this easier	☐
Food addictions — take as many of the steps for breaking food addictions outlined on pages 246–249 during Week 2 of the preparation phase as you can. This will help alleviate the withdrawal symptoms that can occur when you break food addictions.	☐
Enter and track your numbers and lab test results online at www.bloodsugarsolution.com. It will help you change, and help millions of others through patient-driven research.	☐

PART IV

THE SIX-WEEK ACTION PLAN

Never wait for the proper mood to start a thing, nor until the spirit moves you. Make your own mood. Make your own spirit. How? ACT. Do something—anything. Inspiration seldom generates action. Action always creates inspiration.

— Author unknown

The critical ingredient is getting off your butt and doing something. It's as simple as that. A lot of people have ideas, but there are few who decide to do something about them now. Not tomorrow. Not next week. But today.

— Robert Browning

18

Ready. Set. Take Action!

In Part IV, you will gather the tools and knowledge you need to start your journey to health, step-by-step, week-by-week. If you follow the action steps, your health and the quality of your life will be radically transformed.

Unless your mother picked you up at the Sears appliance section, I doubt you came with an owner's manual. We know more about how to keep our cars running for 200,000-plus miles than about how to keep our bodies, minds, and souls healthy for a life-span of 120 years. Ancient cultural knowledge about how to create and maintain health is lost, schools don't teach us, doctors and nutritionists don't learn this in school, and policy makers rely on outdated or flawed science at best and industry influence at worst to guide us. Since you have only one body, I encourage you to learn about how it works and the basic ingredients for health and happiness. The six-week action plan will prepare you with the knowledge you need to safely venture into a supermarket without killing yourself and the tools and techniques to heal your body, mind, and spirit.

Each week you will focus on different aspects of health, such as food, fitness, and mental resilience, and learn how to seek support from friends, social groups, and online communities to supercharge your results. When you keep a journal of your insights, successes, progress, obstacles, food intake, sleep, and exercise, you will strengthen your capacity for creating high-level wellness and wholeness. The menu plan, shopping lists, recipes, snack ideas, and food survival pack included at the end of the book will give you the final tools you need to translate the program into action.

In these six weeks you will also learn how to personalize your prescription for health. Each of us has unique imbalances that have created our state of disease and symptoms. The future of health care is personalized medicine—the personalized prescription of diet, nutrients, lifestyle, and even medications. After testing more than 10,000 patients and gathering thousands of stories, I have also learned to see patterns that connect the dots between different symptoms and diseases and help identify the underlying causes of illness. Some people may have excess inflammation, others may have hormonal disruption or digestive imbalances, and still others may be toxic. You've already started the process of identifying your own imbalances by filling out the quizzes in Part II. These will help you personalize your plan, achieve rapid success, and help guide your medical care, if needed.

Now that you have completed the preparation steps, started your journal and tracking, created a support group, gotten tested, and know whether you need to be on the basic or the advanced plan, it's time to get started with the program.

Before I dive into Week 1, I want to explain a little bit about how to use this part of the book.

In each of the next six chapters, you will find specific action steps to take each week. In Chapter 25 (see page 427), I have provided a summary of the entire program and checklists you can use to guide your progress. These checklists are also available in the online course at www.bloodsugarsolution .com.

You can find additional tools and learn more about our online community and access a weekly curriculum to support you while you are on the program at www.bloodsugarsolution.com.

Many people get overwhelmed with the amount of information they need to learn and the steps they need to take. It's better to layer things in over time, and that's how I have set up the program.

During each week, you will focus on one aspect of the program:

Week 1: Eat Your Medicine: Nutrition Basics

Week 2: Optimize Metabolism with Nutritional Supplements

Week 3: Relax Your Mind, Heal Your Body

Week 4: Fun, Smart Exercise

Week 5: Live Clean and Green

Week 6: Personalize the Program

BASIC OR ADVANCED PLAN: WHAT'S THE DIFFERENCE?

By now, you should know which plan you need to be on. There are only two major differences between the basic plan and the advanced plan. They are:

1. **A more restrictive diet for six weeks.** If you qualify for the advanced plan or you have been diagnosed with diabetes, you will make all of the dietary changes in the basic plan and will **avoid all grains, fruit, and starchy vegetables for six weeks.** This will help **reboot your metabolism** and help your diabesity resolve faster.

2. **A more comprehensive supplement plan.** As you will learn in Week 2, supplements are

extremely helpful in treating diabesity. On the basic plan there are supplements I recommend that everyone take for life. Those who qualify for the advanced plan should take a few additional supplements for a limited period of time.

Understand that many of the steps you are going to take are intended to be long-term changes. The six-week program should set the stage for a healthy life. It's a complete overhaul in the way you eat and live, segmented into accessible weekly chunks. After the six weeks are over, you will simply keep doing most of what you have learned.

To help make these changes easier, you will find a week-by-week summary of the program and action checklist at the end of Chapter 25. This will be your daily reminder of exactly what you are supposed to do to succeed. You can also find a copy of this checklist you can print or use online at www.bloodsugar solution.com.

19

Week 1: Eat Your Medicine: Nutrition Basics

Good nutrition is the foundation of the program. You already have a jump start on this week's action steps from the preparation phase of the program. Here is what you are going to avoid in the next six weeks. These are the staples of our high-processed, hybridized modern diet and they are killing us. I promise you will discover a whole new world of Mother Nature's magnificent food pantry, which will delight your senses, stimulate your palate, and leave you feeling clear and healthy, not to mention automatically thinner.

Avoid:

1. **Sugars in any form whatsoever.** Examples are agave, maple syrup, stevia, and the "latest, greatest" sweetener of the day. You already started

this in the prep week. Keep it up. If you have to ask, "Is this okay?" it isn't.

2. **All flour products (even gluten-free).** These include bagels, breads, rolls, wraps, pastas, etc. They are quickly absorbed and drive insulin sky-high.

3. **All processed food.** This includes all trans fats and high-fructose corn syrup. Again, you started this during the prep week.

4. **All gluten and dairy.** These are the major inflammatory foods in our diet. You will learn more about eliminating them in this chapter.

5. **If you are on the advanced plan, all grains, starchy vegetables, and fruit.** Avoid winter squashes, peas, potatoes, corn, and root vegetables such as rutabagas, parsnips, and turnips, and all fruit, except one-half cup of berries a day, for just six weeks to give yourself a jump start.

After six weeks, I recommend you reintroduce gluten and dairy and see how they affect your weight, blood sugar, and metabolism, and how you feel. You may find they cause weight gain or make you sick. If so, stay off them long term. I explain how to reintroduce these foods later in Chapter 26, "Get Healthy for Life." If you have been on the advanced plan, slowly add back in whole grains and limited amounts of starchy vegetables and fruit (see page 302 for quantities), and watch how they affect your blood sugar, energy and weight.

FOCUS ON FOOD QUALITY

The most important thing you can do to heal your body is focus on **food quality.** Americans spend less than 10 percent of their income on food, while Europeans spend about 20 percent. Quality matters. It is more important than quantity when it comes to calories. If you focus on quality, not quantity, you will feel satisfied while naturally avoiding cravings and attraction to food that won't nourish you. We get the most pleasure from life when we focus on quality — the quality of our relationships, of our work, and of our food. This is not so much about what you can't have but about all the extraordinary tastes, flavors, textures, and foods you *can* explore. The side effects are all good.

There is one simple concept you need to learn about nutrition. It is the most important idea in this book, and it will save your life.

Not All Calories Are Created Equal

Five hundred calories of cookies are not the same as 500 calories of broccoli, an idea that even Weight Watchers and the American Diabetic Association are finally recognizing; they are changing their point system and carb exchanges as a result. If you eat the same amount of calories from broccoli rather than cookies, you will lose weight.

Food is information and it controls your gene expression, hormones, and metabolism. The source of the calories (and the information carried along with the calories) makes a gigantic difference in how your genes, hormones, enzymes, and metabolism respond. If you eat food that spikes your insulin level, you will gain weight. If you eat food that reduces your insulin level, you will lose weight. This is true even if it contains exactly the same number of calories or grams of protein, fat, carbohydrate, and fiber.

Portion Size Matters

When traveling in Europe, I always notice that everything is smaller, including waist sizes. The sandwiches in airports use a small baguette with one thin slice of natural ham, not a giant loaf stuffed with meats and cheeses and sauces, like our sandwiches. The sodas are 6 ounces, not 20 ounces. A cup of coffee is 4 ounces, not a 20-ounce latte laden with sugar. A pasta serving is only 4 ounces, not a giant mound that spills over the edges of our plates. Portion size does matter. Following are serving sizes for common foods:

Important Portion Sizes

- Fruit: 1 medium piece, 1 cup berries, ½ cup mixed fresh fruit, ¼ cup dried fruit
- Starchy vegetables: 1 serving = 1 cup winter squash or ½ sweet potato
- Nonstarchy vegetables: 1 serving = 3 cups salad greens, 1 cup raw, or ½ cup cooked (but these are essentially free foods — binge away on broccoli or asparagus)
- Meat, chicken, fish: 1 serving = 4 ounces
- Whole grains: 1 serving = ⅓ cup cooked
- Beans: 1 serving = ⅓ cup cooked or canned
- Nuts or seeds: 1 serving = ¼ cup or one small handful
- See www.bloodsugarsolution.com for a complete list of serving sizes for different foods.

MASTERING GLYCEMIC LOAD IS MORE IMPORTANT THAN MASTERING CALORIES

Low-glycemic-load diets are the only diets that have been proven to work— these diets don't spike blood sugar and insulin.[1]

In a landmark large-scale study, only one diet showed the capacity for maintaining the most weight loss over time. The study published in the *New*

England Journal of Medicine found that the easiest diet to maintain, and the one that had the biggest impact on preventing weight gain after people had lost weight, was the low-glycemic-load, higher-protein diet.[2] After looking at all diet studies, the Cochrane Database, an independent group of scientists who review all available literature, found that low-glycemic-load diets help you lose weight faster and keep it off.

One of the most important skills you will learn in this book is how to create a meal that has a **low glycemic load.** The glycemic load of a meal tells us how much of and how quickly a fixed quantity of a specific food will raise your blood sugar and insulin levels. The slower these levels rise, and the lower they are, the better.

Think of it this way. If you added 2 tablespoons of flaxseeds and 2 tablespoons of fish oil to your cola, it would raise your blood sugar much more slowly than straight cola. But please, I am not suggesting this as a way to continue drinking your sodas!

It may take a bit of practice to get the glycemic load of your meals as low as possible. For some, testing your blood sugar one hour after a meal can even be helpful. But at the end of the day, controlling the glycemic load of your meals isn't very hard. You need to combine protein; fats; and whole-food, fiber-rich, low-starch carbohydrates from vegetables, legumes, nuts, seeds, and a limited amount of whole grains and low-sugar fruit.

Another way to think about it is to never eat carbs alone. Combine carbs with protein and fat at every meal or snack. Have an apple, but eat some nuts with it. Have a little whole grain, but only with a meal containing some fish or chicken, fat, and veggies with fiber.

If you follow the **10 Rules for Eating Safely for Life** on pages 233–236 and the **10 Tips for Cutting Your Cravings** on pages 246–249, you will be automatically eating a low-glycemic-load diet. You will also be eating this way if you follow the meal plan in Part VI. Eventually, this way of eating will become second nature. The key is to have a slow, even burn of food all day to keep your blood sugar and insulin levels stable.

Take Action! Feed Your Body Right

If the quality rather than the quantity of calories you eat determines the state of your health and your ability to keep weight off, then the question is: Which foods will send the right information to your body?

There are four simple principles you can use to choose quality foods that will heal your body and the planet at the same time. At the end of the book, I provide some resources that will help you find these foods. You will also find additional resources online at www.bloodsugarsolution.com.

The Four Principles for a Healthy Planet and a Healthy You

1. **Eat real food.** Avoid highly processed, factory-manufactured Frankenfoods. Choose fresh vegetables, fruit, whole grains, beans, nuts, seeds, and lean animal protein such as fish, chicken, and eggs.

2. **Clean up your diet.** Look for animal products that are pasture-raised, grass-fed, and antibiotic-, hormone-, and pesticide-free. Go on a low-mercury diet by sticking with small, wild, or sustainably farmed fish.

3. **Go organic.** Pesticides and chemical fertilizers poison your metabolism, your thyroid, your sex hormones, and our planet. Buy as much organic food as your budget allows. Refer to the dirty dozen list for the top offenders and the Clean 15 at www.ewg.org.

4. **Stay local.** Seasonal, local foods you find at farmers' markets or community-supported agriculture projects (CSAs) are healthier, taste better, are typically sustainably grown, and help you recognize the intimate relationship between the ecosystem of your body and the broader ecosystem in which we all live. To find a CSA near you, go to www.nal.usda.gov/afsic/pubs/csa/csa.shtml. To find the closest farmers' market

in your area, try www.bloodsugarsolution.com/localharvest. See the face that feeds you.

If you are part of a support group, you might want to buy things in bulk, such as half a grass-fed lamb, or get shares in a local farm. In this way, you can eat higher-quality food for less money. If you can't make it to farmers' markets or don't have a CSA in your area, you should be able to find everything you need in your local supermarket.

It is possible to heal our planet and our health in one step. What you put on the end of your fork has a broad impact on agriculture, energy consumption, the environment, politics, the economy, and your biology.

CARBOHYDRATES: EAT YOUR MEDICINE

You may not realize this, but there are no essential carbohydrates. There are essential fats (omega-3s) and essential proteins (amino acids), but if you never had any carbohydrates again, you would survive.

But there are a few things that hang out almost exclusively with good-quality carbohydrates that come from plant foods (vegetables, beans, whole grains, fruit, nuts, and seeds). So unless you're going to eat the brains, livers, kidneys, and other organs, and chew the bones of animals like the mostly meat-

sawdust in Wonder Bread doesn't make it healthy. Stick with real food. Remember, if it has a health claim on the label, it is probably bad for you.

Take Action! Boost Phytonutrients

The one thing basically everyone in nutrition agrees on is that eating 5–9 servings of fruits and vegetables a day reduces your risk of chronic illness. One of the reasons these foods are so powerful is because of the phytonutrients they contain.

Different phytonutrients have different properties. Some are natural anti-inflammatories, others are anti-oxidants, and still others support detoxification. Each is important in its own way, and when eaten together in the right proportion, they can have a dramatic impact on health. Think of the supermarket as your pharmacy, and food as your medicine.

Here are some tips for optimizing your phyto-nutrient intake and "eating more medicine."

- **Hunt for natural anti-inflammatories.** Mother Nature has many sources of medicine. Red and purple berries rich in polyphenols, dark green leafy vegetables, orange sweet potatoes, and nuts are all foods that reduce inflammation. Or you can take nature's Advil: the curcumin in turmeric is a COX-2 inhibitor—the same class of anti-inflammatory as ibuprofen.

- **Eat your antioxidants.** These special mitochondria-boosting foods increase energy and reduce oxidation, or rusting. Try anthocyanidins such as dark berries, black rice, and pomegranate; orange and yellow vegetables such as winter squash; dark green leafy vegetables such as kale, collards, and spinach; and resveratrol-containing fruits such as purple grapes, blueberries, bilberries, cranberries, and cherries. Just think color. The deeper the color, the more the antioxidants.

- **Detoxify with diet.** Cruciferous vegetables are especially important for enhancing detoxification. These include broccoli, kale, collards, broccolini, broccoli rabe, Brussels sprouts, cauliflower, bok choy, Chinese cabbage, and Chinese broccoli. Other natural detoxifiers are green tea, watercress, dandelion greens, cilantro, artichokes, garlic, citrus peels, pomegranate, and even cocoa.

- **Have hormone-balancing meals.** Include foods such as miso, tempeh, and tofu (all of which are whole soy foods), and ground flaxseeds.

- **Use herbs.** They are powerful antioxidants, anti-inflammatories, and detoxifiers. Try turmeric, rosemary, ginger, coriander, and others.

- **Eat garlic and onions.** Both lower cholesterol and blood pressure. They are antioxidants, anti-inflammatories, and enhance detoxification. Eat them every day if you can.

- **Try green tea.** This ancient beverage contains anti-inflammatory, detoxifying, and antioxidant phytonutrients. The small amount of caffeine it contains is usually well tolerated by most.
- **Choose dark chocolate.** Okay . . . you can have a little chocolate, but only the darkest, richest type. It should contain at least 70 percent cocoa. Eat no more than 2 ounces a day. Ideally, you should save this for after the first six weeks.

FAT DOES NOT MAKE YOU FAT

While carbs are not "essential," fats are. Without enough of the right type of fats, your biology breaks down at the very root. Fats make up your cell walls. If you don't get enough or you eat too much of the wrong kind, you will not have the building blocks you need for healthy cell membranes, which are needed for optimal insulin function and blood sugar control. Omega-3s are the king among healthy fats. It can take a year to rebuild and remake all your cells and tissues with the right fats, so start right away.

Take Action! Get an Oil Change
Replace the bad fat in your body with good fat:

- **Consume wild or sustainably raised cold-water fish.** These include wild salmon, sardines, herring, small halibut, and sable (black cod). I provide recommendations on where to get high-quality fish in the Resources. I suggest you keep cans of sardines, herring, and wild salmon on hand for quick snacks. See www.bloodsugarsolu tion.com/cleanfish to find safe sustainably raised farmed fish and environmentally safe wild fish. For information on seafood safety, go to www .ewg.org or www.nrdc.org.

- **Eat avocados and olives.** These are sources of good (monounsaturated) fats.
- **Use extra virgin olive oil.** This oil contains anti-inflammatory and antioxidant phytochemicals. It should be your main oil except in high-temperature cooking. Buy the best extra virgin oil your budget allows. **Walnut oil** is very tasty as a dressing on salads, and it's good for you. **Sesame oil** and **sunflower oil** are also healthy oils, and they can be used in high-temperature cooking. Try to find expeller- or cold-pressed unprocessed versions of these two. **Coconut oil** and **butter** contain lauric acid, a powerful anti-inflammatory fat, and can be used instead of butter or for cooking at higher temperatures.
- **Go grass-fed or range-fed.** Animals raised in the pasture, eating the diet they evolved to eat, have healthier fat profiles than feedlot-raised animals.

THE IMPORTANCE OF PROTEIN

Many studies, such as T. Colin Campbell's *China Study*,[3, 4] point to the risks of too much animal protein, although these studies are mostly based on factory-produced animal protein, not the wild species that comprised the diet of our hunter-gatherer ancestors. The wild elk and deer my patients gave me when I was a small-town doctor in Idaho had very different nutritional properties and fats from those of a feedlot cow.

Some people thrive as vegans; others wither. Some feel great when eating animal protein; others get sick and sluggish. You need to find out what works for your body, and this will take some experimentation. My experience with patients with diabesity is that they typically need more good-quality animal protein (grass- or range-fed animals, eggs, or sustainably farmed or caught low-mercury fish).

Whether you choose vegetarian or animal sources, it is essential that you get protein at each meal and snack. Eating protein turns up your metabolic fire and ability to burn calories while reducing your appetite.

Take Action! Eat High-Quality Protein for Blood Sugar and Insulin Balance and Hunger Control

Choose from these high-quality, safe sources of protein.

Vegetarian Sources of Protein

- **Beans or legumes.** They are rich in protein and filled with fiber, minerals, and vitamins that help balance blood sugar. See page 308 for examples of delicious legumes you can choose under "Yellow Carbs."
- **Whole soy products.** These include tempeh, tofu, miso, and natto. These vegetarian protein sources are also rich in antioxidants that can reduce cancer risk, lower cholesterol, and improve insulin and blood sugar metabolism. Don't use processed industrial soy products, such as those found in deli-meat replacements, soy cheese, or typical meal-replacement bars; they are harmful.
- **Nuts.** Keeping nuts in the pantry is essential. They have been proven to help with weight loss and reduce the risk of diabetes.[5] They are also a great snack, full of protein, fiber, minerals, and good fats. Buy raw or lightly toasted unsalted nuts. Avoid nuts that are fried or cooked in oils. The best are almonds, walnuts, macadamia nuts, hazelnuts, and pecans. Stick with one or two handfuls for a snack once or twice a day. They have a tendency to raise blood sugar if you binge on them. Remember a serving is 10–12 nuts or a good handful.
- **Seeds.** Pumpkin seeds, sunflower seeds, and sesame seeds are all high in fiber, protein, vitamins,

and minerals. They are a great snack and addition to vegetable, bean, grain, or salad dishes.

Healthy Animal Products

- **Omega-3 eggs or free-range eggs.** These are one of the few animal products that are low in toxins and high in nutrients and balance blood sugar. They contain lots of DHA and they don't raise your cholesterol; just the opposite. Enjoy up to eight of these kinds of eggs a week. Whole eggs are okay; you don't need to stick to just egg whites. Yolks contain important vitamins and fats needed for brain and mood function.

- **Mercury-free fish, shrimp, and scallops.** These are good sources of high-quality protein as well as omega-3 fats.

- **Organic, grass-fed, and hormone-, antibiotic-, and pesticide-free poultry.** Poultry raised without hormones or antibiotics is recommended. Remove the skin from poultry before cooking. Keep some boneless, skinless breasts in the freezer for a quick dinner.

- **Small amounts of lean, organic, grass-fed, and hormone- and antibiotic-free lamb or beef.** Buy as much grass-fed organic, hormone-free meat as your budget will allow. Buy a whole animal with a group of friends and freeze it and share. Trim all visible fat from the meat before cooking. Remember, red meat is a treat. Lamb is a better choice. Pork is the worst. You can also try buffalo, venison, and ostrich, which are leaner. Eat no more than 4–6 ounces of red meat (the size of your palm) no more than once or twice a week. Excess meat consumption is associated with diabesity,[6] although wild meat such as deer, elk, or kangaroo may reverse it.[7]

- **When choosing meat products, understand your choices and their impact on your health and the planet.** If you eat meat and drive a Prius, you use more energy and harm the planet more than if you are a vegan and drive a Hummer. See the "Meat Eater's Guide" from the Environmental Working Group at www.bloodsugarsolution .com/meateatersguide.

HERBS AND SPICES

Many herbs, spices, and seasonings contain healing properties. Make sure to include plenty of your favorites in your cooking. Keep your pantry stocked with them.

Take Action! Include Healthy Condiments and Seasonings

Here are some that I enjoy:

- Wheat-free tamari (soy sauce).
- Red chili paste.

- Hot sauces to spice things up.
- Tahini, a paste made from ground sesame seeds.
- Kosher salt. Use it for all your salt needs.
- Fresh ground black pepper. Get a grinder.
- Spices. Get a small array of spices to add to foods for flavor. Turmeric, coriander, cumin, rosemary, and whole chili peppers are great to start, but there are dozens of wonderful flavors and exotic spices to explore and include in your cooking.
- Fresh herbs such as rosemary, basil, thyme, and oregano.
- Broth or stock. Make your own or use gluten-free low-sodium versions.
- Canned or boxed foods. Some whole foods, such as tomatoes, artichokes, beans, and sardines, come in cans or boxes. Choose organic and lower-sodium versions when possible.
- Fresh lemon and lime juice.

Journaling Exercise: Making Dietary Changes

How do you feel about the dietary changes I have recommended above? Do you feel resistant to them or are you excited about them? Does this sound like deprivation or renovation? Take a few moments to think about what you have just learned and then answer the following questions in your journal:

- If you have any resistance to the changes above, what are they? Are you afraid you will miss your favorite foods? If so, could you be addicted to these foods?
- Are you one of the many who "hate" veggies? If so, do you believe there are ways you could enjoy them by learning to cook them well and resetting your palate?

HOW SHOULD I EAT AND WHEN SHOULD I EAT?

There are two more important nutritional topics I want to address: how to eat and when to eat. It's not only the quality of your calories that's important. Focusing on when you eat and the composition of your meals can reprogram your metabolism.

Create the Perfect Plate

Composing the perfect meal (or snack) is an essential life skill. And the government's new version of the food pyramid called "my plate" will not guide you correctly (though, I admit, it's an improvement over the food pyramid).

It is most important to avoid eating quickly absorbed carbohydrates alone, as they raise your sugar and insulin levels. And any large meal raises your blood sugar, so smaller meals help keep your blood sugar even.

When you put food on your plate, it should look like this:

- On half of your plate, put low-starch vegetables. (You can refill this part as much as you want. Eat a pound or two of asparagus or broccoli if you like!)
- On one quarter of your plate, put some protein (fish, chicken, eggs, shrimp, meat, nuts, or beans).
- On the other quarter, add either one-half cup of whole grains (ideally brown or black rice or quinoa) or one-half cup of starchy vegetables such as sweet potato or winter squash.

If you have advanced diabesity, you should avoid all grains, starchy vegetables, and fruit until your metabolism resets and you become more insulin-sensitive. That may take 6 weeks to 12 months. Just make vegetables three-fourths of your plate and protein one-fourth.

Eat on Time

We often focus on what to eat, not when we eat it. The best way to gain weight and promote diabesity is to skip breakfast and eat a big meal before bed. I call this the sumo wrestler diet. Other studies show that people who eat small meals frequently through-out the day (3 meals and 2–3 snacks) lose weight compared to people who eat one big meal, even if they eat the exact same number of calories. So eat early and eat often. Keep the fire of your metabolism burning all day, rather than slowing it down during periods of "ministarvation." Always have breakfast, eat every 3–4 hours, and try to schedule meals at the same time every day. Your metabolism will work faster and more efficiently. You will lose weight, have more energy, and feel better.

FOOD ALLERGIES AND SENSITIVITIES: TREATING AND REVERSING DIABESITY

Earlier we reviewed how food allergies and sensitivi-ties trigger inflammation and diabesity. Some foods for some people have the wrong information.

That is why I recommend you avoid two key groups of foods during the program: gluten and dairy, the two primary food allergens that contribute to insulin imbalances. After the first six weeks, you can reintroduce them into your diet, but I strongly advise that you do this part of the program 100 percent, no exceptions, not even a drop of gluten or dairy. You will likely see dramatic results, not just on your weight and diabesity but also on your overall health and well-being. Stopping gluten and dairy can be life-changing for people with diabesity. This is also true for people with type 1 diabetes, because there is a strong correlation between the casein[8] in dairy and the gluten[9] in wheat and the development of the disease.

New studies are now pointing to a connection between a leaky gut and type 2 diabetes, triggered by changes in gut bacteria and irritating proteins found in dairy- and gluten-containing grains. Healing a leaky gut by removing allergens and balancing gut bacteria may help with weight loss, reversing diabesity, and overall healing for many.[10]

Dairy presents a special case because the natural growth hormones in milk stimulate insulin production.[11] There are more than 60 anabolic or growth hormones found naturally in milk—it is designed to make young animals grow. Drinking a glass of milk can spike insulin levels 300 percent[12] and contribute to obesity and pre-diabetes. This is true despite studies funded by the Dairy Council showing that milk helps with weight loss. The question is, milk compared to what? A diet of bagels and Coke, or a healthy phytonutrient, antioxidant-rich, plant-based diet with lean animal protein?

Eliminating gluten and dairy may seem difficult

at first, but after about three days off them, you probably won't crave them anymore. Don't short-change yourself. You can add these back after the six weeks are over and monitor how you feel. Your body will be the best indicator of whether or not you can eat these foods long term.

Take Action! Eat Well for Less

Many people struggle with the cost of good food. Poverty drives obesity and diabetes because subsidized sugar and fat calories are cheap. But I would invite you to keep a careful record of how you spend your food dollars and see if, with some reorganizing of your budget and priorities, you can find more money to spend on real, whole food.

For one week, in your journal track every cent you spend and how you spend every hour of the day. If you understand exactly how you spend your time and money, you can choose what's really important, rather than make unconscious choices that don't serve your health or your life goals. What you learn might surprise you.

How much money do you spend on coffee, gum, sodas, convenience foods, or even cigarettes? How much do you spend eating at restaurants or on fast food or takeout?

Think about how you spend your days. Do you waste time reading tabloids, watching television, surfing the Internet, playing video games, or doing too many errands because you don't plan your time well? Track this in your journal as well.

Then, ask yourself if your time and money are best spent as you are spending them now. Think of money as your life energy. It represents your time in a monetary way. How do you want to spend this life energy? Do you want to spend more of it creating health and vitality? Take some time to write out a response to these questions in your journal.

There is no right or wrong answer. It's just something to think about. You might discover that you have more time and money than you think to invest in yourself—and in the quality of life and health that you deserve.

Once you've thought about your answers to these questions, choose three things to change that can give you more time or money. Write them down in your journal as well. For example, giving up that $2 coffee every day saves you over $700 a year. Or giving up watching just a half hour of television a day gives you an extra 7.6 days a year to plan or cook healthy meals.

We are all overworked, overstressed, and overtaxed. Even so, there are ways of making choices that give us more resources.

Now that I've got you thinking, here are a few secrets for eating well on the cheap—and on the fly.

- **Search out cheaper sources of fresh, whole foods in your neighborhood.** My top choices are stores like Trader Joe's and shopping clubs like Costco or Sam's Club, where you can buy vegetables, olive oil, fruits, nuts, canned beans, sardines, and salmon at much lower prices than regular supermarkets or other retail chains.
- **Think about joining your local food co-op.** Co-ops are community-based organizations that support local farmers and businesses and allow you to order foods and products in bulk at just slightly over the wholesale price. This takes a bit of advance planning but will save you money.
- **Join a community-supported agriculture program.** Buy direct and cut out the middleman. We get organic, mostly seasonal, local vegetables delivered to our house for our family of four for $55 a week, or a little more than $10 a person per week. We don't always get to choose what we get, but it makes us more creative cooks.
- **Develop a repertoire of cheap, easy-to-prepare meals.** Have the ingredients available at home at all times so you don't get stuck eating food that doesn't make you feel well or help you create the health you want. This takes planning but is well worth it. See Chapter 28 for quick, cheap, delicious snacks and pages 242–244 for my three favorite meals made in 30 minutes.

- **Create a "potluck club" at work.** Have coworkers share the responsibility of making lunch for the group once a week or every two weeks. No more buying lunch out, and you get to eat real, whole fresh food and only have to cook a few times a month. Or create a "supper club" with a group of friends; rather than go out to dinner, once a week or once a month rotate dinner parties at one another's homes. You will build community and health at the same time.

Take Action! Have a Plan for Surviving Restaurants

If you eat out, be careful. While I recommend you avoid eating out while on the program, I understand that this is sometimes impossible. Some of you might be obligated to go to business luncheons or social events, for example. In that case, I recommend you follow these guidelines:

1. **Be obnoxious.** You have to be very clear about your needs. If you had a peanut allergy and would die if a drop of peanut butter or peanut oil crossed your lips, you would be sure to let your server know. It may be a slow death, but accepting foods that don't nourish and support you is not being polite. It's being stupid.
2. **Choose the restaurant when you can.** There are many good choices for eating well. Learn

the restaurant choices in your area or when you travel. It is worth doing a little homework. Ethnic is always a good choice. Indian, Japanese, Thai, Mediterranean (Italian, Greek, and Spanish), and Middle Eastern are good options. Stay away from fast-food chains. Enjoy slow-food restaurants that celebrate local, fresh, seasonal ingredients. I am an adviser for a new company, LYFE—Love Your Food Everyday—a low-cost, healthy fast-food restaurant using local, seasonal, organic, grass-fed ingredients to make nourishing and delicious meals. They are just starting up but could reach over the whole country soon.

3. **Tell the server you want no bread on the table and no alcoholic drinks.** Ask for cut-up raw veggies such as crudités. Skip the dips.

4. **Ask for water.** Drink a glass or two before dinner. It will reduce your appetite.

5. **Tell the server you will die if you have any gluten or dairy.** (Not a lie, just a slow death.)

6. **Ask for simple food preparation.** Ask for grilled fish or chicken and a large plate of vegetables steamed, or sautéed in olive oil with a side of sliced lemons. You may have a salad, but ask for extra virgin olive oil and vinegar or sliced lemons instead of dressing.

7. **Skip the starches.** Ask for double vegetables and leave out the potatoes, rice, or noodles.

8. **Stay away from sauces, dressings, and dips.** They are often full of sugar, dairy, and gluten.

9. **Follow "hari hachi bu."** The Okinawans are among the longest-lived people on the planet. They have a simple saying: "hari hachi bu," or 80 percent full. They stop eating when they are gently satisfied. There will always be another meal. Bring leftovers home. Eating too much of the right foods can also spike your insulin.

10. **Ask for berries for dessert.** They are gently sweet and nutrient dense, and after a meal their sugar won't raise your blood sugar or insulin.

Take Action! Create an Emergency Food Pack

If you were insulin-dependent, you wouldn't leave home without your insulin and needle. If you were asthmatic, you wouldn't leave home without your inhaler. If you have a body, you need a life pack—a small hand-held cooler that has your daily needs packed away, something quick to assemble but never to forget. It goes in your car, to work, on trips.

Over time you will find your favorite version of the life pack, but here's an example of what you could include:

- A small bag of raw almonds, walnuts, or pecans
- A small bag of cut carrots or cucumbers
- A small container of hummus (try Wild Garden single-serve packets)
- A can of wild salmon
- A can of sardines
- A container of chickpeas with olive oil, lemon, salt, and pepper
- A healthy whole-food protein bar (see Resources for suggestions)
- A bottle of water

Take Action! Be Prepared for Holidays and Special Events

Sometimes you have to eat someplace where you have no control — a party, an event, a friend's house. You can plan ahead by making special requests, which are happily granted by most. If not, you can do a few things to reduce your stress and preserve your health.

- **Eat before you go to an event.** I will often eat before I go to an event. I am happier, have more fun, and can enjoy talking and interacting if I don't have to focus on eating.
- **Bring an emergency pack.** If you are not sure what the food choices will be, be prepared. Hav-

ing your emergency life pack is a great backup. You can always have something before you go in and after you leave if you are still hungry.

- **Just relax and eat.** Eat things that nourish you such as meat, fish, or chicken. Ask for extra vegetables or a second salad. Or just do your best and relax, and have fun and get back to your routine in the morning.

Take Action! Before You Eat, Breathe and Offer Gratitude for the Meal

Mindful eating is the act of becoming aware of what we eat; how that food looks, feels, and tastes in our mouth; and how it makes us feel afterward. It's the difference between gobbling up junk food or attentively savoring dark chocolate.

When we eat unconsciously, we eat more. Studies allowing people to watch television and eat from bags of chips or popcorn found that the bag always ended up empty, no matter what the size. You taste the first bite of food, but then you drift into mindless eating and don't feel as if you ate anything. It takes 20 minutes for your brain to register that your stomach is full.

The practice of slow, mindful eating is a powerful way to better enjoy your food, lose weight, and improve your metabolism. Here are some steps that will help you eat more mindfully.

- **"Take Five" before a meal.** This is a simple one-minute technique that will lower your stress hormones, which make you store fat when you eat, and get your digestive system ready to metabolize your food. Just take five breaths in through your nose and breathe out through your mouth. Slowly count to 5 on each in-breath and again on each out-breath. That's it.

- **Offer gratitude before the meal.** You can make something up—be thankful for your family, your friends, the earth for providing food, whatever moves you. This is an ancient practice—Christian, Jewish, Muslim, Buddhist, Native American, or even pagan—but it can be completely your own. Just offering thanks is a powerful healing activity that will change your relationship to food. Use this as a chance to reprogram any negative associations you have with food or eating (it will make me fat, sick, tired, etc.).

- **Bring your attention fully to the food.** Stop reading your magazine or book; turn off the television; put down your smartphone. When you sit down to a meal, whether with family and friends or by yourself, place your attention on the food. How does it look on the plate? How does it smell? As you bring that first bite to your mouth, relish the experience. How does it taste? What does it feel like? You will be amazed at how this simple act amplifies your dining experience.

Journaling Exercise: Keeping a Daily Food and Feeling Journal

Every day you are on the program, I recommend you keep track of the foods you eat and how they make you feel. This, in addition to tracking your numbers, will give you the key information you need about how to make healthy food choices in the future. It will help you tune in to the innate wisdom of your body. Does this food make me feel good or bad in my body or mind?

After every meal or snack, do the following:

- **Write down what you ate in as much detail as possible.** Include not only the veggies, whole grains, beans, nuts, and protein you ate, but the herbs, spices, and oils you used as well.
- **Think about how this meal or snack made you feel.** Take notes in your journal. How does your body feel? Have symptoms you've suffered from either increased or decreased? Did the food alter your memory or mood or digestion or congestion?
- **Every evening, think about how your experience with food impacted your day.** Do you see improvements in your energy, your ability to focus?

Does your body feel different? What changes have you experienced? How do these changes make you feel?

Go to www.bloodsugarsolution.com for a downloadable printable cheat sheet on Eat Your Medicine: Nutrition Basics for Everyone and online tools for tracking your daily food and feeling journal.

20

Week 2: Optimize Metabolism with Nutritional Supplements

Nutritional supplements are an essential and effective part of diabesity treatment. Mild diabesity requires moderate nutritional support; more advanced cases, including diabetes, often require more intensive nutrient therapy. I will explain why supplements are so important. I will also review common medications used for diabesity and its complications, such as high blood pressure, high cholesterol, and thick blood, as well as natural alternatives to these medications.

WHAT YOU REALLY NEED: THE TRUTH ABOUT SUPPLEMENTS

Doctors used to think that you got all your vitamins and minerals from food and that any extra was excreted, or worse, was toxic. But the tide is shifting.

Doctors now prescribe over $1 billion in fish oil supplements. Most cardiologists recommend folate, fish oil, and coenzyme Q10. Gastroenterologists recommend probiotics. Obstetricians have always recommended prenatal vitamins.

Emerging scientific evidence has proven the importance of nutrients as essential helpers in our biochemistry and metabolism. They are the oil that greases the wheels of our metabolism. And large-scale deficiencies of nutrients in our population, including omega-3 fats, vitamin D, folate, zinc, magnesium, and iron, have been well documented in extensive government-sponsored research. It may seem like a paradox but obesity and malnutrition often go hand in hand. Processed, high-sugar, high-calorie foods contain almost no nutrients yet require even more vitamins and minerals to metabolize them. It's a double whammy.

There are four main reasons we are nutrient depleted. First, we evolved eating wild foods that contain dramatically higher levels of all vitamins, minerals, and essential fats. Second, because of depleted soils and industrial farming and hybridization techniques, the animals and vegetables we eat have fewer nutrients. Third, processed factory-made foods have *no* nutrients. And fourth, the total burden of environmental toxins, lack of sunlight, and chronic stress leads to higher nutrient needs.

That is why *everyone* needs a good multivitamin,

fish oil, and vitamin D. I also recommend probiotics because modern life, diet, and antibiotics and other drugs damage our gut ecosystem, which is so important in keeping us healthy and thin. Additional nutrients are needed for people with diabesity to reset and correct metabolic imbalances, improve insulin function, balance blood sugar, and reduce inflammation.

I'm sure you are confused by conflicting studies. One day folic acid is good; the next it is found to cause cancer. One day vitamin D is a lifesaver; the next it is found to be not helpful. This media whiplash is enough to make you give up altogether. The problem with these studies is that they treat nutrients as drugs — researchers give one nutrient alone and see what happens. But nutrients work as a team. Broccoli is great for you and can help prevent and cure many diseases, but if all you ate was broccoli, you would get sick and die. Nutrients work together to maintain the proper balance in your body.

In this chapter I will focus on the basic supplements everyone needs to help prevent and reverse diabesity and insulin resistance. Then I will address the additional supplements you need if your self-assessment qualified you for the advanced plan.

Take Action! Be a Smart Supplement Shopper

Drugs are regulated. You know what you are getting when your pharmacist fills your prescription. The government makes sure of it. Supplements are not controlled in the same way. The manufacturers often cut corners. It's a minefield for the average consumer. Here are the potential problems I avoid when choosing supplements for my patients:

1. The form of the nutrient may be cheap and poorly absorbed or used by the body.
2. The dosage on the label may not match the dose in the pill.
3. It may be filled with additives, colors, fillers, and allergens.
4. The raw materials (especially herbs) may not be tested for toxins such as mercury or lead, or may not be consistent from batch to batch.
5. The factory in which it is produced doesn't follow good manufacturing standards, so products may vary greatly in quality.

I use supplements in my practice as a cornerstone of healing and repair, so I have investigated supplement makers, toured factories, and studied independent analyses of their finished products. I have learned there are a few companies I can rely on. At www.bloodsugarsolution.com, I have listed the exact products I have used effectively with thousands of patients. There are other good products on the market, but to make it easy for you, I have provided a complete list (which I may update from time to time as the science advances) of what I recommend—both for the basic and advanced plans.

Whether you follow my product recommendations or not, be sure to pick quality supplements and ones that contain nutrients and compounds research has shown to be helpful in the treatment of diabesity and insulin resistance.[1] Think of them as part of your diet. You want the best-quality food and the best-quality supplements you can buy. Guidance from a trained dietitian, nutritionist, or nutritionally oriented physician or health care practitioner can be helpful in selecting products.

Special Note

Many supplements have multiple uses and benefits and may be listed multiple times throughout the program. For example, alpha lipoic acid works to help balance blood sugar, but it is also important for mitochondrial function and for detoxification. If you find that it is recommended here and again in Week 6 when we discuss personalization, *don't take double the dose.* You will get all the benefits across different systems of the body with the basic recommended dose.

THE BASIC PLAN SUPPLEMENTS

Obesity and diabetes are often paradoxically states of malnutrition. It has been said that diabetes is starvation in the midst of plenty. The sugar can't get in the cells. Your metabolism is sluggish and the cells don't communicate as a finely tuned team. Nutrients are an essential part of getting back in balance and correcting the core problem—insulin resistance. There are two ways in which supplements work—they make your cells more sensitive to insulin and more effective at metabolizing sugar and fats, and special fibers can slow the absorption of sugars and fats into the bloodstream. This leads to a faster metabolism, more balanced blood sugar, improved cholesterol, less inflammation, fewer cravings, more weight loss, and more energy.

Everyone reading this book should get on the basic plan of supplements and stay on them for life. Even if you are "cured" of diabesity, you will need to keep taking them, because you need special vitamins, minerals, and herbs to help compensate for your genetic tendency toward insulin resistance.

Below are the supplements that should be in your daily regimen. The good news is that many of these components can be obtained by taking combination supplements. I suggest you find combination supplements that match my recommendations as closely as possible. Getting these ingredients in the listed dosage ranges is important. At www.bloodsugarsolution.com, I share exactly which supplements I recommend and tell you how to purchase them.

All supplements except the fiber should be taken with a meal, such as breakfast and dinner.

- A high-quality multivitamin and mineral
- 1,000–2,000 IU of vitamin D3 a day with breakfast
- 1,000–2,000 mg of omega-3 fats (should contain a ratio of approximately 300/200 mg of EPA/DHA), once with breakfast and once with dinner
- 100–200 mg of magnesium, once with breakfast and once with dinner
- 300–600 mg of alpha lipoic acid twice a day, once with breakfast and once with dinner
- 200–600 mcg of chromium polynicotinate a day (up to 1,200 mcg a day can be helpful)
- 1–2 mg of biotin, once with breakfast and once with dinner
- 125–250 mg of cinnamon, once with breakfast and once with dinner
- 25–50 mg of green tea catechins, once with breakfast and once with dinner
- 2.5 grams of PGX, a super fiber, 15 minutes before each meal with 8 ounces of water

You can also use hypoallergenic protein powders to add to a morning protein shake.

- 1–2 scoops of rice, soy, hemp, pea, or chia protein powder for breakfast. Follow the directions on the label. This can be added to your UltraShake (see recipes in Chapter 28).

In addition to these, most people should use high-quality probiotics, but this is optional. For more details on the probiotics I recommend, see www.bloodsugarsolution.com.

Notes About Basic Plan Supplements

Let's take a few moments to review specifics about each of these supplements or ingredients and why they are so important in the treatment of diabesity.

High-Quality, High-Potency, Complete Multivitamin

The right multivitamin will contain all the basic vitamins and minerals. Often special formulations for diabesity are available that include many of the ingredients listed for the basic plan above. On *The Blood Sugar Solution* website (www.bloodsugarsolution.com), I review the exact forms and amounts of nutrients that should be in any good-quality multivitamin. I also review specific instructions for testing and monitoring of your nutrient levels that can be done with your physician.

Keep in mind that getting the optimal doses usually requires 2–6 capsules or tablets a day. Some people may have unique requirements for much higher doses that need to be prescribed by a trained nutritional or functional medicine physician.

Note that B complex vitamins are especially important for those with diabesity, as they help protect against diabetic neuropathy, or nerve damage, and improve metabolism and mitochondrial function.

Antioxidants such as vitamin E, C, and selenium are also important as they may help reduce oxidative stress, which is a significant cause of diabesity.

Vitamin D3

Vitamin D deficiency is epidemic, with up to 80 percent of modern humans deficient or suboptimal in their intake and blood levels. Depending on what's in your multivitamin, I recommend taking additional vitamin D.

Vitamin D3 improves metabolism by influencing more than 200 different genes that can prevent and treat diabetes[2] and metabolic syndrome.[3]

There are many important things to keep in mind as you take vitamin D:

1. Take the right type of vitamin D — D3 (chole-calciferol), not D2. Most doctors prescribe vitamin D2. Do not take prescription vitamin D; it is not as effective and not very biologically active.
2. For serious deficiencies, you may need more vitamin D, as much as 5,000–10,000 IU a day for 3 months or more. Do this with your doctor's supervision if needed.
3. Monitor your vitamin D status with your doctor. Get your blood level to 45–60 ng/dl. Check the right blood test, which is 25 OH vitamin D.
4. Give time to fill up your tank. It can take 6–12 months for some people. The average daily dose for maintenance for most people is 1,000 IU–2,000 IU a day.

Omega-3 Fatty Acids (EPA and DHA)

These important fats improve insulin sensitivity, lower cholesterol by lowering triglycerides and raising HDL, reduce inflammation, prevent blood clots, and lower the risk of heart attacks.[4] Fish oil also improves nerve function and may help prevent the nerve damage common in diabetes.[5]

Magnesium

Diets low in magnesium are associated with increased insulin levels, and magnesium deficiency is common in diabetics. Magnesium helps glucose enter the cells and turn those calories into energy for your body.

Some with severe magnesium deficiency may need more than the amount outlined above. Some may need less. If you are concerned you may be severely deficient, discuss the details with your doctor. Diarrhea is often a sign that you are getting too much magnesium. If this occurs, just back off on the dose, and avoid magnesium carbonate, sulfate, gluconate, or oxide. They are the cheapest and most common forms found in supplements but are poorly absorbed. Switch to magnesium glycinate. If you tend to be constipated, use magnesium citrate. People with kidney disease or severe heart disease should take magnesium only under a doctor's supervision.

Alpha Lipoic Acid

Alpha lipoic acid is a powerful antioxidant and mitochondrial booster that has been shown to reduce blood sugar and heal a toxic liver. It may also be useful in preventing diabetic nerve damage and neuropathy. It can improve the clearance of glucose from the blood by 50 percent.[6]

Chromium and Biotin

Chromium is very important for proper sugar metabolism and insulin sensitivity, and can help you make more insulin receptors.[7] Biotin has been shown to enhance insulin sensitivity, lower triglycerides, reduce expression of cholesterol-producing genes, and improve glucose metabolism.[8]

Cinnamon and Green Tea Catechins (ECGC)

A number of herbs, including cinnamon[9] and catechins[10] from green tea, are helpful in controlling blood sugar and improving insulin sensitivity. Green tea can even increase fat burning and metabolism. The best products provide combinations of herbs in one supplement.

PGX (Polyglycoplex)

PGX is a very viscous fiber from a Japanese tuber or root combined with seaweeds into a novel super fiber. It has profound effects on insulin, glucose, and hemoglobin A1c.[11] It reduces the absorption of sugars and fats in your bloodstream and helps control appetite, weight loss, blood sugar, and cholesterol.[12] When taken before meals with a glass of water, it can be a critical component to overcoming diabesity. It can lower your insulin response after a meal by 50 percent while lowering LDL cholesterol by 20 percent and blood sugar by 23 percent. I have had patients lose up to 40 pounds just by using this super fiber.

Protein Shake Powder

I strongly encourage the use of a high-quality, hypoallergenic rice, pea, hemp, chia, or soy protein powder. Some of these powders are anti-inflammatory and support detoxification. Soy protein from whole soy foods with isoflavones can lower blood sugar[13] and cholesterol.[14] A protein shake also serves as an excellent breakfast and snack option, helping balance your blood sugar and heal your liver. See pages 494–496 for great shake recipes.

THE ADVANCED PLAN SUPPLEMENTS

If your diabesity self-assessment quiz qualified you for the advanced plan, you will follow the supplement routine outlined for the basic plan but will add the supplements below. When combined with the basic plan supplements, these herbs will help improve blood sugar balance and insulin sensitivity.

The advanced plan supplements should be taken for at least one year. After one year you should repeat your lab tests with your doctor, repeat the self-assessment quiz, and evaluate your progress. If your numbers are in the ideal ranges and your symptoms better, then you can scale back to the basic plan supplement recommendations.

- 180–360 mg of a combination of acacia (heart-wood extract) and hops extract twice a day, once with breakfast and once with dinner
- 1,000 mg fenugreek seed extract containing a minimum of 70% soluble fiber twice a day, once with breakfast and once with dinner
- 150 mg bitter melon gourd fruit extract twice a day, once with breakfast and once with dinner
- 100 mg gymnema leaf extract standardized to 25% gymnemic acids twice a day, once with breakfast and once with dinner

I use combination products to help my patients achieve these goals at a reasonable cost with a reasonable amount of supplements. Please refer to www .bloodsugarsolution.com to learn more about which products I use with my patients and how to purchase them.

Notes About Advanced Plan Supplements

Let's look at these supplements in more detail.

Acacia and Hops

A new class of herbal supplements from the hops plant regulates critical signaling factors that control your genes. These are called protein kinases. The iso alpha acids in hops (RIAA, or reduced iso alpha acids) and acacia, also known as selective kinase response modulators (SKRMs), have been clinically shown to improve insulin sensitivity and fat metabolism.[15]

Fenugreek, Bitter Melon Gourd, and Gymnema Leaf

For advanced diabesity, I recommend fenugreek, bitter melon gourd,[16] and gymnema leaf.[17] Fenugreek is used in India and the Middle East. It contains 4 hydroxyisoleucine, which assists insulin function and helps lower triglycerides and raise HDL cholesterol. Bitter melon gourd helps reduce blood sugar in diabetes through its phytonutrients. Gymnema is an Ayurvedic herb that lowers blood sugar levels and may help repair or heal the pancreas.

ADDITIONAL SUPPLEMENTS TO SUPPORT CONDITIONS ASSOCIATED WITH DIABESITY

Certain supplements may be useful in treating conditions associated with diabesity. While I *strongly* discourage you from going off any medication without your doctor's supervision, you can integrate these supplements into your regimen to help you overcome the conditions listed below. To learn the specific products I recommend and use with my patients, see www.bloodsugarsolution.com.

Elevated Cholesterol (Alternatives to Statins)

Red Rice Yeast

Red rice yeast powder is derived from *Monascus purpureus,* an organism grown on rice. After centuries of use in traditional Chinese medicine, it was discovered that red rice yeast is useful in helping to maintain a healthful balance of cholesterol and related blood lipids in the body.[18]

- Take 1,200 mg twice a day, once with breakfast and once with dinner.

Plant Sterols

Naturally derived plant sterols can also be useful in maintaining healthy cholesterol levels.[19] Plant sterols are one class of phytonutrients. Taking them in high concentrations can enhance their potency.

- Take one capsule of mixed sterols with 500–700 mg per capsule twice a day, once with breakfast and once with dinner.

High Blood Pressure

The best supplements to help lower blood pressure are fish oil and magnesium, which I have already reviewed, and coenzyme Q10.[20] (To learn about CoQ10 see Chapter 24, Step 6.) They are an important part of treating diabesity. You can also add the following:

Hawthorn Leaf Extract

This herbal remedy has been shown to play an important role in heart muscle function and coronary artery blood flow. It has also been shown to lower blood pressure in diabetics.[21]

- Take 200–300 mg twice a day, once with breakfast and once with dinner.

Blood Thinners

Aspirin is often recommended to thin the blood in patients with diabesity and may be helpful for some, but there is increased risk of stroke and gastrointestinal bleeding. Therefore, I generally recommend natural blood thinners that don't carry that risk.

Nattokinase

This enzyme, found in the traditional Japanese fermented soy food called natto, helps maintain healthy blood flow and supports the body's natural clotting processes.[22] It is also useful in supporting blood vessel health.

- Take 100 mg twice a day, once with breakfast and once with dinner.

Lumbrokinase

Lumbrokinase is among the few fibrinolytic, or blood-thinning supplements, available. It is useful in helping the body maintain normal coagulation processes.[23]

- Take 20 mg twice a day, once with breakfast and once with dinner.

GUIDELINES FOR TAKING SUPPLEMENTS

When taking supplements, there are a few things to keep in mind.

1. Take them with food—with the meal or just before. Taking supplements after a meal may upset your stomach. If you still have an upset stomach, find a doctor who can help correct any digestive problems, which might be the source of intolerance.
2. Take fish oil just before meals to prevent any fish taste from coming up. Or freeze the supplement so the capsule is in your intestine before it dissolves.
3. I recommend the use of capsules whenever possible. They are generally easier to swallow. However, if you have trouble with capsules, open

them and sprinkle the contents onto food or put into shakes. You can crush tablets and mix them with food or a little applesauce. There are also powdered and liquid forms of some nutrients.

THE INTELLIGENT USE OF MEDICATION

There are several different classes of medications that are currently used in the treatment of diabesity. One of the most important studies in medicine, the Diabetes Prevention Program,[24] found that medication did not work nearly as well as lifestyle changes, and this effect lasted even 10 years after the study ended. Patients who follow *The Blood Sugar Solution* may need less and less medication, and many may get off medication completely, or use the natural alternatives I just reviewed. Nonetheless, it's useful to know what's out there.

The only medication that I sometimes find helpful is metformin, or Glucophage. It is well tolerated, has been around a long time, and has been well studied. Most of the other medications cause serious complications or make things worse by boosting insulin levels and increasing the risk of death and heart attacks. Other medications are prescribed for diabesity, but they have limited benefits and significant risks, which I explain below. That is why I stay away from most of them. Nutrition, exercise, supplements, and stress reduction always work much more quickly and dramatically than medication.

Oral hypoglycemic medications fall into this category of medications that can make things worse, not better, by pushing your pancreas to make more insulin. Some of the medications now available are new and have not withstood the test of time. I always think of something I read in a medical editorial years ago: "Be sure and use a new medication as soon as it comes on the market, before the side effects develop." Think Prempro, Avandia, Vioxx, to name a few.

Medications can be used alone or in combination. Here are the main classes of medications used to treat diabetes.

Diabetes Medication

Biguanides, especially metformin (Glucophage), are among the best medications used to improve insulin sensitivity. They can help lower blood sugars by improving your cells' response to insulin.

Thiazolidinedione drugs, including rosiglitazone and pioglitazone (Avandia and Actos), are a new class of diabetes medication that can help improve the uptake of glucose by your cells by making you more insulin sensitive. These medications also reduce inflammation and help improve metabolism by working on the PPAR, a special class of cell receptors that control metabolism, but the costs can be high. Known side effects include weight gain and liver damage. Avandia, the world's number one blockbuster diabetes drug, has been shown to increase the risk of heart attacks, and from 1999 to 2010 it has been responsible for 47,000 cardiac deaths. It can now be prescribed only with special warnings and under certain conditions. Therefore, I am very cautious about prescribing these medications.

Sulfonylureas, which are older medications, include glipizide, glyburide, and glimepiride. I strongly recommend against these medications, because they only reduce your sugar in the short term and can increase insulin production over the long term. In addition, the FDA requires special black box warnings notifying patients that these drugs actually increase the risk of a heart attack, which is what you are trying to prevent in the first place. In short, they treat the symptoms rather than the cause.

Alpha-glucosidase inhibitors, including acarbose and miglitol, can help lower the absorption of sugar and carbohydrates in the intestines. These may be occasionally useful, but I find PGX fiber much more effective in slowing the absorption of sugars into the bloodstream. Touchi extract from black soybeans has been shown in laboratory studies to block alpha-glucosidase, the enzyme responsible for the breakdown of carbohydrates into simpler sugars, and slow the metabolism of certain sugars. I often recommend 300 mg before each meal for my diabesity patients.

Incretins are the new kids on the block. They work by prompting the release of insulin from the pancreas by stimulating glucagon-like peptide-1 (GLP-1) receptors or inhibiting the enzyme DPP-4, which normally breaks down GLP-1. This helps keep blood sugar down. Over 58 percent of those who take the medication experience nausea, and 22 percent have vomiting. Not a fun way to lower your blood sugar. Long-term studies are not available to adequately assess the risks. A large scientific study known as NAVIGATOR[25] showed that it was not effective in reducing risks associated with pre-diabetes, and in fact, a year after being on the medication, insulin and glucose levels were higher than they were before the medication was started. Based on this data, I avoid using these drugs.

Insulin is the last resort, after all other measures have failed, because it can lead to weight gain, increased cholesterol, and higher blood pressure.

Combinations of these medications may be helpful. But as you can see, many come with risks that can easily be avoided and eliminated if you make the necessary dietary and lifestyle changes to treat the underlying causes of your condition.

There are a few other kinds of medication often prescribed to people with diabesity.

Cholesterol-Lowering Medication

Niacin (Niaspan) is a very useful medication. What you may not know is that it is actually vitamin B3. When used in high doses (1,000–2,000 mg) under a doctor's supervision, it can be effective in lowering triglycerides and raising HDL—something statins are not very good at. However, niacin intake should be monitored carefully as it can cause liver damage when taken in high doses. It is my favorite medication to use if we cannot get HDL or triglycerides normalized using dietary and lifestyle measures alone. It also has the benefit of increasing your cholesterol particle size and reducing particle numbers, which statins don't do. It has been shown in studies to reverse cholesterol plaques in arteries.[26] Some studies have shown that combining a low-dose statin with niacin can also reverse plaque. Other studies have shown no benefit when combined with a statin.

Statins (Lipitor, Crestor, Zocor, etc.) have been shown to help lower LDL cholesterol and reduce heart attack risk and death but *only* in high-risk patients. However, they don't significantly improve lipid particle size, lower triglycerides, or raise HDL. They also seem to increase insulin levels and can cause muscle damage and neurologic problems. They actually increase the risk of diabetes by about 9 percent.[27] I find that the natural statins in red rice yeast can work well without the side effects. Statins lower inflammation as an unintended, but good, side effect. However, there are better ways to reduce inflammation, including an anti-inflammatory diet, exercise, fish oil, and even a multivitamin. For more information, see my blogs about cholesterol and statins at www.drhyman.com/cholesterol, including "7 Tips to Fix Your Cholesterol Without Medication," "Do Statins Cause Diabetes?" and "Pharmageddon."

Blood Thinners and Anti-Inflammatories

Aspirin. Many patients with diabesity have inflammation and sticky blood. The recommendation offered by most physicians is to take a baby aspirin (81 mg) every day. This can be helpful but is not without risks. Gastrointestinal bleeding and hemorrhagic stroke can result. Three natural blood thinners are fish oil, nattokinase, and lumbrokinase. See pages 351–352 for more information.

High Blood Pressure Medication

Safely lowering blood pressure is important in diabesity. For most people, simply following *The Blood Sugar Solution* may result in lower blood pressure. But if you need to take high blood pressure medication, there are a few things you should know.

In general, ACE inhibitors such as Altace, ARB blockers such as Diovan, and even diuretics can safely lower blood pressure. The ACE inhibitors and ARB medications can help slow the progression of kidney disease. I would recommend staying away from beta-blockers, however, because they make insulin resistance worse. Studies have shown that they reduce glucose uptake into cells by about 25 percent. Natural alternatives to high blood pressure medication are hawthorn, fish oil, coenzyme Q10, and magnesium. See pages 350–351 for how to use natural alternatives to blood pressure medication.

The key with high blood pressure is to treat the cause. Most high blood pressure is actually caused by insulin resistance. Obstructive sleep apnea, magnesium or potassium deficiency, omega-3 fat deficiency, and environmental toxins such as lead and mercury are other treatable causes of high blood pressure that are often overlooked.

21

Week 3: Relax Your Mind, Heal Your Body

This week we will focus on techniques for hitting your pause button and sinking into deep relaxation.

Stress plays a dramatic role in blood sugar imbalance. It triggers insulin resistance, promotes weight gain around the middle, increases inflammation, and may ultimately cause full-blown diabetes.[1] It is essential to engage in relaxation practices on a regular basis—deep breathing, progressive muscle relaxation, guided imagery, prayer, hot baths, exercise, meditation, yoga, massage, biofeedback, hypnosis, or even making love. Your survival depends on it.

Take Action! Practice Relaxation

Most of us don't know how to relax. Our society doesn't encourage it, and it's a skill we don't take the time to learn. But actively relaxing is an essential life skill if you want to be healthy and happy. Healing, repair, renewal, and regeneration all occur in a state of relaxation. We must activate our parasympathetic nervous system, otherwise known as the relaxation response.[2] How do we do this?

Many cultures have developed techniques for relaxing the mind and healing the body. Here I offer two techniques you can try to help activate your relaxation response.

Belly Breathing

Learning to breathe deeply, sometimes called "belly breathing" or "diaphragmatic breathing," can help you relax almost instantly, and it's a skill you can take with you everywhere you go. I recommend you do this at least five times a day—once upon waking, before every meal, and once before bed. You can do it more often if you like. Try it anytime you are feeling stressed out or overwhelmed.

Learn how to breathe more deeply:

1. If you can, loosen your clothes and get into a comfortable position. Lie on the floor or recline in your office chair or just sit up straight wherever you are.
2. Close your eyes, and get in touch with your breath for a few moments.

3. Now place one hand on your belly and one hand on your chest. Notice whether your chest rises or your belly rises when you breathe. To breathe deeply, your belly should rise more than your chest. If this doesn't happen for you naturally, focus some gentle attention on training your body to do this. Then put your hands gently by your side or on your knees.

4. Now inhale through your nose deeply, into your belly, to the count of 4. Take your time with this.

5. Hold the breath for a count of 2.

6. Exhale through your mouth slowly and steadily to the count of 6.

7. Pause for a count of 1.

8. Repeat the cycle for 10 breaths.

If you want to enhance the activity, you can add a "mantra"—a relaxing word you repeat over and over again—to the exercise. To do this, choose your mantra—it could be the word "relax" or "love" or "peace" or any other word that helps you remember to let go—and repeat it with every exhalation.

You can also extend the period of breathing. Some recommend engaging in diaphragmatic breathing for up to 6–10 minutes a day.

Visualization

As Martin Rossman points out in his book *The Worry Solution,* most stressors today are internal, from our self-talk. You shouldn't believe every stupid thought you have! Our sympathetic nervous system gets triggered by our thoughts, or what we imagine to be true, instead of by real external stressors. One reason for this is that our imagination tends to run away with us. We obsess over problems we can't solve; we imagine the worst-case scenario; we think of the glass as half empty. We believe in and often live up to the negative stories we tell ourselves and often look for evidence to reinforce our self-defeating stories and beliefs about our lives.

If our imagination can be used to make us anxious, it stands to reason it can also be used to calm us down. We can visualize our way to a more peaceful state.

What follows is a simple visualization exercise you can use to help you relax. Memorize it, make a digital recording for yourself, have a loved one read it to you, or use the online version I have created at www .bloodsugarsolution.com.

1. Loosen your clothing and get into a comfortable position. Recline in your chair, or lie on your bed or the floor. Close your eyes, and begin breathing

deeply using the diaphragmatic breathing exercise. Feel your breath come in slowly and go out slowly. Let your body begin to relax. Notice how your muscles begin to unwind and the tension around your eyes and head is released.

2. Now bring to mind a memory of a peaceful, nourishing, relaxing place you have visited. Try to see it in your mind's eye in full detail. You may find yourself visiting the sea, standing under a canopy of redwoods or at the top of a mountain, or sitting in a cathedral. Whatever relaxes you is where you want to be.

3. As you relax into this environment, notice how your body feels. Do your feet and legs feel more relaxed? Is your belly soft? Are your arms heavy and free of tension? How does your chest feel? What about your neck and head? Are these soft and relaxed as well? Take some time to scan through your body and notice where you are holding tension. As you encounter the tension, gently encourage it to release and open up.

4. Take a few moments to tune into your breathing. Is it deep, slow, and powerful? Can you feel your breath fill your whole body? If not, deepen your breath and see if you can allow it to "massage" you from the inside and relax your body.

5. Stay in this place of deep relaxation as long as you like. When you are ready, slowly wiggle

your fingers and toes, open your eyes, stand up, and go about your day. See if you can take the relaxed feeling with you into your day.

For more exercises like this, I strongly recommend Martin Rossman's recorded visualizations. Learn more at http://www.bloodsugar solution.com/the-worry-solution-visualizations.

Take Action! Go on a Media Fast

Linda Stone (www.lindastone.net), a friend of mine who has worked for the CEOs of both Apple and Microsoft, has made some remarkable discoveries about the effects of media on our nervous system. Remember I said that the average American spends 8½ hours in front of a screen every day. The amount of negative and irrelevant information flooding our minds is enormous, and it can make you fat and cause diabetes. It also takes your breath away.

She says that screen time actually distorts your normal breathing. Linda Stone calls it "email apnea." We hold our breath when in front of television and computer screens, and with other media as well, including magazines and radio.

As she says,

The trajectory of our nation's ill health follows the trajectory of the ubiquity of personal technologies as well as our relationship with television. There are at least two things that contribute to email apnea: poor posture and a sense of anticipation. With anticipation, we inhale. Whether the anticipation is a result of email flooding into our inbox, or an emotional television show, the result is the same—we inhale, and most often, we don't fully exhale.

Our breathing patterns are the key to managing our attention, to our feeling of well-being, and most importantly, to nourishing our body with great lymph and blood circulation and with oxygen. Breath holding contributes to a state of fight or flight, to impulsive behavior, to a flood of stress hormones, and to compromised digestion and elimination.

Teaching optimal breathing patterns, particularly in the early years, is as crucial as exercise and proper nutrition.

I recommend a one-week media fast during *The Blood Sugar Solution*.

- No computer (unless needed for work).
- No television or movies.
- No magazines or books except one hour of pleasure reading before bed and this book to help guide you through the program.

- No web surfing, Facebook, Twitter, texting, or smartphone use (other than to get calls), unless you are using the companion tools on the web that support *The Blood Sugar Solution.*

If you are worried you will miss important world events, ask a well-informed friend once a day. You will be surprised at the amount of time you have to do things that support your life and your energy— shop, cook, eat well, exercise, relax, sleep, connect with friends and family. Then decide what media you want to let back into your life.

Journaling Exercise: Write About Your Day

Take 20 minutes every evening to write about your day. Try to write without stopping. If you don't know what to write, just say, "I don't know what to write," until something comes to you. Journaling has proven to be extremely effective in activating the relaxation response.

Take Action! Get Enough Restful Sleep

The research is clear: Lack of sleep or poor sleep damages your metabolism, causes cravings for sugar and carbs, makes you eat more, and drives up your risk of heart disease, diabetes, and early death. Getting enough sleep and sleeping well are essential for health and an easy way to maintain blood sugar balance and lose weight.

The first step is to prioritize sleep. I used to think that "MD" stood for "medical deity" and meant I didn't have to follow the same sleep rules as every other human being. I stayed up late working long shifts, ignoring the demands of my body to rest.

Unfortunately, our lives are infiltrated with stimuli—and we remain stimulated until the moment we get into bed. This is not the way to get restful sleep. Frankly, it's no wonder we can't sleep well when we eat late dinners, answer e-mails, surf the Internet, or do work, and then get right into bed and watch the evening news about all the disaster, pain, and suffering in the world.

Instead we must take a "holiday" in the two hours before bed. Creating a sleep ritual—a special set of things you do before bed to help ready your system for sleep—can guide your body into a deep, healing night's rest.

We all live with a little bit of post-traumatic stress syndrome (or we should say, traumatic stress syndrome, because for many of us there is nothing "post" about it). Much research has been done on the effects of stress and traumatic experiences and images on sleep. If you follow my guidelines for restoring normal sleep, your post-traumatic stress may become a thing of the past.

It may take weeks or months, but these twenty strategies will eventually reset your biological rhythms:

1. **Practice the regular rhythms of sleep.** Go to bed and wake up at the same time each day.

2. **Use your bed for sleep and romance only.** Don't read (except something soothing or calming) or watch television.

3. **Create an aesthetic environment that encourages sleep.** Use serene and restful colors and eliminate clutter and distraction.

4. **Create total darkness and quiet.** Consider using eyeshades and earplugs.

5. **Avoid caffeine.** It may help you stay awake, but this ends up making your sleep worse at night.

6. **Avoid alcohol.** It helps you get to sleep but causes interruptions in and poor-quality sleep.

7. **Get at least 20 minutes of exposure to sunlight a day, preferably first thing in the morning.** The light from the sun enters your eyes and triggers your brain to release specific chemicals and hormones such as melatonin that are vital to healthy sleep, mood, and aging.

8. **Do not eat within three hours of bedtime.** Eating a heavy meal prior to bed will lead to a bad night's sleep.

9. **Don't exercise vigorously after dinner.** It excites the body and makes it more difficult to get to sleep.

10. **Write your worries down.** One hour before bed, write down the things that are causing you

anxiety and make plans for what you might have to do the next day to reduce your worry. It will free up your mind to move into deep and restful sleep.

11. **Take a hot salt/soda aromatherapy Ultra-Bath.** Raising your body temperature before bed helps to induce sleep. A hot bath also relaxes your muscles and reduces tension physically and psychically. By adding 1–2 cups of Epsom salts (magnesium sulfate), ½–1 cup of baking soda (sodium bicarbonate), and 10 drops of lavender oil to your bath, you will gain the benefits of magnesium absorbed through your skin, the alkaline-balancing effects of the baking soda, and the cortisol-lowering effects of lavender, all of which help with sleep.

12. **Get a massage or stretch before bed.** This helps relax the body, making it easier to fall asleep.

13. **Warm your middle.** This raises your core temperature and helps trigger the proper chemistry for sleep. Either a hot water bottle, heating pad, or warm body can do the trick.

14. **Avoid medications that interfere with sleep.** These include sedatives (although used to treat insomnia, they ultimately lead to dependence and disruption of normal sleep rhythms and architecture), antihistamines, stimulants, cold

medications, steroids, and headache medications that contain caffeine (such as Fioricet).

15. **Use herbal therapies.** Try 300–600 mg of passionflower, or 320–480 mg of valerian root extract (*Valeriana officinalis*) 1 hour before bed.

16. **Take 200–400 mg of magnesium citrate or glycinate before bed.** This relaxes the nervous system and muscles. Take magnesium citrate if you tend toward constipation and magnesium glycinate if you tend toward loose bowels.

17. **Try other supplements and herbs.** Calcium, theanine (an amino acid from green tea), GABA, 5-HTP, and magnolia can be helpful in getting some shuteye.

18. **Try 1–3 mg of melatonin at night.** Melatonin helps stabilize your sleep rhythms.

19. **Get a relaxation, meditation, or guided imagery CD.** These can help you get to sleep, or use the technique for breathing and visualization in this chapter when you get into bed.

20. **See your doctor.** If you are still having trouble sleeping, you should be evaluated by your doctor for other problems that can interfere with sleep, such as food sensitivities, thyroid problems, heavy metal toxicity, chronic fatigue, stress and depression, and sleep disorders, which may need to be diagnosed at a sleep lab.

The key is to get good-quality sleep and relax every day—even if just for 5 minutes. Profound, deep relaxation for 30 minutes a day will transform your life. You are welcome to use my guided relaxation CD program called *UltraCalm,* at www.blood sugarsolution.com/ultracalm, to help you hit your pause button.

I have also created a 20-minute guided restorative yoga sequence with audio and pictures available at www.bloodsugarsolution.com. It is a powerful form of deep relaxation and passive stretching that helps reset your nervous system.

22

Week 4: Fun, Smart Exercise

At sixty-four years old, Geoff tipped the scale at 305 pounds. This caused diabetes, heart disease, high blood pressure, and a whole list of other health problems, all treated with medication. At a lecture he heard me say there were very few 300-pound eighty-year-olds walking around, and almost no 300-pound ninety-year-olds. Sheepishly he asked if I could help him. I said yes, but only if he did everything I told him to do (knowing that most people eat half as well and exercise half as much as I recommend). Geoff did everything. Prior to getting on *The Blood Sugar Solution,* his main sport was binge eating. Slowly he built up to 45 minutes of aerobic exercise a day, 30 minutes of strength training 3 times a week, and 15 minutes of stretching a day. A year later he came back 140 pounds lighter, and free of diabetes, heart disease, and medication.

Exercise is probably the most powerful medicine for treating diabesity and other diseases. It is a one-stop-shopping miracle potion. It would save more lives than all the antibiotics and vaccines combined. If it were a prescription medication, we could all buy stock and retire tomorrow. Scientists refer to exercise as a "polypill" because it treats everything.[1]

Here are some of its benefits. Exercise:

- Makes your muscles and cells more insulin sensitive.
- Balances and lowers blood sugar.
- Promotes weight loss and loss of belly fat.
- Regulates your appetite and reduces cravings.
- Lowers blood pressure.
- Lowers triglycerides and LDL (bad) cholesterol.
- Raises good (HDL) cholesterol.
- Reduces inflammation (C-reactive protein and other inflammatory cytokine molecules such as IL-6).
- Improves fatty liver that results from diabesity.[2]
- Boosts the number and function of your mitochondria, leading to a faster metabolism and longer life.

- Improves gene expression, turning on genes that improve insulin sensitivity and reverse diabesity.
- Normalizes sex hormone function in men and women.
- Helps correct and prevent erectile dysfunction in men, often caused by diabesity.[3]
- Improves mood and concentration, creates and improves connections between brain cells, increases energy, and helps sleep and digestive function.

Take Action! Combine Aerobic Conditioning and Strength Training

Recent research in the *Journal of the American Medical Association*[4] found that combining aerobic conditioning (getting your heart rate going for a sustained period) and strength training (building muscle) has the most benefit for diabesity and weight loss.

Aerobic Exercise: Make It Fun

Ideally you should do a minimum of 30 minutes of walking every day. Get a pedometer to track your steps. Wear it every day and set a goal of 10,000 steps a day. See www.bloodsugarsolution.com/fitbit to buy a great step tracker.

More vigorous and sustained exercise is often needed to reverse severe diabesity. Run, bike, dance, play games, jump on a trampoline, or do whatever is fun for you. Sustained aerobic exercise, during which you reach 70–85 percent of your maximum heart rate (see page 376 for how to calculate) for up to 60 minutes, 5–6 times a week is often necessary for getting diabesity under full control. A little is good; more is better. Start with 5 minutes a day and work up. All you need is a pair of sneakers.

Interval Training: Make It Fast

Studies have found you can boost your metabolism, burn more calories all day long, and lose more weight by exercising for *less* time. Interval training—shorter sessions with short speed bursts, or what we call "wind sprints"—is a simple way to supercharge your routine. The key is going anaerobic (meaning your cells switch to burning calories without oxygen for brief periods) and going above your target heart rate for short bursts.

Substituting 30 minutes of interval training 2–3 days a week for your regular aerobic exercise routine can give you more benefits in less time. An example of an interval training regimen might be:

- Do 5 minutes of warm-up.
- Do 10 intervals where you bring your heart rate up to the interval zone (see page 376) for 30 seconds and then back down to the target heart rate zone (see page 376) for 90 seconds.
- Finish with a 5-minute cooldown.

I've come across a powerful interval-training program that many of my readers have used with incredible success. Go to www.bloodsugarsolution.com/pace to find out more.

Strength Training: Make It Strong

Strength training is also important because it helps maintain and build muscle, which can help with your overall blood sugar and energy metabolism. One of the biggest factors in aging and diabesity is muscle loss. The technical word for this is *sarcopenia*. Muscle is where you burn the most calories. If your muscle is flabby and marbled with fat, you become insulin resistant and age faster.

You can build muscle in all sorts of ways—using everything from dumbbells to exercise bands, medicine balls, exercise machines, even your own body weight through martial arts, yoga, or Pilates. Personally I like yoga because I get three in one—strength, stretching, and relaxation. If you do "hot" yoga, you get a sauna and detox, too! You may need help getting started or learning a routine, but make it your own and do it three times a week.

Stay Flexible: Make It Stretch

Keeping flexible with stretching or yoga prevents injury and pain from other types of activity. With some kinds of yoga, you can even achieve aerobic

---

How to Calculate Your Heart Rate Zones

Target Heart Rate Zone is 70–85 percent of your maximum heart rate.

- 220 minus your age _____ = Estimated Maximum Heart Rate (HR)
- Max. HR × 0.70 = Low Zone
- Max. HR × 0.85 = High Zone

Note: If you are taking medications, such as beta-blockers, this equation will not work for you.

Interval Heart Rate Zone is calculated at 85–90 percent of your maximum heart rate.

- Max. HR x 0.85 = Low Zone
- Max. HR x 0.90 = High Zone

   I encourage you to use a heart rate monitor to ensure you are in the "zone." I recommend one at www.bloodsugarsolution.com/heartrate.

---

exercise, strength training, and stretching all in one workout. Try to get in at least 5 minutes of stretching before and after exercise routines, and do 30–60 minutes of whole-body stretching twice a week.

HOW MUCH YOU SHOULD EXERCISE

As a basic minimum, commit to 30 minutes of vigorous walking every day while you are on this program. More is better, and for some of you, increasing your aerobic exercise over time is particularly important. Start by walking every day. Then, if you want or need a more comprehensive exercise regimen (which I strongly encourage), follow these guidelines:

- **Add more vigorous sustained aerobic exercise.** Get your heart rate up to 70–80 percent of its maximum for 60 minutes up to 6 times a week.
- **Try interval training.** Try shorter sessions (30 minutes) 2–3 times a week with regular speed bursts to supercharge your aerobic program and get fit faster.
- **Make yourself stronger with strength training.** Whether it's resistance training with weights or a yoga routine, integrate strength training 2–3 times a week.
- **Stay flexible.** Stretch for at least 5 minutes before and after exercise routines and try to do 30–60 minutes of full-body stretching twice a week for 20 minutes.

For more detailed instructions, suggestions, and resources for how to incorporate exercise into your life and build a routine that works for you, please see www.bloodsugarsolution.com. There are many great programs, ideas, and ways to get moving. But just get moving!

Take Action! Explore Play

I have a confession to make. I hate to exercise. Play, absolutely, but exercise, ugh. You will almost never find me in the gym.

I do many different things that keep me fit, and I encourage you to explore all the things you enjoy and save traditional exercise for those times when you just can't find a way to play.

Here are my favorite ways to play:

- Turn down the shades, turn up your favorite tunes, and dance with abandon.
- Play a game (tennis, squash, tag, capture the flag, basketball, soccer, volleyball).
- Join a sports league where you can do regular games with others of your skill level.
- Find a friend to jog or dance with. Use your small group as a chance to connect and exercise together.
- Do something outside in nature—walk, hike, bike, roller blade, or ski. It will nourish your body and your soul.

- Do seasonal exercise — cross-country ski or snowshoe in the winter; swim in a pond or walk on the beach in the summer. Keep it varied and interesting.
- Go to classes. Group exercise makes it easier — spinning, yoga, dance, zumba, etc.
- Do something different every day or at least every week.

Journaling Exercise: Why Don't You Exercise?

What are your excuses for not exercising?

- I don't have enough time.
- I don't like exercise.
- I don't know how.
- I am too tired to exercise.
- I am embarrassed.
- I have injuries or fears of getting hurt.
- It's cold outside; it's hot outside.
- It costs too much to join a gym or get a trainer.
- I was made fun of in gym class at school.
- It's too much work.
- I don't like to sweat.
- I am worried I am going to have a heart attack or stroke.

Are these excuses based in reality, or is there something you can do about them? More often than not, there is something else going on—lack of motivation, negative associations, or low self-esteem. Inertia is hard to overcome, and there may be some initial painful feelings and beliefs, but once you start, you will wonder why you ever resisted it.

23

Week 5: Live Clean and Green

Environmental toxins are bad for your body and the planet. Unfortunately our food, water, air, homes, and body care products are often the source of hidden toxins. The link between environmental toxins, obesity, and diabetes, as well as many chronic and inflammatory diseases, is no longer in question. The best we can do is to reduce the burden on our bodies and our communities. We often think of how we can create sustainable environmental practices to prevent the destruction of our planet's ecosystems and the extinction of species. But the little secret is that we are also part of the ecosystem, and our bodies have become toxic waste dumps. **If we were food, we would not be safe to eat.**

Most of the 80,000-plus new chemicals and toxins on the market since 1900 have never been proven safe. We use something, then decades later it is proved not to be safe (for example, cigarettes, DDT or dioxins, phthalates in water bottles, or bisphenol A in baby bottles and cans). The more prudent approach is not to use something unless it has first been proven safe. That won't happen in our current regulatory environment, so I follow the precautionary principle, otherwise known as better safe than sorry!

It is useful to think of sources of toxins and work on simple things we can do to reduce our exposure from each of the five major sources:

1. Food
2. Water
3. Metabolic toxins (internal waste products)
4. Hidden environmental chemicals and metals in body care and household products
5. Electromagnetic radiation or frequencies (EMFs)

Take Action! Eat Organic, Grass-Fed, Sustainable, Clean Food

Avoid the most common sources of chemicals and toxins in our diet as much as possible. The more demand there is for clean food, the cheaper and more available it will become.

Fruits and vegetables. Buy organic, local, and seasonal when possible. When not possible, avoid the most contaminated foods (go to www.ewg.org for an up-to-date list of the Dirty Dozen and the Clean Fifteen). Avoid conventionally grown fruits and vegetables with the highest toxin load. Here are the ten worst offenders: peaches, apples, sweet bell peppers, celery, nectarines, strawberries, cherries, lettuce, grapes, and pears. Choose only organic versions of these high-pesticide-residue fruits and vegetables.

Meat and poultry. Buy meat from animals raised without hormones, antibiotics, or pesticides and that are free-range or grass-fed when possible. Animal fat is a reservoir for storing pesticides and other toxins. The quality of fat in animals that are raised naturally is radically different from that of animals raised in feedlots, both in terms of the fatty acid profile and the toxic profile. Choose the best-quality meat you can afford.

Fish. Avoid large predatory fish and river fish, which contain mercury and other contaminants in unacceptable amounts; these include swordfish, tuna, Chilean sea bass, large halibut, tilefish, and shark. For low-mercury and low-toxin wild fish, I suggest salmon, sardines, herring, shrimp, and scallops. Stay away from endangered fish. Use the Natural Resources Defense Council's wallet card when choosing fish (http://www.nrdc.org/health/ effects/mercury/walletcard.PDF). When possible, eat fish either farmed or caught with sustainable, restorative, regenerative practices. Check out www .bloodsugarsolution.com/cleanfish to find out which brands and companies to choose from.

Take Action! Drink Clean Water

Your body is made mostly of water. Your cells are bathed in it. It is what you use to excrete many toxins. As one professor said to me in medical school, "The solution to pollution is dilution."

Water is the best beverage (and until recently, mostly what humans drank). Drinking clean, fresh, pure water—six to eight glasses a day—has many benefits. Often we think we are hungry when we are thirsty, or we are tired when we are really dehydrated.

If your urine is dark or yellow, you aren't drinking enough water. It should be clear or light yellow (except right after you take your vitamins, because riboflavin, vitamin B2, makes your urine bright yellow). If you are constipated, it is often because your stools are dehydrated. If you eat fiber but don't drink enough water, your stools turn to cement.

Forty years ago, when I was a teenager on canoe trips in the Canadian wilderness, I would stick my face right in a lake or stream and suck up delicious, pure water. Today I wouldn't dare. The average freshwater rivers and lakes contain over thirty-eight contaminants, including harmful microbes, pesticides, plastics, metals, chlorine, fluoride,[1] medications, and other toxins. Ever wonder where all that Prozac or Premarin goes once it's excreted in people's urine? Every deep aquifer in America is contaminated with petrochemicals from pesticides that have seeped into the ground from our industrial farming practices. Tap water is not safe to drink. In some areas of the country, a new natural gas mining technique called fracturing releases toxic chemicals into the water. People can light their tap water on fire with a match.

Bottled water is often not much better. Most is unregulated, and some water that could be good, such as reverse osmosis–filtered water, is distributed in plastic bottles that may contain phthalates or bisphenol A, toxic petrochemicals.

The best option is to filter your own water and carry it with you in stainless steel bottles. There are many filtering options. The two best are simple **carbon filters** (such as Brita) or a **reverse-osmosis filtering system,** which puts the water through a multistep process to remove the toxins. There is an initial cost to installing it, but it is cheaper over the long run. See www.bloodsugarsolution.com/reverse-osmosis-water-filter for water filter suggestions.

Take Action! Get Your Fluids Moving and Rid Yourself of Metabolic Toxins

Your body is smart. It knows how to detox. You just have to make sure you help it do its job. Every moment of every day your body is mobilizing, transforming, and excreting toxins through your urine, liver, sweat, and breath. If you didn't breathe, you would go unconscious from carbon dioxide in 4 minutes and die. If you didn't pee, you would die in a week or so from uremic poisoning, and if your liver stopped working and you couldn't excrete toxins, you would die in about a month. If you don't sweat, through exercise or saunas, you can't get rid of all the stored petrochemicals and metals your body accumulates in a lifetime.

So you need the quadruple "P" treatment to keep your body detoxing.

1. **Pee.** Drink six to eight 8-ounce glasses of water a day to have clear urine.
2. **Poop.** Have one to two bowel movements a day. (See Chapter 24, Step 4, or www.bloodsugarso lution.com if you are constipated.) Extra magnesium citrate, vitamin C, and fiber (such as ground flaxseeds, with eight glasses of water a day) will cure most constipation.

3. **Perspire.** Sweat regularly and profusely through exercise and the use of steam baths or saunas. (See the guidelines for saunas in Chapter 24, Step 5.) You can also use my favorite technique to heat up and sweat, the UltraBath.

4. **Pranayama (Sanskrit for breathing).** Learn and practice deep breathing using the belly breathing technique (see Chapter 21).

Take Action! Avoid Hidden Environmental Chemicals and Metals

Most of us are unaware of the extent of our daily exposures to environmental chemicals, plastics, and heavy metals; or of molds in our food, water, air, homes, workplaces, and from our hobbies. We don't think twice about the cleaning products we use in our homes, the fertilizers we use in our gardens, or the lotions or makeup we use on our skin.

Below is a list of common daily exposures to chemicals. We can't eliminate all risk or exposure, but awareness helps. We can change the important things — our household cleaners, our body care products, or the main sources of indoor air pollution. Please see the Resources section or www.blood sugarsolution.com to find the cleanest products and alternatives on the market.

For Your Home

- Decorate your home with houseplants—they help detoxify the air.
- Reduce dust, molds, volatile organic compounds (off-gassing from synthetic carpets, furniture, and paints), and other sources of indoor air pollution by using HEPA/ULPA filters and ionizers. You can find my favorite at www.bloodsugarsolu tion.com/air-filters.
- Clean heating systems and monitor them for release of carbon monoxide, the most common cause of death by poisoning in America.
- Look for nontoxic household products (especially drain and oven cleaners, dishwashing detergent, furniture oils and waxes, carpet cleaners). See a list of products I like at www.bloodsugarsolution .com/household-products.
- Minimize exposure to bright and fluorescent-lit areas as much as possible. Substitute subdued full-spectrum/natural incandescent or LED bulbs or candlelight whenever you can.

For Your Body

- Don't "nuke" your food. The microwave produces more AGEs (advanced glycation end products) in the food and creates more oxidative stress, inflammation, and diabesity.[2] Warming may be okay, but not cooking.

- Avoid water from plastic bottles, which contain phthalates. Filter your tap water or drink water from glass or stainless steel bottles.

- Avoid charbroiled foods—foods that are grilled over charcoal. They contain cancer-causing polycyclic aromatic hydrocarbons.

- Don't buy or use toxic personal care products (aluminum-containing underarm deodorant, antacids, and shampoos). See a list of clean cosmetics and personal care products at www.bloodsugarso lution.com/personal-care-products.

- Stop using creams, sun block, and cosmetics that contain paraben, petrochemicals, lead, or other toxins. Drugs and chemicals are well absorbed through your skin. If you wouldn't eat it, don't put it on your skin.

- Avoid excess exposure to environmental petrochemicals and toxins (garden chemicals, dry cleaning, car exhaust, secondhand smoke).

I encourage you to read *Raising Healthy Children in a Toxic World: 101 Smart Solutions for Every Family* by Dr. Phillip Landrigan from Mount Sinai Hospital in New York, an important book on reducing your environmental exposures by one of the leading authorities on the biological effects of toxins. It's not just about kids but about healthy adults, too. I also recommend *Green Housekeeping* by Ellen Sandbeck, about how to keep a healthy home. You won't make all these changes overnight, but commit to changing one thing each week.

Take Action! Minimize Your Electromagnetic Radiation Exposure

An emerging concern for our health is the hidden effects of electromagnetic radiation or electromagnetic frequencies (EMFs).[3] We live in a wireless, connected, linked-up world surrounded by invisible waves of energy that have not been proven safe over time.

The evidence is controversial, but more is coming in every day, including a recent study in the *Journal of the American Medical Association* that found increases in glucose metabolism in the brain during cell phone use that could not be explained by the heat from the phone.[4] Increasingly data link these EMFs to cancer and other health conditions.[5] Billions of people use cell phones and wireless technology, and they are not going away, but if we focused on new technologies to diffuse or reduce emissions or protect ourselves, we may mitigate the risks. Remember that *the absence of evidence is not evidence of absence.* Just because it hasn't been proven harmful doesn't mean it is safe.

Here are things you can do to minimize your risk of harmful effects from EMR.

- Children and pregnant women should avoid talking on cell phones.
- Do not keep your cell phone near your head or use it to play games, movies, etc. Turn it off when it is not in use.
- Try to keep your cell phone at least six to seven inches away from your body while it is on or when you are talking, texting, or downloading.
- Use air tube headsets or speaker mode when talking. Wireless and wired headsets may still conduct radiation.
- Keep your cell phone away from your hip. The bone marrow in your hip produces 80 percent of the body's red blood cells and is especially vulnerable to EMR damage. The close proximity to your genitals may also affect fertility.
- Replace as many cordless and WiFi items as you can with wired, corded lines (phones, Internet, games, appliances, devices, etc.).
- Sit as far back from the computer screen as possible; flat screens are preferable. Use wired Internet connections, not WiFi—especially for laptops.

- Keep a low-EMR sleep, home, and personal zone.
  1. Move your alarm clock radio at least three feet from your head or use a battery-powered clock; six feet is the recommended distance for you to be from all electronic devices during sleep.
  2. Avoid waterbeds, electric blankets, and metal frames, which attract electromagnetic frequencies. Futons and wood-framed beds are better than metal-coiled mattresses and box springs.
  3. When using electric stoves, cook on back burners instead of front as much as possible.

To learn more about the dangers of electronic pollution and how to protect yourself, read *Zapped: Why Your Cell Phone Shouldn't Be Your Alarm Clock and 1,268 Ways to Outsmart the Hazards of Electronic Pollution* by Ann Louise Gittleman.

24

Week 6: Personalize
the Program

Six weeks of healthy eating alone are enough to heal
chronic symptoms for many people. As you have added
in supplements, relaxation techniques, and exercise,
and you have begun eliminating toxins from your environment, I am sure you have seen additional improvements in your health. If you are in the 80 percent of
people who have great results in the first six weeks of
the program, then that is all you will need to follow.
But if you don't feel better, or haven't lost weight, or
your blood sugar is not in better balance, then you
may be in the 20 percent who have deeper imbalances
in the seven core systems of your body. This chapter
will guide you through a process of finding your
unique imbalances and correcting them. It is the closest you can come to being treated by a functional
medicine doctor without actually seeing one.

I will help you personalize *The Blood Sugar Solution* program with additional steps I call **self-care.** For most people, that will be enough. However, some will need to follow up with **medical care**— further testing and treatment that I outline in *How to Work with Your Doctor to Get What You Need* at www.bloodsugarsolution.com.

Here's how to personalize your self-care. The big secret is that most health problems don't require the attention of a doctor. You can fix them yourself if you have the right information. By following these additional steps, you will experience a process I use successfully every day with my patients.

Go back to Part II of the book and take the diagnostic quizzes in each step now. If you took them before, take them again at this stage as it's likely your healthy eating and lifestyle plan has already impacted your biology and you may not score the same way you did. You will use your current scores to personalize your plan. Here's how:

1. Complete the quizzes, then note if you qualified for self-care or medical care in any of the body's key systems.
2. Record your scores in the chart below.
3. Stay on *The Blood Sugar Solution* program for an additional six weeks as you integrate the steps in this chapter for the step (or steps) where

your score still indicates self-care or medical care.

KEY QUIZ SCORES

Quiz Name	Score	Self-Care or Medical Care
Step 1: Boost Your Nutrition		
Magnesium Quiz		
Vitamin D Quiz		
Essential Omega-3 Fats Quiz		
Step 2: Regulate Your Hormones		
Thyroid Quiz		
Sex Hormones Imbalance Quiz		
Step 3: Reduce Inflammation		
Inflammation Quiz		
Step 4: Improve Your Digestion		
Digestion Quiz		

(Continued)

Quiz Name	Score	Self-Care or Medical Care
Step 5: Maximize Detoxification		
Toxicity Quiz		
Step 6: Enhance Energy Metabolism		
Energy Metabolism Quiz		
Oxidative Stress or Rusting Quiz		
Step 7: Soothe Your Mind		
Stress and Adrenal Fatigue Quiz		

Note: You can take all of your quizzes online and track your progress at www.bloodsugarsolution.com.

HOW TO USE THIS CHAPTER

You may be surprised at how much your scores have changed in six short weeks. If so, this is a good indication you are on the road to healing.

However, if you do not see improvement in all areas, it may mean you have deeper imbalances that require a little extra help.

If your score for any step still indicates self-care or medical care, go to the relevant sections in this chapter. For example, if you scored above 7 on the Inflammation Quiz, you would go to "Step 3, Reduce Inflammation," and add the steps outlined there to your plan. Try these additional steps for six weeks, then retake the quiz. If after this you still don't see the results you want or you still qualify for medical care, it may be time to seek the help of a practitioner experienced in functional or integrative medicine. I have outlined some of the testing options and treatments you and your doctor might consider for each step. More information can be found in *How to Work with Your Doctor to Get What You Need*.

If you qualify for self-care or medical care in more than one step, simply stay on the program for an additional six weeks and add the recommendations for each step you scored high on. Start by addressing one step at a time in the order I note below. Add recommendations for each new step every three days.

1. Improve Your Digestion. The gut is often the source of health problems and inflammation. Start here and extraordinary results may occur.
2. Reduce Inflammation.
3. Boost Your Nutrition.
4. Maximize Detoxification.
5. Regulate Your Hormones.

6. Enhance Energy Metabolism.

7. Soothe Your Mind.

Though this process may take some time, I encourage you to follow these steps. The results are worth it.

In the sections that follow, there are further options for correcting key systems, including more intensive dietary changes, additional supplements, and even medication. I have kept my recommendations to a few suggestions for each step; however, further treatment could be carried out with the help of an experienced practitioner. Some advanced and innovative tests may be needed, and you may find that the average physician will not order them. *How to Work with Your Doctor to Get What You Need,* at www.blood sugarsolution.com, will help you find the right practitioner and understand what additional tests or treatments may be needed.

Of course, we invite you to team up with our doctors, nutritionists, and health coaches at **The Ultra-Wellness Center** in Lenox, Massachusetts (www .ultrawellnesscenter.com). We have been working together for 15 years to help thousands regain their health and solve complex chronic health problems.

Now, here are the steps you need to take to personalize the program and rebalance each of the seven steps.

STEP 1: BOOST YOUR NUTRITION

The most important tool you have to heal yourself is your fork. Food is the most essential medicine. When used intelligently and deliberately, it is powerful enough to heal most chronic illnesses. Yet for some, even the healthiest diet may not be enough to overcome certain nutritional deficiencies.

The nutrition recommendations in Week 1 — how, when, and what to eat — and the supplements outlined in Week 2 are designed to work together to heal diabesity.

However, for those whose score indicates they are deficient in omega-3 fats, vitamin D, or magnesium, more of the foods noted below should be included.

Magnesium Deficiency

If you scored over 3 on the Magnesium Quiz, focus on eating the following foods.

- Dark green leafy vegetables
- Legumes — beans of all varieties
- Nuts, especially almonds

Also, add one (not both) of the following:

- 300 mg of magnesium citrate twice a day, once with breakfast and once with dinner

- 240 mg of magnesium glycinate twice a day, once with breakfast and once with dinner

Use magnesium citrate if you tend toward constipation (reduce the dose if you get loose bowels). Use magnesium glycinate if you have normal bowels or tend toward loose stools or diarrhea.

Vitamin D Deficiency

If you scored over 3 on the Vitamin D Quiz, eat more of the following:

- Mackerel, herring
- Porcini or shiitake mushrooms

Besides taking a supplement of vitamin D3, the best way to ensure adequate blood levels is to get 15 minutes of full-body sun exposure between 10 am and 2 p.m. daily, without sunscreen (although I would recommend sunscreen on your face). This works only in the summer, so I recommend you take additional vitamin D to optimize your level. Most people require an additional 2,000 to 5,000 units of vitamin D3 a day.

Omega-3 Fat Deficiency

If you scored over 4 on the Essential Omega-3 Fats Quiz, make sure to include plenty of the following foods in your diet every day:

- Sardines, herring, wild salmon, mackerel
- Flaxseeds, walnuts

In addition to my recommendations in the basic or advanced supplement plan, add the following:

- An extra 1,000 mg of EPA/DHA twice a day. I use a high-concentrate form containing 720 mg of EPA/DHA per 1,000 mg of fish oil capsule. Most fish oils contain only 300 mg of EPA/DHA per capsule. This means fewer pills, more benefit.

STEP 2: REGULATE YOUR HORMONES

In Chapter 21, "Relax Your Mind, Heal Your Body," I focused on how to get your stress hormones back in balance. Here we will focus on balancing the thyroid and sex hormones, critical for optimal weight and blood sugar balance.

Enhance Your Thyroid
Self-Care Plan

Low thyroid function affects 1 in 10 men and 1 in 5 women, half of whom are *not* diagnosed. To make matters worse, many patients on thyroid hormone replacement are not adequately treated. If your thyroid is low, you can't adequately balance your blood sugar and your cholesterol or lose weight. That is why using a whole-foods diet, nutritional supplements, and optimizing thyroid hormone replacement are critical in resolving diabesity.

If you scored over 3 on the Thyroid Quiz, boost your thyroid with the following foods:

- Seaweed or sea vegetables (for iodine)
- Fish, especially sardines and salmon, for iodine, omega-3 fats, and vitamin D
- Dandelion greens for vitamin A
- Smelt, herring, scallops, and Brazil nuts for selenium

Certain foods can potentially interfere with thyroid function. Gluten, for instance, can cause auto-immune thyroid disease. Luckily, this has already been eliminated as part of *The Blood Sugar Solution*.

Soy foods have been linked to problems in thyroid function. Studies show that when eaten in the traditional forms (tofu, tempeh, miso, edamame) and amounts, they have no effect on thyroid function.[1] The real problem is with what I call FrankenSoy—a by-product of soybean oil extraction—which is made into soy hot dogs, protein bars, and other assorted junk food. Soy in this form has been shown to disrupt thyroid function. Avoid these foods.

I would also avoid fluoride[2] because it competes with iodine during the production of thyroid hormones, leading to potential difficulties in thyroid production. Buy toothpaste that isn't fluoridated and filter your water as outlined in Chapter 23.

Medical Care Plan

Doctors do not always do complete testing for thyroid function. They check something called TSH but not other numbers such as free T3, free T4, and antithyroid antibodies. This means, they may miss subtle thyroid imbalances. And to treat imbalances, they use only the inactive thyroid hormone (T4) found in Synthroid or Levoxyl. Most people respond better to a combination of the active (T3) and inactive (T4) hormone called Armour thyroid.

Guidelines for effective thyroid testing and natural thyroid hormone replacement are provided in *How to Work with Your Doctor to Get What You Need* (www.bloodsugarsolution.com). If you have significant thyroid problems or are already on thyroid medication, I recommend that you read my report or watch my webinar on *The UltraThyroid Solution* (www.bloodsugarsolution.com/ultrathyroid).

Regulate Your Sex Hormones
Self-Care Plan

If you scored over 9 if you are a woman and over 4 if you are a man on the Sex Hormones Imbalance

Quiz, the following foods can help get the hormones back in balance for both men and women:

- Whole traditional soy foods such as tofu, tempeh, miso, natto, and edamame, which contain isoflavones.
- Ground flaxseeds, 2 tablespoons a day, which contain lignans.

In addition to the basic supplement plan, women should take the following:

- **Evening primrose oil.** This is an essential anti-inflammatory omega-6 fat (GLA, or gamma-linoleic acid). Take 1,000 mg twice a day, once with breakfast and once with dinner.
- **Chasteberry fruit extract** (*Vitex agnus-castus*). This may help balance the hormones released by the pituitary gland and can help regulate menstrual cycles and relieve PMS (premenstrual syndrome).[3] Take 100 mg twice a day, once with breakfast and once with dinner.
- **Saw palmetto.** This is most often used for prostate health; however, it is also important for blocking an enzyme that causes increased testosterone. It can reduce facial hair and acne in women. Take 320 mg twice a day, once with breakfast and once with dinner.

Men should take the following in addition to the basic supplement plan:

- **Arginine.** This is an amino acid that, like Viagra, creates nitric oxide, without the headaches and blue visual spots. Take 700 mg twice a day, once with breakfast and once with dinner.
- **Tribulus fruit.** This Ayurvedic herb helps boost sexual function. Take 1,000 mg twice a day, once with breakfast and once with dinner.
- **Ginseng.** This Chinese herb also helps boost sexual function. Take 200 mg of an extract standardized to 8% (16 mg) ginsenosides twice a day, once with breakfast and once with dinner.

Medical Care Plan

Sometimes bioidentical hormone treatment is necessary. I often recommend topical testosterone cream or gel for men with low testosterone levels. It helps them build up muscle, lose weight, improve insulin sensitivity, have more energy and a better sex drive, and better erections. In advanced diabesity, nerve or blood vessel damage can occur and medication such as Viagra can be helpful. Women also may benefit from additional support such as hormone replacement therapy. Guidelines for sex hormone testing and natural bioidentical hormone replacement are provided in *How to Work with Your Doctor to Get What You Need.*

STEP 3: REDUCE INFLAMMATION

The two biggest causes of inflammation that lead to diabesity are, first, our high-sugar, processed food, inflammatory diet, and sedentary lifestyle, and second, hidden food sensitivities or allergens, most commonly gluten and dairy. Remember the domino effect of sugar—it causes insulin to spike, which leads to the storage of belly fat. Those belly fat cells produce tons of inflammatory molecules that inflame your whole system, leading to more insulin resistance and weight gain. Environmental toxins and microbes and stress also trigger inflammation.

The Blood Sugar Solution is designed to be a powerful anti-inflammatory program. A whole-foods, low-sugar, high-omega-3 fat, phytonutrient-rich diet, exercise,[4] multivitamins,[5] fish oil, vitamin D, and stress reduction are all powerful natural anti-inflammatories.

But for some, inflammation will persist, and that means you need to hunt for the cause, either by yourself or with your doctor. The most common and obvious causes are diet and lack of exercise. But there are many factors, and at times specialized testing and treatment are needed to find hidden causes such as a virus, parasite, or bacteria that might not cause immediately obvious symptoms; mold in your surroundings (hidden in walls, in damp basements, or in moldy bathrooms); a medication you are taking, such as the birth control pill; or toxins such as mercury or pesticides.

Self-Care Plan

If your Inflammation Quiz score was over 6, take the following additional steps:

- Follow a more comprehensive elimination/reintroduction diet after the six weeks are over. In addition to gluten and dairy, eliminate eggs, yeast, corn, peanuts, citrus, and soy, the other common foods that trigger sensitivities and inflammation. For a step-by-step plan for following the elimination diet, please refer to my book *The UltraSimple Diet* (www.bloodsugarsolution.com/ultrasimple-diet) or the related DVD program, *Kick-Start Your Metabolism in 7 Days: The UltraSimple Plan to Quickly and Safely Lose up to 10 Pounds* (www.bloodsugarsolution.com/ultrasimple-challenge).
- Add herbs such as turmeric, rosemary, and ginger to your cooking.
- Take an anti-inflammatory herbal supplement. Curcumin, the yellow spice found in curry, is the best anti-inflammatory. You can purchase anti-inflammatory herbal supplements in combinations such as turmeric, ginger, and rosemary. Take 200 mg twice a day, once with breakfast and once with dinner.

Medical Care Plan

If you qualified for medical care on your quiz, see *How to Work with Your Doctor to Get What You Need* (www.bloodsugarsolution.com) for further testing and treatment options for inflammation, allergies, hidden infections, and toxins.

STEP 4: IMPROVE YOUR DIGESTION

One of the most surprising discoveries of the last decade is the link between gut problems, obesity, and diabetes. It seems odd, but scientists have found that two major problems in the gut drive weight gain and diabetes: a leaky gut and bad bugs. You learned about this in Chapter 11. When the lining of the intestine is injured by medication, poor diet, food allergens, irritating food proteins such as gluten and dairy, and imbalances in the gut ecosystem, then undigested food particles and proteins are absorbed and trigger inflammation, which, as you now know, causes weight gain and insulin resistance.

Fixing your digestive system is something that many people can do on their own with a few simple steps. Not only can this help you lose weight and reverse diabesity, but it can also help you fix many other chronic health problems, including fatigue, mood disorders, headaches, arthritis and autoimmune diseases, and more.

If your gut is healthy, you can keep bad bacteria out and prevent allergens from leaking through your intestinal barrier. This will lower inflammation, help control your appetite, and prevent bad bugs from extracting more calories from your food. That means that you end up with more food on your lips and less on your hips!

Here are some things you can try. But for those of you who have very bad bacterial overgrowth or weird bugs such as parasites, worms, or yeast, medical testing and treatment will be necessary to kill the bugs.

Self-Care Plan

If you scored above 8 on the Digestion Quiz, here's what you can do:

- For six weeks, eliminate foods from your diet that ferment and produce gas in your gut (beans, grains, and all sugars, including all artificial sweeteners, especially sugar alcohols). This will starve the bad bugs.
- Eat slowly, chew your food, and sit down when you eat. These all help support healthy digestion.
- Take digestive enzymes and hydrochloric acid supplements to help break down your food and

prevent allergies and fermentation of starches (see below).

- Take probiotics (healthy bacteria) to put good bugs back in your gut and reduce inflammation (see page 413).
- Take the gut-repairing nutrients l-glutamine and quercetin, in addition to your basic supplements (see page 414).
- If your symptoms are not better and you continue to score high on the Digestion Quiz after six weeks on the self-care plan, follow the medical care plan outlined in *How to Work with Your Doctor to Get What You Need* (www.bloodsugarsolution.com).

Gut-Healing Supplements

Here is what I suggest:

ENZYMES

- Take 2 capsules of a broad-spectrum, plant-based digestive enzyme 3 times a day, once with each meal. The product should contain enzymes that break down proteins, fats, and carbohydrates.

HYDROCHLORIC ACID SUPPORT

Too much stomach acid can cause reflux and other symptoms, but too little can cause bloating, an inability to break down food or active digestive enzymes, and an overgrowth of yeast and bacteria.

If you are taking an acid-blocking medication, this may, in fact, be part of the problem. See if diet changes and other recommendations in *The Blood Sugar Solution* help your reflux, and work with your doctor to get off that medication.

I usually recommend that betaine or hydrochloric acid supplements be used carefully, under the supervision of a health care practitioner. However, if you follow the guidelines below, they can be very helpful while your gut is healing.

- Start with 1 capsule or tablet at the beginning of each meal. Increase the dose by 1 capsule per meal until you have a warm feeling in your stomach. Then drop back down to the dose just before the warm feeling occurred. Stay on it for 1–2 months then stop and see how you feel.

PROBIOTICS

These essential ingredients support intestinal health. Our poor-quality diet, overuse of medication, and stress all alter our normal, healthy intestinal flora or bacteria. Abnormal flora can trigger toxin release into the body and generate local inflammation and weight gain,[6] both of which trigger systemic inflammation. I believe that given all the stresses on our guts, probiotics are needed for the vast majority of people for long-term health.

Preparations include freeze-dried bacteria packaged in powder, tablet, or capsule form. It is important to take a combination product with multiple species of organisms. If you are dairy-sensitive, seek out dairy-free brands.

- Take at least 10–20 billion organisms of a broad-spectrum probiotic twice a day, once with breakfast and once with dinner.

Gut-Repairing Nutrients

Zinc, omega-3 fats, vitamin A, and other gut-healing nutrients are part of the basic plan, but a few other things can be very helpful.

L-glutamine, a nonessential amino acid, is the food for the cells that line your intestine. It generally comes in powder form and is often combined with other compounds that facilitate gut repair. Quercetin is a potent anti-inflammatory that is helpful in restoring balance in the gut.

- Take 2,500 mg of l-glutamine twice a day, once with breakfast and once with dinner.
- Take 500 mg of quercetin twice a day, once with breakfast and once with dinner.

Medical Care Plan

Testing for gut problems and fixing them is one of the most powerful things I do in my practice. Unfortunately most conventionally trained physicians do not know how to diagnose common problems such as a leaky gut or food sensitivities, or do the right tests to identify bacterial or yeast overgrowth, parasites, or worms. In *How to Work with Your Doctor to Get What You Need* (www.bloodsugarsolution.com), I explain the testing and treatment for gut problems. There are safe and effective medications for bacterial overgrowth, parasites, and yeast that can help people get better faster. If you scored over 13 on the Digestion Quiz or feel you might have a problem (even though you don't have digestive symptoms), seek out a functional medicine practitioner.

STEP 5: MAXIMIZE DETOXIFICATION

Toxins are often invisible. They are in our air and water, and in the food we eat. Slowly, daily, inevitably, our bodies accumulate more and more toxins. A high body burden of toxins can prevent you from losing weight, or worse, damage your metabolism and lead to a weight loss plateau.

Living clean and green is a cornerstone of creating health, losing weight, and preventing diabetes. You learned how to do that in Chapter 21. However, some people have accumulated such a high body burden of persistent organic pollutants (pesticides, PCBs, phthalates, flame retardants, etc.) and heavy metals (mercury, lead, arsenic, etc.) that they need additional support for detoxification using detox-boosting foods, supplements, herbs, saunas, and sometimes chelating medication to get rid of heavy metals (to be done under a doctor's supervision). If you qualified for self-care or medical care on the Detoxification Quiz in Chapter 11, then you should add these next steps to your program.

Self-Care Plan

Our bodies have a natural intelligence and are designed to help us mobilize and transform toxins. Given today's toxic environment, it is important that you learn how to boost your body's own detoxification system.

It's not that difficult.

If you scored over 6 on the Toxicity Quiz:

- Eat more cruciferous vegetables (broccoli, kale, collards, cabbage, etc.), garlic, green tea, turmeric, and whole eggs. They contain phytonutrient detox-boosting compounds. Add them to your diet daily. Other great detox foods are cilantro, celery, parsley, dandelion greens, citrus peels, pomegranate, and rosemary.

- Take glutathione-boosting and detox-boosting supplements NAC, milk thistle, and vitamin C (see below).
- Sweat regularly using saunas (see below).

Detoxification-Boosting Supplements

You can take all three of these supplements, or just take NAC, which I think is the most important.

- **N-acetyl-cysteine, or NAC.** This amino acid dramatically increases glutathione. It is even used in the emergency room to treat liver failure from Tylenol overdose. Take 600 mg twice a day, once with breakfast and once with dinner.
- **Milk thistle.** This herb has long been used in liver disease and helps boost glutathione levels. Take 175 mg of a standardized extract twice a day, once with breakfast and once with dinner.
- **Buffered ascorbic acid (vitamin C).** This vitamin is especially useful during periods of increased detoxification. Take 1,000 mg twice a day, once with breakfast and once with dinner. Too much vitamin C may cause diarrhea. If this happens for you, simply reduce the dose.

Hyperthermic Therapy or Heat Therapy

People all over the world have used sauna and heat therapies for hundreds of years to purify mind and body. Recently the Environmental Protection Agency found sauna therapy helpful for supporting excretion of heavy metals (lead, mercury, cadmium, and fat-soluble chemicals such as PCBs, PBBs, and HCBs).[7] It also improves quality of life in patients with type 2 diabetes.[8] It helps lower blood pressure, lower weight, and reduce stress. I think of it as the lazy man's way to exercise.

Follow these guidelines for safe detoxification. More intensive detoxification protocols should be used only in conjunction with a physician or health care practitioner.

- If you are on multiple medications or have a chronic illness, check with your doctor before starting heat therapy, and start slowly.
- Drink at least 16 ounces of purified water before entering the sauna or steam bath.
- Drink another 16 ounces after the sauna or steam.
- Begin with 3 and build up to 5–7 saunas per week.
- Start with 10 minutes during your first treatment and increase by 5 minutes during each subsequent treatment until you reach a maximum of 30–45 minutes. You should take cold dips or rinses in a shower every 10 minutes. Keep the sauna or steam temperature under 150 degrees.

- For more intensive detoxification, use heat therapy daily for six weeks; use once a week as maintenance therapy afterward.

- If you take saunas or steam baths more than 3–4 times a week, I recommend an additional multimineral supplement to replace what you sweat out. This contains not vitamins but extra minerals such as zinc, magnesium, potassium, sodium, and calcium, which you lose during sweating.

- Infrared saunas work at lower temperatures. They can be more effective and better tolerated than regular saunas. I have a Sunlighten sauna our whole family uses. (See www.bloodsugarsolution .com/sunlighten-saunas.)

- Get the toxins off your skin after the sauna or steam. Use a hot shower with soap and even a skin brush.

- Some people have symptoms from the release of toxins, including skin rashes, headaches, fatigue, nausea, irritable bowel, confusion, or memory problems. If you experience any of these side effects, take buffered vitamin C or get the help of a functional medicine or integrative practitioner.

Medical Care Plan

If your score suggests that you should seek medical care, your practitioner may test you for heavy metals such as mercury and lead, and recommend additional detoxification strategies, including supplements, intravenous nutrients, and chelation.

I have found that over 80 percent of the patients coming to my practice (who admittedly are sicker than average) have elevated levels of mercury, and 40 percent have very elevated levels. But the body hides these metals in organs and tissues, and so regular blood tests aren't accurate. I recommend a special test called a chelation challenge with medication such as DMSA or DMPS, which pulls out hidden stored mercury and other metals and gives a better picture of your total body burden. If you have elevated levels, there are medical treatments to help clear metals from your body. In *How to Work with Your Doctor to Get What You Need* (www.bloodsugarsolu tion.com), I explain the tests that can assess your body's own detoxification system and levels of persistent organic pollutants and heavy metals. I also explain treatment options. This is often a critical step in helping people lose weight and correct diabesity.

STEP 6: ENHANCE ENERGY METABOLISM

By following the basic plan in *The Blood Sugar Solution*, you will already be doing things to enhance your metabolism—eating a plant-based antioxidant-rich diet, exercising, reducing toxic exposures, and lowering inflammation. By supplementing with mitochondrial-protective and antioxidant compounds, we can preserve and restore our energy metabolism to optimal function.

If you scored above 6 on the Energy Metabolism Quiz, follow the steps below.

Supplements to Boost Energy and Reduce Oxidative Stress

Most people with diabesity have poorly functioning mitochondria and need help burning calories and fat. A number of special nutrients become essential under conditions of stress, toxicity, and aging. Taken as supplements, they can dramatically improve energy production and mitochondrial function, as well as protect the mitochondria from damage. Alpha lipoic acid has been well studied[9] and is the most important mitochondrial nutrient for weight loss, blood sugar control, and diabetic neuropathy. That is why I included it in the basic plan of supplements, but higher doses are often needed for more advanced diabesity. Here is what you should add to your regimen.

- 300–600 mg of alpha lipoic acid twice a day, once before breakfast and once before dinner.
- 300–500 mg of l-carnitine twice a day, once with breakfast and once with dinner. L-carnitine helps

fat burning in the mitochondria.[10] It can also help diabetic neuropathy.

- 100 mg of CoQ10 once a day with breakfast. Coenzyme Q10 helps lower fasting insulin and glucose levels, and improves blood pressure and antioxidant status.[11]

- 400 mg of resveratrol twice a day, once with breakfast and once with dinner. Resveratrol, found in dark purple grapes, improves insulin function[12] through its effect on sirtuins, the master metabolism-control genes.[13] It is also being studied as a compound that may slow aging.

- New research has found that "branched chain amino acids" can be helpful in improving mitochondrial function, creating new mitochondria, and improving insulin sensitivity.[14] They also help improve muscle size, physical endurance, and motor coordination and even extend lifespan in animal studies. The research is based on a product I use that comes from Germany. The doses used are one packet (5.5 grams) twice a day dissolved in water. At www.bloodsugarsolution.com, I explain how to use this and where you can find it.

Medical Care Plan

A functional medicine doctor can check your mitochondrial function and oxidative stress through a urine test that measures organic acids. He or she may recommend additional supplements such as D-ribose, creatine, glutathione, and arginine. To learn more about testing and treatment for your mitochondria, see *How to Work with Your Doctor to Get What You Need* at www.bloodsugarsolution.com.

STEP 7: SOOTHE YOUR MIND

Stress finds you. You don't have to look for it. It is an unavoidable part of life. But deep and profound relaxation and calming of the nervous system do not happen automatically. We are not taught the antidote for our chronic stress. We try to look for it—we drink alcohol, numb our emotions with sugar and junk food, zone out in front of the television or computer screen. But these are maladaptive behaviors. They actually make the problem worse. We have no idea where to find or how to push our pause buttons. But this is key to health.

We have unabated, unremitting stress. Our cortisol levels stay elevated. That's bad news because high cortisol makes you gain belly fat and lose muscle, makes you hungry and crave sugar, and causes diabetes.

Everybody has a different pause button. Seek out yours. There are many wonderful resources and programs available to help you achieve this goal. This is key to long-term metabolic health. We have to make it part of our daily lives.

If you scored over 7 on the Stress and Adrenal Dysfunction Quiz, the following steps may help you find balance again.

Self-Care Plan

- If you haven't created or joined a group to support you, do it now—it can be an online group, but ideally it is with people you share your life with. See Chapter 16 on getting healthy together by harnessing the power of community. To learn how to create or join your own group, go to www .bloodsugarsolution.com.

- Identify and reduce the causes of social, psychological, and physical stressors in your own life. Review the journaling exercise on pages 227–228 about energy gain and energy drain. Use the exercises in Chapter 21, "Relax Your Mind, Heal Your Body," or seek the help of professional psychotherapeutic or medical professionals as needed.

- Try life coaching. It is a way of making your life more integrated and overcoming obstacles to thriving. I recommend the Handel Group to help you turn information into transformation. See www.bloodsugarsolution.com/handelgroup to find a coach.

- Incorporate one or two additional ways to push the pause button besides belly breathing, guided visualization, restorative yoga, or stretching, such as

UltraBaths or saunas (see pages 370 and 417–419). You can also use my guided relaxation CDs, *Ultra-Calm* (www.bloodsugarsolution.com/ultracalm) for guided breathing exercises, imagery, and more.

- Try stress-balancing herbs such as cordyceps, rhodiola root extract, and Asian ginseng root extract (see page 426).

I have found many ways to hit my pause button, and have used many with my patients. You have to find what works for you. But please, find something and do it! In the Resources section at www .bloodsugarsolution.com, I provide more detailed recommendations.

Stress-Reducing Supplements and Herbs

Stress can deplete the nutrients needed for deep relaxation of the nervous system, including magnesium, the B vitamins, and vitamin C. When you follow the basic supplement plan, you will make sure to have enough on board.

Certain plant compounds known as adaptogens help modulate and balance the stress response, correcting some of the negative effects of chronic stress.[15] I most often recommend a combination supplement of cordyceps, rhodiola root extract, and Asian ginseng root extract.[16] When taken with meals, ginseng can lower blood sugar and improve insulin function.

You can add the following stress-reducing supplements to your regimen if you are imbalanced in this area:

- 400 mg of cordyceps (containing cordycepic acid and adenosine) twice a day, once with breakfast and once with dinner.
- 50 mg of rhodiola root extract (standardized to 1% [0.5 mg] salidroside) twice a day, once with breakfast and once with dinner.
- 200 mg of Asian ginseng root extract (standardized to 8% [16 mg] ginsenosides) twice a day, once with breakfast and once with dinner.

Medical Care Plan

Some of my patients need more support for handling chronic stress. They may need therapy, coaching, or even medication as a short-term bridge to get through the toughest parts of life. I refer them to a good psychotherapist, psychiatrist, or life coach. See Resources and *The Blood Sugar Solution* website (www.bloodsugarsolution.com) for more information on finding the appropriate help.

25

The Blood Sugar Solution: Weekly Overview

Here I provide a brief summary of the main points outlined each week of the program as well as checklists you can use as you progress. Each week, review the summary, and then use the corresponding checklist to walk through the daily action items you need to complete. You can find printable or trackable versions of all this at www.bloodsugarsolution.com.

WEEK 1: EAT YOUR MEDICINE: NUTRITION BASICS

The basics of good nutrition are simple: It comes down to what you should avoid and what you should include. Here is a brief reminder of each.

What to Avoid

1. All sugars in any form whatsoever.
2. All flour products (even gluten-free).
3. All processed food.
4. All gluten and dairy.
5. All grains and starchy vegetables and fruit (except for ½ cup berries a day) if you are on the advanced plan.

What to Include

1. High-quality foods.
2. Low-glycemic-load meals.
3. Phytonutrient-rich foods.
4. Slow carbs, not low carbs.
5. Omega-3 fats and other healthy fats.
6. High-quality protein.
7. Herbs and healing spices.
8. Three square meals and two snacks.
9. Mindful eating.

WEEK 1 DAILY CHECKLIST

Wake up 1 hour before breakfast. Engage in a physical activity you enjoy such as a walk or yoga.	☐
Breakfast. Try a protein shake, eggs, or use one of the breakfast recipes in the meal plan.	☐

WEEK 1 DAILY CHECKLIST

Journaling. Record what you ate and how you felt. ☐

Midmorning snack. A handful of nuts and a piece of fruit are a great snack. ☐

Journaling. Record what you ate and how you felt. ☐

Lunch. Try one of the quick meals I provide on pages 242–244 or in the meal plan. ☐

Journaling. Record what you ate and how you felt. ☐

Midafternoon snack. Experiment with something different. How about half an avocado with lemon juice, salt, and pepper, or hummus and veggies? Find great snacks in the meal plan. ☐

Journaling. Record what you ate and how you felt. ☐

Dinner. Again, you can try one of the quick meals outlined on pages 242–244 or in the meal plan. ☐

Journaling. Record what you ate and how you felt. Think about how your experience with food impacted your day. What improvements do you see in your energy, your ability to focus? How does your body feel different? How do these changes make you feel? ☐

WEEK 2: OPTIMIZE METABOLISM WITH NUTRITIONAL SUPPLEMENTS

Supplements are an essential and effective part of diabesity treatment, and they are necessary for most of us to stay healthy for life. Though supplementation can seem confusing on the surface, there are really only a few things you need to remember:

1. We are nutrient-depleted.
2. Everyone should take a good multivitamin, fish oil, vitamin D, and magnesium. Most also need a probiotic.
3. People with diabesity need more support.
4. Those on the basic plan should take alpha lipoic acid, chromium polynicotinate, biotin, cinnamon, green tea catechins, and PGX.
5. In addition, those on the advanced plan should take acacia extract (heartwood), hops extract, fenugreek seed extract, bitter gourd fruit extract, and gymnema leaf.
6. PGX should be taken before meals; everything else should be taken in divided doses with breakfast and dinner.

WEEK 2 DAILY CHECKLIST

Wake up 1 hour before breakfast. Engage in a physical activity you enjoy. ☐

Breakfast. Try a protein shake, eggs, or use one of the breakfast recipes in the meal plan. ☐

Supplements. Take appropriate morning supplements with breakfast. ☐

Journaling. Record what you ate and how you felt. ☐

Midmorning snack. Refer to the recipes on pages 500–504 for options. ☐

Journaling. Record what you ate and how you felt. ☐

Lunch. Try one of the quick meals I provide on pages 242–244 or in the meal plan. ☐

Journaling. Record what you ate and how you felt. ☐

Midafternoon snack. Refer to the recipes on pages 500–504 for options. ☐

Journaling. Record what you ate and how you felt. ☐

Dinner. Use one of the quick meals outlined on pages 242–244 or in the meal plan. ☐

(Continued)

WEEK 2 DAILY CHECKLIST

Supplements. Take appropriate evening supplements with dinner. ☐

Journaling. Record what you ate and how you felt. Think about how your experience with food impacted your day. What improvements do you see in your energy, your ability to focus? How does your body feel different? How do these changes make you feel? ☐

WEEK 3: RELAX YOUR MIND, HEAL YOUR BODY

Relaxation is essential for long-term health. Stress plays a dramatic role in blood sugar balance, and relaxation helps reverse this. You should practice relaxation daily to heal your body and mind. To do this, simply:

1. Find time to relax deeply every day.
2. Practice belly breathing 5 times a day.
3. Try the visualization exercise once this week.
4. Go on a one-week media fast.
5. Try some of the 20 tips for better sleep.

WEEK 3 DAILY CHECKLIST

Wake up 1 hour before breakfast. Engage in a physical activity you enjoy. ☐

Morning relaxation. Begin your day with belly breathing. You can do visualization or a restorative yoga sequence if you have time. You can also do this before dinner or before bed. ☐

Breakfast. Try a protein shake, eggs, or use one of the breakfast recipes in the meal plan. ☐

Supplements. Take appropriate morning supplements with breakfast. ☐

Journaling. Record what you ate and how you felt. ☐

Midmorning snack. Refer to the recipes on pages 500–504 for options. ☐

Journaling. Record what you ate and how you felt. ☐

Right before lunch. Do belly breathing. ☐

Lunch. Try one of the quick meals I provide on pages 242–244 or in the meal plan. ☐

Journaling. Record what you ate and how you felt. ☐

Midafternoon snack. Refer to the recipes on pages 500–504 for options. ☐

(Continued)

WEEK 3 DAILY CHECKLIST

Journaling. Record what you ate and how you felt. ☐

Right before dinner. Do belly breathing. ☐

Dinner. Try one of the quick meals outlined on pages 242–244 or in the meal plan. ☐

Supplements. Take appropriate evening supplements with dinner. ☐

Journaling. Record what you ate and how you felt. Think about how your experience with food impacted your day. What improvements do you see in your energy, your ability to focus? How does your body feel different? How do these changes make you feel? ☐

Relaxation before bed. Do belly breathing, and try another deep relaxation technique such as the UltraBath or restorative yoga. ☐

WEEK 4: FUN, SMART EXERCISE

The role of exercise in health, weight loss, and blood sugar balance is clear. We have bodies. We need to use them to be healthy. The good news is that we don't have to pound away on the treadmill to get fit. Following a few simple tips will help you make exercise fun and effective:

1. Walk daily.
2. Track your heart rate.
3. Count your steps with a pedometer.
4. Try interval training.
5. Add strength training.
6. Stretch.
7. Play!

WEEK 4 DAILY CHECKLIST

Wake up 1 hour before breakfast. Engage in a physical activity you enjoy. ☐

Morning relaxation. Begin your day with belly breathing. You can also do visualization or a restorative yoga sequence if you have time. ☐

Stretch. Do 30–60 minutes of full-body stretching at least twice a week. ☐

Breakfast. Try a protein shake, eggs, or use one of the breakfast recipes in the meal plan. ☐

Supplements. Take appropriate morning supplements with breakfast. ☐

Journaling. Record what you ate and how you felt. ☐

Midmorning snack. Refer to the recipes on pages 500–504 for options. ☐

(Continued)

WEEK 4 DAILY CHECKLIST

Journaling. Record what you ate and how you felt. ☐

Right before lunch. Do belly breathing. ☐

Lunch. Try one of the quick meals I provide on pages 242–244 or in the meal plan. ☐

Journaling. Record what you ate and how you felt. ☐

Midafternoon snack. Refer to the recipes on pages 500–504 for options. ☐

Journaling. Record what you ate and how you felt. ☐

Late afternoon: Do 30 minutes of exercise nearly every day (start with fast walking). ☐

Right before dinner. Do belly breathing. ☐

Dinner. Try one of the quick meals outlined on pages 242–244 or in the meal plan. ☐

Supplements. Take appropriate evening supplements with dinner. ☐

Journaling. Record what you ate and how you felt. Think about how your experience with food impacted your day. What improvements do you see in your energy, your ability to focus? How does your body feel different? How do these changes make you feel? ☐

WEEK 4 DAILY CHECKLIST

Relaxation before bed. Do belly breathing, and try another deep relaxation technique like the UltraBath or restorative yoga.   ☐

WEEK 5: LIVE CLEAN AND GREEN

Toxins are a growing concern. As environmental pollutants continue to be released, it's not only our planet but our bodies that are impacted. Heal your body and the planet at the same time by taking a few simple steps:

1. Eat organic, grass-fed, sustainable, clean food.
2. Drink clean, filtered water.
3. Flush your body fluids; remember the 4 "P's" (pages 388–389).
4. Avoid hidden environmental chemicals and metals.
5. Reduce exposure to electromagnetic radiation frequencies (EMF).

WEEK 5 DAILY CHECKLIST

Wake up 1 hour before breakfast. Engage in a physical activity you enjoy. ☐

Morning relaxation. Begin your day with belly breathing. You can also do visualization or a restorative yoga sequence if you have time. ☐

Stretch. Do 30–60 minutes of full-body stretching at least twice a week. ☐

Drink filtered water. Drink at least eight 8-ounce glasses a day. ☐

Get your fluids moving. Remember the 4 "P's" (pages 388–389). ☐

Breakfast. Try a protein shake, eggs, or use one of the breakfast recipes in the meal plan. ☐

Supplements. Take appropriate morning supplements with breakfast. ☐

Journaling. Record what you ate and how you felt. ☐

Midmorning snack. Refer to the recipes on pages 500–504 for options. ☐

Journaling. Record what you ate and how you felt. ☐

Right before lunch. Do belly breathing. ☐

Lunch. Try one of the quick meals I provide on pages 242–244 or in the meal plan. ☐

WEEK 5 DAILY CHECKLIST

Journaling. Record what you ate and how you felt. ☐

Midafternoon snack. Refer to the recipes on pages 500–504 for options. ☐

Journaling. Record what you ate and how you felt. ☐

Late afternoon. Do 30 minutes of exercise nearly every day (start with fast walking). ☐

Right before dinner. Do belly breathing. ☐

Dinner. Try one of the quick meals outlined on pages 242–244 or in the meal plan. ☐

Supplements. Take appropriate evening supplements with dinner. ☐

Journaling. Record what you ate and how you felt. Think about how your experience with food and detoxifying impacted your day. What improvements do you see in your energy, your ability to focus? Does your body feel different? How do these changes make you feel? ☐

Relaxation before bed. Do belly breathing, and try another deep relaxation technique such as the UltraBath or restorative yoga. ☐

WEEK 6: PERSONALIZE THE PROGRAM

It may sound complicated, but it's actually very simple. To personalize the program, you just need to follow two principles:

- Take out the things that cause imbalance (stress, toxins, allergens, microbes, poor diet).
- Add in the things that create balance (real food, nutrients, hormones, sleep, rhythm, clean air and water, movement, love, connection, meaning, and purpose)

When you do this, the body naturally restores balance on its own.

In Chapter 24, I outlined all the steps you need to take to personalize the program. To use that chapter effectively, simply:

1. Retake the key quizzes in Part II.
2. Record your scores. You can use the chart on pages 397–398 or the one I have provided at www.bloodsugarsolution.com.
3. Follow the advice in Chapter 24 for any step when your score indicates self-care or medical care. For many of you, just following the first six weeks of the program will correct most of the imbalances.

4. Continue the program, with the additional steps, for another six weeks.

WEEK 6 DAILY CHECKLIST

Wake up 1 hour before breakfast. Engage in a physical activity you enjoy. ☐

Morning relaxation. Begin your day with belly breathing. You can also do visualization or a restorative yoga sequence if you have time. ☐

Stretch. Do 30–60 minutes of full-body stretching at least twice a week. ☐

Drink filtered water. Drink at least eight 8-ounce glasses a day. ☐

Get your fluids moving. Remember the 4 "P's" (pages 388–389). ☐

Personalize the program. Add the necessary personalization steps from Chapter 24. ☐

Breakfast. Try a protein shake, eggs, or use one of the breakfast recipes in the meal plan. ☐

Supplements. Take appropriate morning supplements with breakfast. ☐

Journaling. Record what you ate and how you felt. ☐

(Continued)

WEEK 6 DAILY CHECKLIST

Midmorning snack. Refer to the recipes on pages 500–504 for options. ☐

Journaling. Record what you ate and how you felt. ☐

Right before lunch. Do belly breathing. ☐

Lunch. Try one of the quick meals I provide on pages 242–244 or in the meal plan. ☐

Journaling. Record what you ate and how you felt. ☐

Midafternoon snack. Refer to the recipes on pages 500–504 for options. ☐

Journaling. Record what you ate and how you felt. ☐

Late afternoon: Do 30 minutes of exercise nearly every day (start with fast walking). ☐

Right before dinner. Do belly breathing. ☐

Dinner. Try one of the quick meals outlined on pages 242–244 or in the meal plan. ☐

Supplements. Take appropriate evening supplements with dinner. ☐

WEEK 6 DAILY CHECKLIST

Journaling. Record what you ate and how you felt. Think about how your experience with food and personalizing the program impacted your day. What improvements do you see in your energy, your ability to focus? Does your body feel different? How do these changes make you feel? □

Relaxation before bed. Do belly breathing, and try another deep relaxation technique such as the UltraBath or restorative yoga. □

NEXT STEPS: GETTING HEALTHY FOR LIFE

Now that you have made it through the whole program, what's next? In Chapter 26, you will learn how to maintain the changes you have made and stay healthy for life. You will also learn how to handle common obstacles and what to do when things aren't improving.

26

Get Healthy for Life

When the program is over, you may want to go out and celebrate by indulging in your favorite foods — pizza, chocolate cupcakes, a beer, or a few glasses of chardonnay. This is a temptation you should resist. After being on a diet like this, overloading your system with bad foods can cause severe reactions. If you can't resist temptation, take it slowly and choose what you want carefully. It might be one of the most profound (and painful) lessons you will ever get regarding the power of food.

In this chapter, I've outlined how you can modify the program to create a sustainable diet and lifestyle for the long term.

WHAT TO DO ABOUT FOOD

You should stick with all of the basic nutrition principles you learned in Chapter 19 for life. This means keeping sugar, flour, and processed foods to a minimum; including high-quality, whole-food carbs, protein, and fats at every meal; composing your meals according to the 50-25-25 principle (50 percent vegetables, 25 percent lean high-quality protein, and 25 percent whole grains); timing your meals in a way that makes sense for your biology by eating protein for breakfast and not eating 2–3 hours before bedtime; and limiting your intake of addictive substances such as caffeine and alcohol.

There are only two foods you need to consider reintegrating: gluten and dairy. You have two options.

Option 1: Stay Off Dairy and Gluten

You can stay off gluten and dairy for as long as you wish. Despite what Big Food may tell you, you don't need either of these foods to stay healthy. If avoiding gluten and dairy feels good to you, keep them out of your diet or choose them as a small treat from time to time.

After you have reset your metabolism and established a pattern of eating and self-care that nourishes you, flexibility will become important. Moderation in all things is still great advice. Even if you choose to avoid gluten, dairy, or other foods long term, it's likely there will be times in your life when you want to eat them or when eating them is unavoidable. Assuming they do not cause a life-threatening reaction for you, and you aren't one of the rare people for whom they trigger a spiral of overeating, this is absolutely fine.

Your inner wisdom is the critical factor. Listen to your body. Staying in balance and finding a rhythm are the keys to a healthy metabolism and lifelong health.

Option 2: Reintegrate Dairy and Gluten

Most people will likely want to try and reintegrate dairy and gluten into their diet, and I encourage you to at least test these foods to confirm whether or not they have been contributing to your symptoms. The key is to do this slowly and systematically:

1. Start with dairy.
2. Eat it at least 2–3 times a day for 3 days.
3. Track your reactions for at least 72 hours. (I'll explain how in a moment.)
4. If you have a reaction, stop dairy immediately.
5. Wait 3 days.
6. Now try gluten. Follow the same process you did for dairy: Eat it 2–3 times a day for 3 days, track your reactions for at least 72 hours, and quit if you notice a reaction.

What kind of reactions should you expect? Everyone is different and many subtle reactions may occur, but here are some of the most common:

- Weight gain
- Cravings
- Fluid retention
- Nasal congestion
- Chest congestion
- Headaches
- Brain fog
- Difficulty remembering things
- Mood problems (depression, anxiety, or anger)
- Sleep problems
- Joint aches
- Muscle aches
- Pain
- Fatigue
- Changes in your skin (acne)
- Changes in digestion or bowel function (bloating, gas, diarrhea, constipation, reflux)

Reactions like these may happen immediately after you consume the food or may not crop up for 72 hours. If you don't experience a reaction within 72 hours, you should be safe.

If you do experience a reaction, I recommend you eliminate the offending food from your diet for twelve weeks. For most, this is enough time for the inflammation in your system to cool down and your gut to heal. After that, it's likely you will be able to consume the food again, but it's prudent to keep it to a minimum (perhaps no more than once or twice a week at most) so that you don't reinitiate the same cycle of illness.

If you still react after eliminating the food from your diet for twelve weeks, you should stay off that food for life, or see a physician, dietitian, or nutritionist skilled in managing food allergies.

Tracking your symptoms is relatively simple. Just use the food log below or download it at www.blood sugarsolution.com.

DATE	FOOD INTRODUCED	SYMPTOMS

Remember, if you still test high on the Inflammation Quiz after twelve weeks on the program (six weeks of the basic plan and an additional six with the personalization steps integrated), it may mean you have sensitivities to more than just gluten and dairy. In this case, I recommend a more extensive elimination-reintroduction program like the one outlined in *The UltraSimple Diet* (www.bloodsugar solution.com/ultrasimple-diet). In that book and the associated DVD home-study program, *Kick-Start Your Metabolism in 7 Days: The UltraSimple Plan to Quickly and Safely Lose Up to 10 Pounds* (www.blood sugarsolution.com/ultrasimple-challenge), I provide a comprehensive set of guidelines for eliminating and reintegrating all the major food allergens so you can determine exactly which foods you are sensitive to.

WHAT TO DO ABOUT SUPPLEMENTS

I strongly encourage you to stay on the basic supplement plan for life. If we lived in a world free of toxins; ate only real, whole foods; had no chronic stress and relaxed as much as we needed to; got enough exercise; and had strong connections to our community, we wouldn't need supplements. But we don't live in that world anymore, and that's why 99 percent of Americans are nutrient deficient. Stick to the supplement plan and you will provide your body with many of the raw materials it needs for long-term health.

If you are on the advanced plan, you will need to stay on the advanced supplement plan for at least a year. After one year you should repeat the lab tests you took before you started the program, repeat the self-assessment quiz, and evaluate your progress. If

---

A Special Note for Those on the Advanced Plan

If you are on the advanced plan, you may reintroduce whole grains and fruit into your diet after the program. If you had personalization steps to complete, wait until you have completed twelve weeks on the program (the six-week basic plan and another six with personalization included). When you do add these foods back, stick to small portions (no more than one-half cup of each per day). You should also monitor your weight and blood sugar carefully as you add them. If you find yourself slipping, eliminate these foods until you have fully reset your metabolism.

---

your numbers are in the ideal range and your symptoms are better, you can scale back to the basic supplement plan.

If you added supplements as part of the personalization steps in Chapter 24, continue taking these for 3–6 months and recheck your quiz scores. You may need those supplements long-term. However, if your quiz scores are no longer in the self-care or medical care category, you can stop taking them. If you are still having trouble, seek out the help of a functional medicine practitioner.

WHAT TO DO ABOUT RELAXATION

If you need to ask what to do about the relaxation techniques in this program, you probably haven't been using them! Daily relaxation is critical for long-term health. Keep stress and its damaging effects at bay by continuing with the relaxation strategies you have incorporated into your life and adding new ones over time.

WHAT TO DO ABOUT EXERCISE

Exercise is another part of the program you will want to continue for life. In fact, over time you will probably want (and need) to amplify your exercise program. If you haven't been moving your body, just 30 minutes of daily walking will make a big difference. However, as you start to lose weight and get in shape, you will need more exercise to maintain the gains you have made and improve your health.

Work on integrating interval and strength training into your exercise program (see Chapter 21). And definitely don't forget to play—explore new and exciting ways to move your body. You may be one of those people who hates to exercise, but I feel certain you can find activities that are not only nourishing but fun!

Living clean and green is one of the best ways to

protect your health, the health of our planet, and our children's future. Follow the advice in Chapter 23, and integrate as many as you can over time.

WHAT TO DO ABOUT PERSONALIZATION

After you have worked through the steps in Chapter 24 for an additional six to twelve weeks, retake the self-assessment for any of the steps in which you originally had an imbalance. Many of you may find that you no longer have imbalances and consequently don't need to continue the suggestions in the self-care plan or medical care customizations. If that's the case, you can choose to stop the personalization.

If you do still qualify for self-care or medical care, you should continue the steps you have been taking. You may also choose to seek the help of a functional or integrative medical practitioner to assist you in integrating additional treatments into your plan. See more information on additional tests and treatment plans in the online guide *How to Get What You Need from Your Doctor* (www.bloodsugarsolution.com).

WHAT TO DO ABOUT TESTING

Finding and working with a doctor is important during the program. You should monitor your lab tests every 2–3 months, repeating your abnormal lab tests. Eventually you can scale back this testing regimen to once every 6 months or once a year. With time, you will learn how your body works and how to work with it rather than against it, and you will need less and less medical supervision and care.

WHAT TO DO IF THE PROGRAM ISN'T WORKING

Let me state the obvious. Getting and staying healthy in our modern world is a heroic feat. It is a subversive and revolutionary act. We have to navigate dangerous food landscapes, resist carefully designed temptations at every turn, fight marketing that goes right after our primitive hard-wired survival impulses, and fend off food pushers, saboteurs, and a thousand distractions online, on television, and in the other media.

You need to cultivate your survival skills and a plan of attack against these obstacles to success. If you can identify and preempt these land mines, you will become less discouraged and have more dramatic results.

There are five reasons why the program might not work:

1. Problems with Diet

Often, people think they are eating a low-sugar, low-refined-flour, low-carbohydrate diet when in fact they aren't. Things can sneak in, such as a little too much sugary fruit or a high-carbohydrate breakfast such as oatmeal. These foods may be thought of as healthy, but they can cause problems for many. Go on the advanced plan and see what happens. No grains, no fruit, no starchy veggies for six weeks.

Carefully monitoring and analyzing your diet is critical. Reading labels is essential. Even better — eat only fresh food without labels.

2. Inadequate or Inefficient Exercise

If you have never exercised, small amounts of exercise create large benefits at the initial stage of conditioning. However, as you progress and get healthier, you need a higher intensity of exercise to achieve the same benefit. For example, someone who is 300 pounds and has never taken a walk in his life can walk a block and get an extreme workout, whereas a marathon runner would need to run 10 miles at a 5-minute pace to get an equivalent workout.

As you get into shape, increase your exercise intensity and duration, and add interval training to continue your improvements in weight, blood sugar, and insulin. Chapter 22 guides you on how to do interval training. If you haven't started strength training, start now — 20 minutes, 2–3 times a week.

3. **Hidden Food Sensitivities and Gluten Intolerance or Celiac Disease**

Eliminating gluten and dairy for six weeks is a key strategy in the foundation of *The Blood Sugar Solution*. However, sometimes people have other food allergies or sensitivities, and a more comprehensive elimination diet is needed. In my book *The Ultra-Simple Diet*, an elimination program is outlined to identify the degree to which food sensitivities or allergies may be driving inflammation.

4. **Toxic Overload**

For many people, an accumulation of toxins from substances such as petrochemicals and heavy metals cause problems. This could be due to overexposure, genetic predispositions that make it difficult to detoxify these chemicals, or both. If this is the case for you, you may need heavy metal detoxification protocols and saunas. It is then critical to boost detoxification through various supplements, including n-acetylcysteine, milk thistle, and vitamin C. This is part of the personalization steps in Chapter 24.

Note that heavy metal detoxification is a medical procedure that requires the guidance of an experienced medical professional.

5. Imbalances in the Seven Steps

The personalization steps outlined in Week 6 are essential for many people to fully heal. Because we don't hear much about the need to focus on our specific biochemical and metabolic imbalances from our doctors or the media, many believe that this part of the program can safely be skipped. This is not the case.

The basic diet and lifestyle program outlined in *The Blood Sugar Solution* is enough to help 80 percent of the people suffering with diabesity. However, some need further intervention.

Make sure you carefully work through the quizzes and self-care steps in this book. If you do, and you still don't see the results you hope for, it's likely to be time to seek out the help of a practitioner trained in functional or integrative medicine. You may have deeper imbalances—such as bugs in your digestive tract, low thyroid function, or other imbalances that are driving your health problems. Treating these underlying conditions is critical for complete healing.

Now that you are on the road to health, I invite you to join a movement so we can create a healthier world together.

PART V

TAKE BACK OUR HEALTH

If you want to travel swiftly, go alone. If you want to travel far, go together.

— African proverb

27

Get Healthy Together: Creating a Social Movement

Our health has been hijacked from us, taken from us slowly, quietly, over the past century. Our current food, social, family, school, work, faith-based, and community environments, health care institutions, and government policies make it hard for us to make healthy choices. We are presented with choices that foster bad habits. But together, getting and staying healthy is possible given the right information, tools, support, and collective action to **take back our health.**

Our food choices are influenced by government subsidies for agricultural mass production of poor-quality fats and sugars. The government food pyramid reflects industry interests, not science, although the 2010 Dietary Guidelines report and the new "my plate" initiative take a step in the right direction, recommending a plant-based, whole-foods diet with less meat, sugar, and refined foods. On the other hand, the Food and Drug Administration (FDA) has not protected us from harmful pharmaceutical influence. Avandia, the number one diabetes drug in the world, has been allowed to stay on the market in the United States, even after it has been shown to cause 47,000 deaths from heart disease since it was introduced in 1999.

During the health care reform process, Dr. Dean Ornish, founder of the Preventive Medicine Research Institute; Dr. Michael Roizen, Chief Wellness Officer of the Cleveland Clinic; and I helped Senators Harkin, Wyden, and Cornyn introduce the *Take Back Your Health Act of 2009*, designed to reimburse patients with heart disease, diabetes, and pre-diabetes for intensive lifestyle treatment. Net savings in direct health care costs were estimated at $930 billion over 10 years. The bill was left on the cutting room floor of the Senate in last-minute horse trading. Afterward, in a two-hour meeting with Senator Harkin, I insisted that our only goal was to have policy reflect science. He paused for a moment and remarked, "That would make too much sense."

Health is a human right that is neglected and undervalued. It is time to take it back.

No single change will help us take back our

health. Pharmaceutical companies continually promise the next breakthrough on diabetes, obesity, and heart disease, yet we inevitably end up disappointed by new drugs' meager benefits or disillusioned by their unexpected harm. The food and diet industry promise slick new quick fixes: just eat this one thing or do this one super exercise and your problems and pounds will melt away. But there will never be one quick fix.

It is the hundreds of little choices we make every day that will transform our collective health—and have some good side effects such as preventing economic collapse, climate change, and environmental degradation; reinvigorating families, communities, and faith-based organizations; and reversing the epidemic of obesity and chronic disease weighing down our planet. By making choices as individuals, families, and communities, we can force change. Demand for healthier food, for example, has convinced the giant retailer Walmart to offer organic and lower-sugar and -fat products. It's that kind of pressure that forces change in large swaths of the economy (including food growers and producers) and reduces the toxic burden on the environment.

Through our collective action and online tools such as those at www.takebackourhealth.org, we can communicate with our elected representatives and link to resources to help us create change at the local and national levels. Here are some specific steps we can take or demand through our words, actions, and votes.

Contribute your own ideas at www.takeback ourhealth.org and help build the movement for all of us to take back our health.

Take Action! It Is Time to Take Back Our Health for Our Bodies

One in two Americans has pre-diabetes or diabetes. One in three children born today will have diabetes. Chronic lifestyle-preventable and -treatable diseases kill 50 million people a year. It is time to take action.

- **Follow the six-week plan in** *The Blood Sugar Solution.* Create health through food, supplements, exercise, stress management tools, and reduced exposure to toxins. Balance your body's systems.
- **Vote every day with your fork**. What you put on your fork has the most impact on your health, our economic prosperity, and the health of the environment.
- **Cut down on screen time.** Invest more time in self-care, learning how to cook, taking a walk, dancing in your living room, trying yoga, practic-

ing deep breathing exercises, or connecting with your loved ones or friends.

Take Action! It Is Time to Take Back Our Health for Our Families

You have total control over what you bring into your home, and what you choose to do there. Small changes can have a big impact on your family's health and happiness and on the food industry, agriculture, and marketing practices.

- **Eat at home.** In 1900, 2 percent of all meals were eaten outside the home. In 2010, 50 percent were eaten away from home. One in five eat breakfast from McDonald's. Family meals happen about three times a week, last less than 20 minutes, and are spent watching television or texting while each family member eats a different microwaved "food" made in a different factory. We complain of not having enough time to cook, but Americans spend more time watching cooking shows on The Food Network than actually preparing their own meals.
- **Eat together.** No matter how modest the meal, create a special place to sit down together, and set the table with care and respect. Family meals are

a time for empathy and generosity, a time to nourish and communicate. Research shows that children who have regular meals with their parents do better in every way, from better grades to healthier relationships to staying out of trouble, and are 42 percent less likely to drink, 50 percent less likely to smoke, and 66 percent less likely to smoke pot. Regular family dinners protect girls from bulimia, anorexia, and diet pills. Family dinners reduce the incidence of childhood obesity. In a study on household routines and obesity in American preschool-aged children, kids as young as four had a lower risk of obesity if they ate regular family dinners, had enough sleep, and didn't watch television on weekdays. Taking back our family dinners will help us learn how to find and prepare real food quickly and simply, teach our children how to connect, and build security, safety, and social skills, meal after meal, day after day.

- **Reclaim your kitchen.** Throw out foods with high-fructose corn syrup, hydrogenated fats, and sugars or fat as the first or second ingredient on the label. Fill your kitchen with real, fresh, whole, local foods whenever possible. Join a community-supported agricultural network to get a cheaper supply of fresh vegetables, or shop at nearby farmers' markets.

- **Plant a garden.** It's the tastiest, most nutritious, most environmentally friendly food you will ever eat. You can create a small garden in a box on your roof or porch if you have limited space.
- **Conserve, compost, and recycle.** Bring your own shopping bags to the market and recycle your paper, cans, bottles, and plastic. Start a compost bucket (and find out where in your community you can share this rich fertilizer).

Take Action! It Is Time to Take Back Our Health in Our Communities

We live in communities without sidewalks, or where it is not safe to walk down the street, or where we must walk five miles to find a vegetable. Many live in communities where the only "grocery store" is the convenience store at a gas station. We must navigate miles of aisles in grocery stores filled with different variations of sugar, fat, salt, and coloring disguised as food, all of which are scientifically proven to cause disease and premature death. There are ten McDonald's restaurants within ten miles of my house, and I live in a remote country location.

- **Get healthy together.** Small groups are the catalyst that will make everything easier. Create your own group of friends, coworkers, church, mosque, synagogue, or community members to support your journey to wellness. Learn how at www.takebackourhealth.org.

- **Create virtual groups.** Learn how to start a group on Facebook or other social networks at www.takebackourhealth.org.
- **Start a dinner or cooking club.** Take turns with other families or friends to cook healthy, tasty meals once a week.

Take Action! It Is Time to Take Back Our Health from Media and Food Industry Marketing Practices

The average kid spends seven and a half hours a day in front of a screen watching billions of dollars in advertising for foods of the poorest nutritional quality.[1] Overweight kids eat 50 percent of their meals in front of the television. Teaching our children every day about healthy nutrition cannot compete with the marketing onslaught. Thomas Frieden, MD, director of the Centers for Disease Control, recommends that we prohibit food marketing to children.

- **Restrict all media marketing of liquid calories, fast food, junk food, and processed food, especially to children.** Our senses are inundated with food industry marketing practices that mostly succeed in convincing us that their health-sapping options are easy, fun, and affordable and will make us stronger and happier. We have taken the bait. One billion cans of Coca-Cola are consumed every day around the world. In communities without health care, education, running water, or enough food, there is Coke! Food marketing directed at children should be banned (through the Federal Trade Commission). This has been done in over 50 countries across the globe, including Australia, the United Kingdom, the Netherlands, and Sweden. We should follow suit.

- **Restrict unproven health claims on labels.** Foods with health claims on the label are often the least healthy. Adding a little fiber to a sugary cereal doesn't make it healthy. Will Vitamin Water or Gatorade, made cool by Kobe Bryant and Lebron James, make our kids super athletes or just super fat? The FDA should restrict health claims.
- **Do a media fast.** Avoid all media for a week (or two) with your family, or create a media fast group at work or school.

Take Action! It Is Time to Take Back Our Health in Our Schools

Schools have become hazardous zones full of empty calories, junk food, and stripped-down physical education programs. When most school kitchens have only deep fryers, microwaves, and displays for candy and junk food at the checkout counters, how can children stay healthy? When the food served is as addictive as heroin or cocaine, who is accountable? General Jack Keane, former Vice Chief of Staff of the U.S. Army, shared with me that 70 percent of the applicants for the military are unfit to serve. The school lunch program was started in 1946 because military recruits were too thin to serve in the military; now, in part because of our school lunch program, our children are too fat to serve.

- **Help reinvent school lunch programs.** The Healthy, Hunger-Free Kids Act of 2010 removes junk food from schools by applying nutrition standards to *all* foods sold in schools (including vending machines in hallways), and supports access to fresh produce through farm-to-school networks, the creation of school gardens, and the use of local foods. It doesn't solve the void in education for self-care and nutrition, but it is a beginning. Watch the movie *Two Angry Moms* to learn how to take back the lunchroom.
- **Support schools as safe zones.** Give students access only to foods that promote health and optimal brain functioning.
- **Support changes in zoning laws.** Prevent fast-food and junk-food outlets from operating next to schools.

- **Support "eat only in lunchroom" policies for schools.** Studies have shown that when school districts prohibit eating in hallways and classrooms, children lose 10 percent of their body weight without ANY other change in diet or exercise.
- **Build school gardens.** Teach children about the origins of food and let them experience the sensory delight of real, garden-fresh fruits and vegetables.
- **Support the integration of self-care and nutrition curriculum into schools.** Work with your local or regional school boards to introduce programs like Mehmet Oz's HealthCorps into schools around the country.
- **Bring back basic cooking skills to schools.** Make these skills part of a curriculum that includes essential life tools.

Take Action! It Is Time to Take Back Our Health in Our Workplaces

Workplaces are dangerous environments. Bowls of chips, fridges full of sugar-laden caffeinated sodas, cafeterias with hardly a vegetable in sight, drawers full of candy, and high-stress environments all fuel our ill health. E-mail and BlackBerries tether us mentally and physically to work 24/7. One large company human resources director told me they were planning on blocking employees' access to e-mail when they went on vacation.

When Starbucks spends more on health care than on coffee beans and General Motors spends more on health care than on steel, something has to change. Corporations have the most to gain by investing in creating healthier environments, building wellness programs, and allowing for default choices that support health.

- **Identify and train wellness champions in the workplace.** These individuals can lead support groups for employees to get healthy together by following *The Blood Sugar Solution* online course.
- **Improve workplace food culture by improving snack areas and cafeteria offerings.** Provide more real, fresh food and less processed, sugary food. Support workplace lunch potlucks to share the burden and cost of creating healthy lunches and strengthen community within organizations.
- **Develop incentives (including financial) for employees to participate in wellness programs.** Safeway's Steve Burd implemented financial incentives for healthy lifestyle change for his employees called Healthy Measures.[2] If this type of program was implemented nationally, it would shave $550 billion a year off our health care bill.

- **Support the development of work-based self-care and group support programs.** Companies are starting to understand that solving the problem of poor health is not a cost or liability but an investment opportunity. *Presenteeism,* being *at* the job but not *on* the job, costs companies two to three times its direct medical costs, mostly from lost productivity owing to obesity and depression-related symptoms such as fatigue, brain fog, and low motivation. Globally, companies lose $2 trillion a year in productivity from lifestyle-preventable conditions. Workplace wellness efforts can yield 1,000–2,000 percent returns on investment. The World Economic Forum created a Wellness App to show companies how much they can save by creating wellness programs (http://wellness.weforum.org).

Take Action! It Is Time to Take Back Our Health in Our Places of Worship

Do you not know that your body is a temple of the Holy Spirit, who is in you, whom you have received from God? You are not your own; you were bought at a price. Therefore honor God with your body. (*1 Cor. 6:19–20*)

Pastor Rick Warren of Saddleback Church, a congregation of 30,000, made a radical assertion as we launched The Daniel Plan (see Chapter 16). God wants us to be healthy. In his sermon, he pointed out that in the world's major Western religious traditions — Judaism, Christianity, and Islam — there are teachings on ethics, compassion, and spirituality, supporting the mind and spirit. But in synagogues, churches, temples, and mosques around the world, health and the body are rarely discussed. No rabbi, priest, minister, pastor, or imam encourages care of the body as well as the soul. Church and temple functions are centers of community activity, yet they provide an abundance of poor-quality, calorie-rich, starchy, sugary foods that help their members get to heaven early.

- **Encourage care of the body as well as the soul.** Social change often begins in faith-based organizations — abolition, civil rights, and human rights. But health is the most neglected of all human rights. The community, connections, and social networks that already exist within faith-based organizations can support health of the mind, spirit, *and* body.
- **Add "body study" to Bible study groups.** Incorporate "body" and soul into small support and study groups within faith-based communities. You can study a healthy lifestyle curriculum like The Daniel Plan (www.danielplan.com).

- **Create a culture of wellness within faith-based organizations.** Encourage healthy food at gatherings and events. Create fitness activities to do together. Follow some of the examples we used at Saddleback Church (www.danielplan.com).

Take Action! It Is Time to Take Back Our Health in Our Democracy

I was invited along with other experts in prevention and wellness to the White House Forum on Prevention and Wellness in June 2009. As part of our effort to create true health care change, we advocated for an interagency council to support, coordinate, and develop health promotion and wellness movements across all government agencies. In June 2010, President Obama established the National Council on Prevention, Health Promotion, and Public Health, and Senator Tom Harkin nominated me for a presidential appointment to a 25-person group to advise the administration and the new council. This is a step in the right direction. But there is more we can do.

Send letters and e-messages to your elected representatives to support health initiatives such as:

- **Eliminating unhealthy foods from all schools, child care, and health care facilities, and all government institutions.** The government must establish rigorous standards for school nutrition consistent with current science (through the USDA). Similarly, we need to create nutrition programs for other public and government-run institutions such as the military, Veterans Affairs, the Indian Health Service, and community health centers.

- **Supporting lobby reform.** We must change campaign finance laws so that corporate political donations from entities such as Big Food, Big Farming, and Big Pharma can no longer control the political process.

- **Subsidizing the production of fruits and vegetables.** Change the Farm Bill. Agricultural policies should support public health and encourage the production of fruits and vegetables, not commodity products such as corn and soy. Eighty percent of government subsidies presently go to soy and corn, which are used to create much of the junk food we consume. We need to rethink subsidies and provide more for smaller farmers and a broader array of fruits and vegetables.

- **Incentivizing supermarkets to open in poor communities.** Poverty and obesity go hand in hand. One reason for this is the food deserts we see around the nation. Poor people have a right to high-quality food, too. We need to create ways to provide it to them.

- **Building the real cost of industrial food into the price.** Include its impact on health care costs and lost productivity.
- **Taxing sugar.** We tax cigarettes and alcohol, and this helps pay for prevention and treatment programs. Sugar is at least as addictive, if not more so. Scientists suggest a penny-an-ounce tax on sugar-sweetened beverages. This would reduce sugar consumption, obesity, and health care costs, and provide revenue to support programs for the prevention and treatment of obesity and chronic disease.
- **Creating a public health advertising campaign.** Let's make being healthy cool and sexy and expose the subversive practices of Big Food, Big Farming, and Big Pharma. Use the advertising techniques that best speak to the emotional needs of the consumer and our children.
- **Supporting the creation of a health corps.** Our goal should be to train 1 million health workers and champions in communities around the country by 2020. Through the act of getting healthy together, we can create a double revolution — change the medicine we do (lifestyle and functional medicine) and change how we do medicine (in small support groups). This new workforce of community health workers would "accompany" and support individuals in making better food

and lifestyle choices and cleaning up their homes, workplaces, schools, faith-based organizations, and environment.

Take Action! It Is Time to Take Back Our Health from the "Sick Care" System

Marcia Angell, former editor in chief of the *New England Journal of Medicine,* wrote a scathing critique of the infiltration of Big Pharma into medical research, education, and health and drug policy.[3] Aside from the $30 billion a year spent on marketing pharmaceuticals to physicians (known as "continuing medical education"), Big Pharma has turned many academic researchers into hired hands. Though leaders from academic medical centers are provided grants to do research "contracted for" by Pharma, the research is often designed, executed, and ghostwritten by the funders. The conflict-of-interest statements of authors on research articles now often run several pages long. These authors not only receive grants but also sit on corporate advisory boards, receive large speaking fees, and enter into patent and royalty agreements with Pharma.

It would appear that our evidence-based medicine isn't based on very good evidence. We have the power to change that.

- **Fix perverse financial incentives in health care reimbursement.** In New York City, a very successful diabetes prevention and treatment program was implemented. It resulted in fewer complications, hospitalizations, and amputations. But the program was stopped by the hospital because its revenue dropped. Cutting off a diabetic toe and receiving $6,000 from Medicare is better than being reimbursed $100 for a nutrition consult. The system profits from having more sick and fat patients.

- **Support real health care reform.** We need to change not only insurance regulation, but also the type of medicine we do (lifestyle and functional medicine) and how we deliver health care (in small groups, in communities, and in health care organizations). During the health reform process in Washington, DC, Dean Ornish, Michael Roizen, and I were asked what organization we represented. We replied simply that we didn't represent anyone but the patients or anything but the science. They accepted it, but looked perplexed. No wonder. During health care reform, the pharmaceutical industry had three lobbyists for every member of Congress and spent over $600,000 a day to make sure their needs were represented in the legislation.

- **Mandate nutrition and lifestyle medicine training in medical schools and residency programs.** As we know, all of the major drivers of disease and health care costs are lifestyle-preventable factors. If these factors were addressed, we could eliminate 90 percent of the heart disease and diabetes. Yet only one in four medical schools has a nutrition course, and only 28 percent of schools meet the minimum 25 hours of nutrition education recommended by the National Academy of Sciences.[4] Most of those nutrition hours address diseases of nutritional deficiency such as scurvy and rickets. If we were successful in reducing heart disease by half or reducing diabetes (along with its complications) by 80 percent, hospitals would go bankrupt, Pharma would see their profits plummet, and many physicians would be forced to start "institutes of lifestyle medicine," not more heart surgery hospitals.

- **Support and develop a modular scalable nutrition curriculum.** If food is our most powerful medicine, then educating health care professionals about nutrition is essential. We must develop and provide funding to support a nutrition curriculum built for people in the health care industry. This will address the lack of supply of adequate experts. (We could scale existing programs such as those provided by the Institute for Functional Medicine.)

- **Provide reimbursement for lifestyle treatment of chronic disease.** Despite the support of nearly all the major medical societies who joined in publishing a review of the scientific evidence for lifestyle medicine, for the prevention and *treatment* of chronic disease,[5] this approach is still not part of medical training or practice. We need to have lifestyle treatments like the one outlined in this book paid for if they are going to become a part of mainstream medical practice.

- **Develop more funding for nutritional science.** Congress should mandate greater funding for nutritional science, and examine and test innovative treatment models. Responsibility for dietary policy should be placed with an independent scientific group such as the Institute of Medicine instead of with the politically and corporately influenced U.S. Department of Agriculture. In the 1980s, they advised a low-fat diet food pyramid with at least 8–11 servings a day of bread, rice, pasta, and cereal, which coincided with the rapid increase in obesity and diabetes. It was lethal to mix politics and health recommendations.

- **End irresponsible relationships between medicine and industry.** Public health organizations such as the American Heart Association and the American Dietetic Association should avoid partnerships, endorsements, or financial ties with industry that compromises their independence and credibility. Coca-Cola sponsoring events at the American Dietetic Association, or the American Heart Association promoting sugary cereals as heart healthy because they have a few grains of whole wheat—is this credible?

Take Back Our Health: Be Part of the Movement, Be Part of the Conversation

Any one act by any one individual or organization will not be enough to create change. I am reminded of what Mother Teresa once said: *"There are no great acts; only small acts done with great love."*

One step, one choice, one change at a time. One word, one action, one vote at a time.

Go to www.takebackourhealth.org to take the first step, join the movement, and learn how we can and must get healthy together.

Reversing the Diabesity Epidemic

One in three children born in America today will become diabetic if current trends continue. One in two Americans will have diabesity by 2020, and 90 percent won't know it. This is the world's biggest health epidemic, but it is nearly 100 percent preventable.

We don't need more research. The 10-year follow-up of the Diabetes Lifestyle Prevention Trial and the current Look Ahead Trial using intensive group lifestyle treatment prove that lifestyle intervention in groups is much more effective than medication in preventing diabetes. It is also the most powerful treatment if you already have diabetes or pre-diabetes.

The science is clear. We have enough information to solve this problem now, but no one is calling for action or mobilizing a global campaign to address it. We fight AIDS, malaria, and tuberculosis all across the globe. But when confronted with a problem that causes more deaths than all those infectious diseases combined, we are silent.

My hope is that each of you will transform your biology from diabesity to vibrant optimal health. Then you will understand the power you have to change your genes and your health by changing what and how you eat, supporting your biochemistry and metabolism with supplements, moving your body, learning to deeply relax, and living clean and green.

You have the power to avert health problems by learning how to support your body so it can function optimally.

You also have the power to become part of a movement to "Take Back Our Health"—a clear solution using the power of food and lifestyle to prevent, reverse, and even cure most chronic illness, the cause of endless personal suffering and an unsustainable burden to our global economies and social fabric. We don't need new discoveries. We just have to apply what we already know, so that our children and their children can live in a world free from diabesity, healthy and fully engaged with life.

The Blood Sugar Solution is a personal plan for you to get healthy, for us to get healthy together in our communities, and for us to take back our health as a society.

And it starts with each one of us.

PART VI

THE BLOOD SUGAR SOLUTION MEAL PLAN AND RECIPES

Let food be thy medicine, and medicine be thy food.

— Hippocrates

28

Your Six-Week Meal Plan

While the guidelines you've been given throughout this book are enough for you to get and stay on *The Blood Sugar Solution* program successfully, many people like to have a bit more guidance regarding what to eat.

With the assistance of Deb Morgan, culinary inspiration and leader extraordinaire behind the Kripalu Kitchen, I've developed two weeks' worth of daily menus you can rotate over the course of the program. In reality, you can use any of the recipes for any day of the program. However, I've structured daily menus to keep the program nice and simple.

To make it even simpler, follow the menus as outlined for the first 14 days. After two weeks of using these recipes, you will have a good sense of what your body craves and how to nourish it properly. At that stage, you can mix and match recipes and daily menus for the remaining four weeks.

For each week's recipes, I have created a comprehensive shopping list that will make it easy to shop for all the food you need to make these delicious and nourishing meals (see pages 560–563).

Depending on your food preferences and cultural traditions, substitutions are possible. For example, vegan and vegetarian options can be substituted for those with animal proteins; simply replace the animal protein in the recipes with tofu, tempeh, or other forms of vegan protein. You will get the same benefits as long as you stick to high-fiber, nutrient-dense foods.

All the recipes are permitted on the basic program, and most are appropriate or can be adapted for the advanced program as noted. I have also provided tips for amazing do-it-yourself salads (see pages 557–559). There are also many more recipes online, including kid-friendly recipes, at www.bloodsugar solution.com.

Following this plan should make healing from diabetes more fun and delicious. Enjoy!

WEEK 1 MENU

Day 1

Breakfast: Selections can vary; refer to
             Breakfast Recipes.
Snack: Selections can vary; refer to
             Snack Recipes.

Lunch: Salmon Salad in Steamed Collard
          Wraps (see pages 504–506).
Dinner: Lentil and Chicken Stew over
          Roasted Quinoa with Kale and
          Almonds (see pages 525–527).

Day 2

Breakfast: Selections can vary; refer to
           Breakfast Recipes.
Snack: Selections can vary; refer to
           Snack Recipes.
Lunch: White Bean Salad with Walnut Pesto
           Chicken (see pages 506–507).
Dinner: Fish and Vegetables in Parchment
           with Pecan Wild Rice and Goji Berry
           Pilaf (see pages 527–529).

Day 3

Breakfast: Selections can vary; refer to
           Breakfast Recipes.
Snack: Selections can vary; refer to
           Snack Recipes.
Lunch: Quinoa Avocado Salad with
           Black Beans over Arugula (see
           pages 508–509).
Dinner: Turkey and Spinach Meat Loaf with
           Millet Cauliflower Mash (see pages
           530–531) and Braised Greens with

Red Onion and Sun-Dried Tomatoes
(see page 532).

Day 4

Breakfast: Selections can vary; refer to
Breakfast Recipes.

Snack: Selections can vary; refer to
Snack Recipes.

Lunch: Split Pea and Rosemary Soup and
Spicy Roasted Squash (see pages
509–511).

Dinner: Asian Tofu Snap Pea Stir-Fry with
Sesame Peanut Sauce over Brown
Rice (see pages 532–534).

Day 5

Breakfast: Selections can vary; refer to
Breakfast Recipes.

Snack: Selections can vary; refer to
Snack Recipes.

Lunch: Chicken Vegetable Soup with Rice
(see pages 511–512).

Dinner: Mediterranean Shrimp over Grilled
Polenta (see pages 534–536).

Day 6

Breakfast: Selections can vary; refer to
Breakfast Recipes.

Snack: Selections can vary; refer to Snack Recipes.

Lunch: Quinoa-Crusted Quiche (see pages 513–514).

Dinner: Black Bean Soup, Toasted Cumin Rice, and Garlic Kale and Cauliflower (see pages 536–538).

Day 7

Breakfast: Selections can vary; refer to Breakfast Recipes.

Snack: Selections can vary; refer to Snack Recipes.

Lunch: Tofu Fried Rice (see pages 514–515).

Dinner: Salmon Pecan Cakes with Peach Chutney and Sautéed Swiss Chard with Slivered Almonds (see pages 538–541).

WEEK 2 MENU

Day 1

Breakfast: Selections can vary; refer to Breakfast Recipes.

Snack: Selections can vary; refer to Snack Recipes.

Lunch: Shrimp and Avocado Salad over Arugula (see pages 515–516).

Dinner: Coconut Curry Chicken and Vegetables over Brown Rice (see pages 541–542 and 534).

Day 2

Breakfast: Selections can vary; refer to Breakfast Recipes.

Snack: Selections can vary; refer to Snack Recipes.

Lunch: Hearty Garden Vegetable Soup with Pinto Beans (see pages 516–517).

Dinner: Coriander and Almond-Crusted Scallops, Whipped Yams, and Sautéed Spinach and Watercress (see pages 542–544).

Day 3

Breakfast: Selections can vary; refer to Breakfast Recipes.

Snack: Selections can vary; refer to Snack Recipes.

Lunch: Rice and Chickpea Salad with Balsamic Vinaigrette (see pages 518–519).

Dinner: Braised Lamb and Pomegranate Molasses over White Beans with Lemon Broccoli (see pages 545–546).

Day 4

Breakfast:	Selections can vary; refer to Breakfast Recipes.
Snack:	Selections can vary; refer to Snack Recipes.
Lunch:	Curry Egg Salad in Lettuce Wraps with Roasted Asparagus (see pages 519–520).
Dinner:	Quick Mexicana Chili with Quinoa, Baked Corn Tortilla Strips, and Lacinato Kale with Roasted Squash (see pages 547–549).

Day 5

Breakfast:	Selections can vary; refer to Breakfast Recipes.
Snack:	Selections can vary; refer to Snack Recipes.
Lunch:	Red Lentil Stew (see pages 520–521).
Dinner:	Grilled Salmon with Cilantro Mint Chutney, White Bean and Corn Salad, Grilled Summer Vegetables (see pages 550–553).

Day 6

Breakfast:	Selections can vary; refer to Breakfast Recipes.

Snack: Selections can vary; refer to
            Snack Recipes.

Lunch: Sun-Dried Tomato Turkey Burgers
            (see page 522).

Dinner: Tofu and Cashew Stir-Fry over Bas-
            mati Rice (see pages 553–554).

Day 7

Breakfast: Selections can vary; refer to
            Breakfast Recipes.

Snack: Selections can vary; refer to
            Snack Recipes.

Lunch: Chicken and Black Bean Wraps in
            Steamed Collard Greens with Avo-
            cado and Salsa (see pages 523–524).

Dinner: Sunday Night Bouillabaisse (see
            pages 554–556).

29

Recipes and Shopping Lists

BREAKFAST RECIPES

THE ULTRASHAKE

This shake provides essential protein for detoxification, omega-3 fatty acids from flax oil, fiber for healthy digestion and elimination, and antioxidants and phytonutrients from berries and fruit. It will sustain you, balance your blood sugar, and help you control your appetite throughout the day.

You will find three shake variations here; you may alter any recipe to your taste preference.

See www.bloodsugarsolution.com for instructions on where to order my favorite protein powders.

NOTE: Use flaxseeds in up to two shakes a day, no more. If you are on the advanced plan, omit the fruit from these recipes.

RICE PROTEIN SHAKE

Serves 1   Prep time: 5 minutes   Cook time: none

This satisfying shake is the easiest to make and digest.

- 2 scoops rice protein powder (or follow directions for the serving size of the product you pick)
- 1 tablespoon organic combination flax and borage oil
- 2 tablespoons ground flaxseeds
- ice (made from filtered water), if desired
- 6–8 ounces filtered water
- ½ cup fresh or frozen noncitrus organic fruit (such as cherries, blueberries, raspberries, strawberries, peaches, pears, or bananas)
- Optional: ¼ cup nuts, soaked overnight (such as almonds, walnuts, pecans, or any combination)

Place all ingredients in a blender and thoroughly combine.

FRUIT AND NUT SHAKE

Serves 1   Prep time: 5 minutes   Cook time: none

This recipe uses silken tofu instead of rice protein. This is a nice creamy shake.

- ¼ cup drained silken tofu
- ½ cup plain, unsweetened gluten-free soy milk (such as Silk)

- 1 tablespoon organic combination flax and borage oil
- 2 tablespoons ground flaxseeds
- ½ cup fresh or frozen noncitrus organic fruit (such as cherries, blueberries, raspberries, strawberries, peaches, pears, or bananas)
- ice (made from filtered water), if desired
- 2–4 ounces filtered water
- Optional: ¼ cup nuts soaked overnight (such as almonds, walnuts, pecans, or any combination)

Place all ingredients in a blender and thoroughly combine.

NUT SHAKE

Serves 1   Prep time: 5 minutes   Cook time: none

This shake is designed to be soy-free.

- ½ cup plain, unsweetened gluten-free almond or hazelnut milk
- ¼ cup nuts soaked overnight (such as almonds, walnuts, pecans, or any combination)
- 1 tablespoon organic combination flax and borage oil
- 2 tablespoons ground flaxseeds
- ½ cup fresh or frozen noncitrus organic fruit (such as cherries, blueberries, raspberries, strawberries, peaches, pears, or bananas)

- ice (made from filtered water), if desired
- 2–4 ounces filtered water

Place all ingredients in a blender and thoroughly combine.

POACHED EGGS OVER SPINACH

Serves 4   Prep time: 2 minutes   Cook time: 3–4 minutes
Program: basic and advanced plans

- ½ cup water
- 1 cup tomato, diced
- 6 cups chopped or baby spinach (stems removed)
- 4 organic large eggs
- pinch of sea salt and/or pepper
- ½ tablespoon fresh thyme
- Splash of extra virgin olive oil

Into a sauté pan over medium high heat, place the water, tomato, and spinach. Try to make small indentions in the spinach and then gently crack the eggs on top. Sprinkle with salt, pepper, and fresh thyme. Cover; allow to cook until eggs are done to your liking. The spinach should be wilted and the water evaporated. Serve topped with olive oil.

Nutritional Analysis per Serving: calories 81,
carbohydrates 4.7 g, fiber 1.6 g, protein 7.2 g,
fat 4.7 g, cholesterol 186 mg, sodium 99 mg,
calcium 87 mg.

SCRAMBLED TOFU

Serves 4   Prep time: 5 minutes   Cook time: 10 minutes
Program: basic and advanced plans

- 1 pound firm tofu
- 2 tablespoons extra virgin olive oil
- ½ small onion, chopped
- 1 teaspoon curry powder
- 2 cups Swiss chard, finely chopped
- ½ carrot, grated
- ½ teaspoon dried oregano
- ½ teaspoon dried basil
- ½ tablespoon wheat-free tamari

Rinse the tofu, pat dry, then crumble and set aside. In a large sauté pan over medium heat, heat the olive oil and sauté the onions until they start to brown, about 5 minutes. Add the curry powder and stir. Add the tofu to the onions and stir to combine well. Add the remaining ingredients and stir until heated through, allowing the chard to wilt.

Nutritional Analysis per Serving: calories 155, carbohydrates 5.1 g, fiber 2.0 g, protein 10.2 g, fat 11.6 g, cholesterol 0 mg, sodium 184 mg, calcium 260 mg.

SESAME GINGER TOFU

Serves 4   Prep time: 5 minutes   Cook time: 15 minutes
Program: basic and advanced plans

- 1 pound tofu
- 1 tablespoon sesame oil
- 1 teaspoon ginger, minced
- 1 teaspoon garlic, minced
- ¾ tablespoon wheat-free tamari
- 1 tablespoon mirin or cooking wine
- ½ tablespoon brown rice vinegar
- 2 tablespoons sesame seeds

Rinse the tofu, pat dry, and cut into small cubes. Heat a sauté pan over medium heat and add the sesame oil. Carefully place the tofu in the pan and sauté for about 5 minutes, turning the tofu occasionally to brown on all sides. Combine the remaining ingredients, pour over the tofu, and stir. Bring to a boil and reduce heat. Simmer about 6–8 minutes until the liquid has reduced so that the tofu is lightly glazed.

Nutritional Analysis per Serving: calories 147, carbohydrates 5.5 g, fiber 1.7 g, protein 10.5 g, fat 10.4 g, cholesterol 0 mg, sodium 236 mg, calcium 297 mg.

Avocado and Herb Omelet

Serves 2   Prep time: 5 minutes   Cook time: 7 minutes
Program: basic and advanced plans

- 3 eggs
- 1 tablespoon water or unsweetened soy milk
- pinch of sea salt
- 1 tablespoon extra virgin olive oil
- ½ teaspoon fresh thyme
- 1 tablespoon fresh basil, chopped
- ½ ripe avocado, sliced
- black pepper, to taste

Crack the eggs into a bowl and whisk with either the water or soy milk. Add the sea salt. Heat a small sauté or omelet pan over medium heat, then add the oil to the pan. Once the oil is hot (be careful not to allow it to smoke), pour in the eggs. Using a flexible spatula, lift the edge of the egg from the side of the pan and allow the wet egg to roll to the bottom of the pan. When the eggs are firm, lay fresh herbs and sliced avocado on one half of the omelet. Turn off heat and fold the egg over to serve. Top with black pepper to taste.

Nutritional Analysis per Serving: calories 236, carbohydrates 5.0 g, fiber 3.5 g, protein 9.4 g, fat 20.7 g, cholesterol 279 mg, sodium 213 mg, calcium 52 mg.

SNACK RECIPES

HONEY ALMOND BUTTER SPREAD

Makes four 1-tablespoon servings   Prep time: 3 minutes
Cook time: none   Program: basic plan

- ¼ cup raw almond butter
- 1 tablespoon raw honey
- pinch of cardamom

Combine all ingredients. Use as a dip with apples, pears, or raw vegetables.

NOTE: If you are on the advanced plan, use this dip only with veggies.

Nutritional Analysis per Serving: calories 115, carbohydrates 7.7 g, fiber 0.6 g, protein 2.4 g, fat 9.2 g, cholesterol 0 mg, sodium 2 mg, calcium 45 mg.

MINTY HUMMUS

Makes eight 2-tablespoon servings   Prep time:
10 minutes   Cook time: none   Program: basic
and advanced plans

- ½ cup almonds
- 1 (15-ounce) can chickpeas, drained and rinsed
- 1 tablespoon sesame seeds, toasted
- 2 garlic cloves
- 2 tablespoons fresh mint leaves
- ¼ cup fresh lemon juice

- 1 teaspoon cumin
- pinches of sea salt and pepper
- ½ cup water

Blend the almonds, chickpeas, sesame seeds, and garlic in a food processor until well mashed. Add remaining ingredients, blend until smooth. Serve with raw vegetables or apple slices.

Nutritional Analysis per Serving: calories 239, carbohydrates 34.9 g, fiber 10.3 g, protein 11.9 g, fat 6.8 g, cholesterol 0 mg, sodium 14 mg, calcium 95 mg.

DEVILED EGGS

Serves 6   Prep time: 5 minutes   Cook time: 15 minutes
Program: basic and advanced plans

- 6 eggs
- 1 tablespoon extra virgin olive oil
- 1 tablespoon dill pickle, minced
- ½ teaspoon paprika
- pinch of sea salt

Place the eggs in a pot of cold water and bring to a rolling boil, then turn the heat to medium. Hard-boil the eggs for 12–15 minutes, depending on their size; an extra-large egg will take up to 17 minutes. Turn off the heat, allowing the eggs to sit in hot water for 2 minutes, then gently remove them from the water and set aside to cool. When the eggs are cool, peel and cut in half lengthwise. Gently scoop out the center yolk.

In a small bowl, mash the cooked egg yolks with a fork, and mix in the olive oil, pickle, paprika, and salt. Scoop the yolk mixture back into the egg white halves and sprinkle with a little more paprika. Store covered in the refrigerator. The eggs will remain fresh for at least 5 days. Enjoy as a snack or an addition to a salad.

Nutritional Analysis per Serving: calories 84, carbohydrates 0.5 g, fiber 0 g, protein 5.6 g, fat 6.6 g, cholesterol 186 mg, sodium 120 mg, calcium 22 mg.

POACHED PEARS AND CASHEW CREAM

Serves 4   Prep time: 10 minutes plus cashew soaking time
Cook time: 15 minutes   Program: basic plan only

FOR THE CASHEW CREAM

- 1 cup raw cashews
- 1 tablespoon raw honey
- 2 drops vanilla extract

Cover the cashews with water and soak overnight. Drain the cashews, reserving the water. Place the cashews, honey, and vanilla in a blender and blend, adding small amounts of the soaking water until the mixture is smooth. Set aside.

FOR THE PEARS

- 2 pears
- 1 cinnamon stick
- ¼ cup fresh mint, plus more for garnish

Peel the pears, cut in half lengthwise, and remove the seeds. Place the pear halves in a saucepan cut side down and add enough water to cover. Add the cinnamon stick and mint. Bring to a boil. Reduce heat and simmer 6–8 minutes until the pears are tender but not mushy. Allow the pears to sit in cooking water with the heat off for 4–5 minutes, then remove them from the cooking liquid and allow to cool completely or serve slightly warmed. Serve topped with cashew cream.

Nutritional Analysis per Serving: calories 276, carbohydrates 32.2 g, fiber 4.7 g, protein 5.9 g, fat 16.0 g, cholesterol 0 mg, sodium 8 mg, calcium 43 mg.

ROASTED NUTS AND SEEDS

*Serves 4   Prep time: 1 minute to prep, 5 minutes to cool
Cook time: 10 minutes   Program: basic
and advanced plans*

- ½ cup walnuts
- ½ cup almonds
- ¼ cup pepitas (pumpkin seeds)
- ¼ cup sunflower seeds
- 2 tablespoons sesame seeds

503

TO ROAST THE NUTS

Heat oven to 350°F. Place the nuts on a dry baking sheet. Bake for approximately 8–9 minutes, checking often. The nuts are done when they start to change color and impart a nutty fragrance. Remove from the hot baking pan and cool. Store in a sealed container in a cool, dry place, and the nuts will remain fresh for up to 2 weeks.

TO ROAST THE SEEDS

Heat a dry skillet to medium and add the seeds. Stir continuously until the seeds start to brown. Pumpkin seeds will even pop a little. Remove from heat immediately and cool before storing.

Combine and store in a sealed container in a cool, dry place, and the seeds will remain fresh for several weeks.

Nutritional Analysis per Serving: calories 254, carbohydrates 7.3 g, fiber 3.6 g, protein 9.8 g, fat 22.8 g, cholesterol 0 mg, sodium 3 mg, calcium 118 mg.

LUNCH RECIPES

SALMON SALAD IN STEAMED COLLARD WRAPS

Serves 4   Prep time: 15 minutes   Cook time: 45 minutes
Program: basic and advanced plans

- 1 cup wild rice, rinsed
- 3 cups water

- 4 medium collard leaves
- 1 (7.5-ounce) can unsalted salmon
- 2 tablespoons red onion, minced
- 1 tablespoon extra virgin olive oil
- 1 garlic clove, minced
- 1 tablespoon capers
- 6 cherry tomatoes, sliced

TO COOK THE WILD RICE

Place the wild rice in a small pan. Add 1 cup water and bring to a boil. Reduce to medium-low, cover, and simmer for 45 minutes. Drain excess water from the rice through a small strainer.

TO PREPARE THE COLLARD GREENS

Bring 2 cups of water to a boil in a large sauté pan. Place the collard greens in the water, cover, and turn off heat. Allow to sit 1 minute, then rinse the collard greens under cold water.

Drain the juice from the canned salmon. Place the salmon (skin and small bones included) in a medium bowl and use a fork to flake the salmon. Add the onion, oil, garlic, cooked rice, and capers.

Lay out each steamed collard leaf on a plate and divide the salmon and sliced tomatoes among the four plates. Feel free to add a little of your favorite premade sugar-free salad dressing or an extra splash of olive oil. Roll the collard greens as you would a tortilla and enjoy.

NOTE: Omit the rice from this recipe if you are on the advanced plan.

Nutritional Analysis per Serving: calories 324, carbohydrates 39.0 g, fiber 5.5 g, protein 19.9 g, fat 10.9 g, cholesterol 33 mg, sodium 112 mg, calcium 66 mg.

WHITE BEAN SALAD

Serves 4   Prep time: 10 minutes   Cook time: 5 minutes
Program: basic and advanced plans

- 1 tablespoon extra virgin olive oil
- ½ small red onion, diced
- 2 cloves garlic
- 2 tablespoons sun-dried tomatoes (in summer, use fresh grape tomatoes)
- 1 (15-ounce) can cannellini beans, drained
- 2 cups sliced fresh greens of your choice (good choices are kale or chard, or a combination of greens)
- pinch of sea salt
- pepper to taste

In a sauté pan, heat the olive oil on medium heat and then add the onions, garlic, and sun-dried tomatoes. Sauté until the onions begin to brown. Remove from heat and cool. Place the drained beans in a medium bowl. Add the onion mixture, fresh greens, salt, and pepper. Garnish with Walnut Pesto Chicken (see below) and enjoy.

Nutritional Analysis per Serving: calories 411, carbohydrates 69.4 g, fiber 27.5 g, protein 26.6 g, fat 4.6 g, cholesterol 0 mg, sodium 115 mg, calcium 220 mg.

WALNUT PESTO CHICKEN

Serves 4 when added to the White Bean Salad   Prep time: 10 minutes   Cook time: 5 minutes   Program: basic and advanced plans

- ¼ pound skinless boneless chicken
- pinch of sea salt
- 1 tablespoon grape seed or extra virgin olive oil
- 2 tablespoons extra virgin olive oil
- ¼ cup raw walnuts
- 2 cups fresh basil leaves
- 2 garlic cloves
- pinch of sea salt

Slice the chicken into thin strips. Toss with salt. Heat 1 tablespoon of grape seed or olive oil in a sauté pan or griddle over medium-high heat. Cook the chicken on each side until cooked through. Set aside on a paper towel to cool.

Grind the walnuts in a food processor until fine. Rinse the basil and pat dry. Add the basil, garlic, and salt to the processor. With the processor running, drizzle in 2 tablespoons of olive oil until desired consistency is reached. Toss with the chicken strips. Unused pesto can be kept in the fridge for up toa week.

Nutritional Analysis per Serving: calories 161, carbohydrates 1.6 g, fiber 0.8 g, protein 9.2 g, fat 13.5 g, cholesterol 18 mg, sodium 112 mg, calcium 30 mg.

QUINOA AVOCADO SALAD WITH BLACK BEANS OVER ARUGULA

Serves 4   Prep time: 5 minutes   Cook time: 25 minutes
Program: basic and advanced plans

- 1 cup quinoa
- 1¾ cups water
- ½ red bell pepper, diced
- 2 scallions, thinly sliced
- ¼ cup pumpkin seeds, toasted
- 2 tablespoons extra virgin olive oil
- ¾ tablespoon fresh lime juice
- pinch of sea salt
- 4 cups baby arugula
- 1 fresh ripe avocado, sliced
- 1 (15-ounce) can black beans, drained and rinsed
- 2 tablespoons fresh cilantro

Rinse the quinoa and drain. Place in a saucepan with the water. Cover and bring to a boil. Reduce to low heat. Let simmer for 12 minutes. Turn off heat and let sit, covered, for another 8 minutes until all the water is absorbed.

Remove the quinoa from the pan and fluff with a fork onto a plate to cool. When cool, add the pepper, scallions, and pumpkin seeds. In a small bowl, combine the olive oil, lime juice, and salt. Toss with the quinoa.

To serve, place arugula on a plate, spoon the quinoa salad on top, then garnish with fresh sliced avocado, a spoon of drained black beans, and a sprinkle of cilantro.

Optional: Add slices of grilled chicken breast seasoned with a pinch of salt and pepper.

NOTE: If you are on the advanced plan, omit the quinoa.

Nutritional Analysis per Serving: calories 361, carbohydrates 36.4 g, fiber 7.7 g, protein 10.2 g, fat 20.8 g, cholesterol 0 mg, sodium 103 mg, calcium 77 mg.

SPLIT PEA AND ROSEMARY SOUP

Serves 6   Prep time: 5 minutes   Cook time: 1 hour
Program: basic and advanced plans

- 1 tablespoon extra virgin olive oil
- 1 small onion, diced
- 2 cloves garlic, chopped
- 1 cup carrots, diced
- ½ cup celery, diced
- 1 cup green split peas, rinsed

- 6 cups water or vegetable stock
- 2 tablespoons fresh rosemary, chopped
- 1 teaspoon sea salt
- 2 cups fresh peas
- pepper to taste

Heat the olive oil in a large soup pot over medium heat. Add the onions, garlic, carrots, and celery, and lightly sauté for about 5 minutes. Add the split peas and water or stock and bring to a boil. Turn heat down to low and add the rosemary. Simmer until the split peas are tender, about 40 minutes. Add salt. Continue to cook until the beans are very tender. For a smoother soup, blend all or part of it. Add the fresh peas and simmer just until the peas are tender, about 5 minutes, being careful not to overcook. Adjust the salt, if needed, and add pepper to taste. Serve with Spicy Roasted Squash (see below), unless you are on the advanced plan, in which case you should choose another side dish.

Nutritional Analysis per Serving: calories 182, carbohydrates 29.2 g, fiber 11.7 g, protein 11.0 g, fat 3.0 g, cholesterol 0 mg, sodium 336 mg, calcium 67 mg.

SPICY ROASTED SQUASH

Serves 4   Prep time: 5 minutes   Cook time: 25 minutes
Program: basic plan only

- 4 cups peeled butternut squash, cut into wedges
- 1 tablespoon extra virgin olive oil

- pinch each of paprika, chili powder, and cayenne
- pinch of sea salt

Preheat oven to 375°F. In a large bowl, toss the squash with the olive oil, spices, and salt. Place on a baking sheet and bake for 25 minutes, turning halfway through the cooking time. The squash is done when tender.

Nutritional Analysis per Serving: calories 93, carbohydrates 16.4 g, fiber 2.8 g, protein 1.4 g, fat 3.5 g, cholesterol 0 mg, sodium 44 mg, calcium 75 mg.

CHICKEN VEGETABLE SOUP WITH RICE

*Serves 6   Prep time: 5 minutes   Cook time: 50 minutes
Program: basic plan only*

- 1 tablespoon sesame oil
- 1 small carrot diced
- 2 stalks celery, diced
- 1 small onion, diced
- 2 organic skinless chicken breasts, bone in
- 1 teaspoon sea salt
- pinch of black pepper
- 2 cups green cabbage, thinly sliced
- 1 bay leaf
- 1 teaspoon dried sage
- 1 teaspoon dried thyme
- 6 cups water

- 2 teaspoons apple cider vinegar
- ½ cup long-grain brown rice, rinsed
- ¼ cup fresh parsley, chopped

Heat the sesame oil in a large soup pot on medium heat. Add the carrot, celery, and onion, and sauté until the onions become translucent. Push the vegetables to the side of the pot, lay the chicken breasts in the center, and sprinkle with salt and pepper. Sear for a minute on each side. Stir the vegetables back around the chicken. Add the cabbage, bay leaf, herbs, water, and cider vinegar. Bring to a boil then turn down heat and simmer for 30 minutes, until the chicken is cooked through.

Remove the chicken from the pot. Bring to a boil and add the rice. Reduce to medium, cover, and cook for 10 minutes until the rice is tender. Meanwhile, pull the chicken meat from the bones. When the rice is cooked, add the chicken back to the soup, adjust the seasoning, add the parsley, and serve.

Nutritional Analysis per Serving: calories 187, carbohydrates 15.9 g, fiber 1.4 g, protein 19.5 g, fat 4.5 g, cholesterol 49 mg, sodium 377 mg, calcium 45 mg.

QUINOA-CRUSTED QUICHE

Serves 8   Prep time: 10 minutes   Cook time: 45 minutes
Program: basic plan only

- 1½ tablespoons extra virgin olive oil
- 1 small onion, diced
- 1 small carrot, diced
- 1 red bell pepper, diced
- ¼ cup quinoa, rinsed
- 2 cups broccoli, small florets
- 10 eggs, beaten
- 1½ cups unsweetened soy milk
- 2 tablespoons fresh thyme leaves
- ½ teaspoon salt
- pinch of black pepper

Preheat oven to 350°F. In a medium sauté pan, heat the olive oil on medium heat and add the onions, carrots, and peppers. Sauté until the vegetables are tender and the onions start to brown. Remove from heat and cool a few minutes.

In a large bowl combine the cooked vegetables with the remaining ingredients. Lightly oil a 9 × 13-inch baking dish and pour in the mixture. Place in the oven and bake for 40 minutes or until the eggs are set. Allow to cool 5 minutes before serving.

Nutritional Analysis per Serving: calories 195, carbohydrates 15.6 g, fiber 2.8 g, protein 11.5 g, fat 9.9 g, cholesterol 233 mg, sodium 254 mg, calcium 144 mg.

TOFU FRIED RICE

Serves 4   Prep time: 5 minutes   Cook time: 45 minutes for rice plus 10 minutes for final recipe   Program: basic plan only

- 1¼ cups brown rice, rinsed
- 2½ cups water
- 2 tablespoons sesame oil
- 1 pound firm tofu, rinsed and cubed
- 1 small onion, diced
- 1 small carrot, diced
- 1 tablespoon garlic, minced
- 1 tablespoon ginger, minced
- 1½ tablespoons wheat-free tamari
- 1 tablespoon brown rice vinegar
- 1 tablespoon white wine
- 2 cups frozen green peas
- 2 scallions, sliced

Place the rice in a saucepan, and add the water. Bring to a boil, cover, and reduce to simmer on low for 40 minutes until the rice is cooked through and the water is gone.

In a large sauté pan or on a griddle, heat the sesame oil over medium-high heat. Add the tofu and sear for a minute on each side. Gently remove the tofu from the pan and set aside. In the same pan, add the onions and carrots and sauté until tender, then add the garlic and ginger and sauté a few minutes more. Add the rice and mix together. Allow to sit until the rice starts to get a little crusty on the bottom.

In a small bowl, combine the tamari, vinegar, and wine. Pour over the rice and then stir to combine. Allow the rice to get slightly crusty again, then stir. Add back the tofu, add the peas and scallions, and stir gently to combine. Continue to sauté until the peas are warmed through, then serve.

Nutritional Analysis per Serving: calories 398, carbohydrates 53.5 g, fiber 7.2 g, protein 18.0 g, fat 13.2 g, cholesterol 0 mg, sodium 406 mg, calcium 308 mg.

SHRIMP AND AVOCADO SALAD OVER ARUGULA

Serves 4   Prep time: 15 minutes   Cook time: 4 minutes
Program: basic and advanced plans

- ½ pound shrimp, peeled and deveined
- pinch of sea salt
- ½ teaspoon chili powder
- 1 tablespoon extra virgin olive oil
- ½ red bell pepper, diced
- 4 shoots scallions, sliced
- 3 tablespoons fresh cilantro

- 1 ripe avocado, cubed
- 1 cup grape or cherry tomatoes, halved
- 1 tablespoon lime juice
- 4 cups arugula

Rinse the shrimp and pat dry. Sprinkle with salt and chili powder. Heat ½ tablespoon of the olive oil in a skillet on medium heat. Carefully place the shrimp in the pan and sear on each side for about 2 minutes until cooked through. Remove from heat and set aside to cool.

Combine all vegetables in a serving bowl and toss with the remaining olive oil and lime juice. Gently fold in the shrimp and serve over the arugula sprinkled with a little extra virgin olive oil.

Nutritional Analysis per Serving: calories 198, carbohydrates 11.5 g, fiber 4.8 g, protein 14.0 g, fat 11.7 g, cholesterol 111 mg, sodium 202 mg, calcium 85 mg.

HEARTY GARDEN VEGETABLE SOUP WITH PINTO BEANS

Serves 6   Prep time: 10 minutes   Cook time: 30 minutes
Program: basic and advanced plans

- 2 tablespoons extra virgin olive oil
- ½ small onion, diced
- 1 tablespoon garlic, minced
- 1 tablespoon tomato paste
- 1 teaspoon celery, fennel, or cumin seeds

- 2 stalks celery, sliced
- 1 small carrot, diced
- 1 small turnip, peeled and diced
- 2 cups kale or collard greens, chopped
- 1 large tomato, chopped
- ½ teaspoon sea salt
- 1 (15-ounce) can pinto beans
- 1 cup fresh or frozen corn
- 5 cups water
- 2 tablespoons fresh basil or 2 teaspoons dried basil
- salt and pepper to taste
- splash of balsamic vinegar or lemon juice

In a large soup pot, heat the oil over medium heat and sauté the onions and garlic until they sweat. Add the tomato paste and stir to coat the onions. Add the celery, fennel, or cumin seeds, then the carrots and turnips. Sauté for a few minutes to soften.

Add the greens and tomato, sauté 1 minute, then add the salt. Add the pinto beans with their liquid, corn, water, and basil. Bring to a boil, then turn down to low and simmer for 15 minutes.

Add salt and pepper to taste and a splash of balsamic vinegar or lemon juice.

Nutritional Analysis per Serving: calories 340, carbohydrates 55.9 g, fiber 13.3 g, protein 17.6 g, fat 6.0 g, cholesterol 0 mg, sodium 200 mg, calcium 143 mg.

RICE AND CHICKPEA SALAD WITH BALSAMIC VINAIGRETTE

Serves 6   Prep time: 10 minutes   Cook time: 30 minutes
Program: basic plan only

- ¾ cup brown rice, rinsed
- 1½ cups water
- ½ green bell pepper, diced
- ½ red bell pepper, diced
- ½ small carrot, grated
- 3 scallion shoots, sliced
- ¾ cup grape or cherry tomatoes, halved
- 1 small stalk celery, diced
- 1 (15-ounce) can chickpeas, drained
- ¼ cup parsley, chopped
- 2 tablespoons extra virgin olive oil
- 1 tablespoon balsamic vinegar
- ½ teaspoon dried oregano
- 2 tablespoons fresh basil
- ¼ teaspoon sea salt
- dash of black pepper

Place the rice in a medium pan with the water. Bring to a boil, reduce heat, cover, and simmer on low until tender, about 25 minutes.

Meanwhile, combine the vegetables and parsley in a medium bowl. Set aside.

To make the vinaigrette, whisk together the olive oil, vinegar, herbs, salt, and pepper.

When the rice is cooked, you can either toss everything together for a warm salad or cool the rice on a platter, and then combine all the ingredients for a lovely cold summer salad.

Nutritional Analysis per Serving: calories 151, carbohydrates 23.5 g, fiber 2.0 g, protein 2.5 g, fat 5.3 g, cholesterol 0 mg, sodium 102 mg, calcium 31 mg.

CURRY EGG SALAD IN LETTUCE WRAPS WITH ROASTED ASPARAGUS

Makes 8 wraps   Prep time: 10 minutes   Cook time: 10 minutes   Program: basic plan only

- 8 Romaine lettuce leaves
- 8 stalks asparagus, trimmed
- 1 tablespoon extra virgin olive oil
- pinch of sea salt
- 8 hard-boiled eggs
- 1 stalk celery, minced
- 2 scallions, chopped
- ¼ cup Vegenaise
- 1½ teaspoons curry powder
- 1 teaspoon stone-ground mustard
- squeeze of lemon juice
- ¼ teaspoon sea salt

Preheat oven to 375°F. Rinse and pat dry the Romaine leaves. Set aside. Rinse and pat dry the asparagus. Toss with the olive oil and salt. Place the asparagus in a baking pan and bake for 8–10 minutes until tender. Set aside to cool.

Chop the hard-boiled eggs into small cubes and place in a medium bowl. Add the remaining ingredients and stir to combine. Spread the egg salad on the Romaine leaves. Cut each asparagus stalk in half. If they are especially large, cut them lengthwise as well. Add the equivalent of one stalk of roasted asparagus to each wrap and roll up.

Nutritional Analysis per Serving: calories 135, carbohydrates 2.7 g, fiber 1.2 g, protein 6.6 g, fat 11.2 g, cholesterol 189 mg, sodium 203 mg, calcium 44 mg.

RED LENTIL STEW

Serves 6   Prep time: 5 minutes   Cook time: 45 minutes
Program: basic and advanced plans

- 2 tablespoons extra virgin olive oil
- ½ onion, diced
- 2 tablespoons garlic, minced
- 2 teaspoons black mustard seeds
- 1 teaspoon cumin
- 1 teaspoon turmeric
- ½ teaspoon coriander

- 1 small carrot, diced
- 2 cups cauliflower, small florets
- 1¼ cups red lentils, rinsed
- 6 cups water
- 1 cup tomato, diced
- 2 cups broccoli, small florets
- ½ teaspoon sea salt
- 1 tablespoon lemon juice
- chopped fresh parsley or cilantro for garnish

Heat the olive oil in a large soup pot on medium heat. Sauté the onions and garlic until tender. Add the mustard seeds and stir until they begin to pop. Add the other spices and sauté 1 minute. Add the carrot and cauliflower and stir to coat. Add the lentils and water and bring to a boil. Reduce to low and simmer until the lentils are soft, about 25 minutes. Add the tomato, broccoli, and salt and continue to simmer 5 more minutes. Just before serving, stir in the lemon juice and sprinkle with parsley or cilantro.

Nutritional Analysis per Serving: calories 223, carbohydrates 32.1 g, fiber 14.8 g, protein 12.8 g, fat 5.6 g, cholesterol 0 mg, sodium 350 mg, calcium 75 mg.

Sun-Dried Tomato Turkey Burgers

Makes 4 patties   Prep time: 15 minutes   Cook time: 8 minutes   Program: basic and advanced plans

- 3 tablespoons sun-dried tomatoes
- 1 teaspoon extra virgin olive oil
- 1 pound organic ground turkey meat
- 1 tablespoon balsamic vinegar
- 2–3 tablespoons fresh basil, chopped
- 1 tablespoon garlic, minced
- 1½ teaspoon Dijon mustard
- pinch of sea salt
- pinch of black pepper

Cover the sun-dried tomatoes in warm water and soak until soft. This will take about 10 minutes, depending on how soft your tomatoes are to start with. Drain and chop the tomatoes into small pieces. Combine with the remaining ingredients and form into 4 patties. Grill, pan-sear, or bake in the oven at 375°F until done, about 8 minutes. Serve over a large salad.

NOTE: Flavors melt together as they sit so feel free to mix up the ingredients ahead of time. As long as you started with fresh turkey (not frozen), uncooked patties can be frozen for future use.

Nutritional Analysis per Serving: calories 198, carbohydrates 2.1 g, fiber 0 g, protein 22.8 g, fat 11.3 g, cholesterol 66 mg, sodium 156 mg, calcium 11 mg.

Chicken and Black Bean Wraps in Steamed Collard Greens with Avocado and Salsa

Serves 4   Prep time: 15 minutes   Cook time: 10 minutes
Program: basic plan only

- ½ tablespoon ground cumin
- 2 teaspoons paprika
- pinch of cayenne pepper
- pinch of sea salt
- ½ pound boneless, skinless chicken breast
- 1 tablespoon extra virgin olive oil or grape seed oil
- 1 tablespoon fresh lemon or lime juice
- 2 cups water
- 4 large collard greens
- 1 (15-ounce) can black beans, drained
- 1 ripe avocado, sliced
- hot sauce (optional)

FOR THE SALSA

- 2 medium-ripe tomatoes, diced
- 1 tablespoon red onion, diced
- 1 tablespoon garlic, minced
- ½ tablespoon olive oil
- 1 tablespoon fresh cilantro, chopped
- 1 tablespoon fresh lemon juice
- pinch of sea salt

In a large bowl, combine the cumin, paprika, cayenne, and salt. Slice the chicken into thin strips and coat in the olive oil or grapeseed oil, then toss in the spices.

Heat a large skillet on medium heat and lightly coat with additional oil as needed. Lay the chicken strips in the hot pan and sear on all sides until cooked through, about 5 minutes depending on the thickness of the chicken, sprinkle with lemon or lime juice, and set aside to cool.

Place the water in a sauté pan and bring to a boil. Add the collard greens, cover, and cook for 1 minute, then remove and rinse under cold water to cool.

To prepare the salsa, combine all the salsa ingredients in a small bowl and stir.

To make the wraps, layer the chicken strips, black beans, avocado slices, and fresh salsa on the collard greens. Roll the greens, tucking in the edges. Add the hot sauce for extra heat.

Nutritional Analysis per Serving: calories 267, carbohydrates 11.1 g, fiber 5.5 g, protein 19.2 g, fat 17.2 g, cholesterol 50 mg, sodium 205 mg, calcium 65 mg.

DINNER RECIPES

LENTIL AND CHICKEN STEW

Serves 4   Prep time: 10 minutes   Cook time: 55 minutes
Program: basic and advanced plans

- 2 tablespoons sesame oil
- 1 small onion, diced
- 2 stalks celery, diced
- 2 small carrots, diced
- 2 garlic cloves
- 1 tablespoon tomato paste
- 2 large organic skinless chicken breasts, bone in
- 1 tablespoon za'atar spice mix*
- 1 teaspoon sea salt
- ¼ cup cooking wine (white or red)
- 1 cup French lentils
- 5 cups water or stock
- 2 tablespoons extra virgin olive oil

In a large pot, heat the sesame oil on medium heat and then sauté the onions, celery, and carrots until soft. Add the garlic and tomato paste and continue to sauté a few minutes. Add the chicken, za'atar (or other herbs), and salt and sauté a few minutes until the vegetables begin to stick to the pan.

Deglaze the pan with the wine (to do this, splash the wine on the bits that have stuck to the pan during sautéing, then scrape the pan to release the bits and the flavor). Add the lentils and water or stock. Bring to a boil, reduce heat to medium-low, cover, and simmer for 45 minutes, until the chicken is cooked through and the lentils are soft. During cooking, the chicken may fall off the bones. Remove the bones before serving.

Splash the olive oil on top of the chicken just before serving. Serve with Roasted Quinoa with Kale and Almonds (see below).

> *NOTE: Za'atar is a Middle Eastern spice made with sumac, thyme, and sesame seeds. If your local food stores do not carry it, simply substitute equal parts thyme, oregano, and sesame seeds.

Nutritional Analysis per Serving: calories 467, carbohydrates 34.8 g, fiber 16.0 g, protein 39.8 g, fat 17.2 g, cholesterol 73 mg, sodium 112 mg, calcium 78 mg.

ROASTED QUINOA WITH KALE AND ALMONDS

Serves 4   Prep time: 5 minutes   Cook time: 25 minutes
Program: basic plan only

- 1 tablespoon sesame oil
- 1 cup quinoa, rinsed
- 2 cups kale, chopped into small pieces
- 1¾ cups water
- ½ cup roasted almonds (see page 504), chopped or slivered

Heat the sesame oil on low in a medium saucepan. Add the quinoa. Bring to medium heat and sauté for 3–4 minutes, until the quinoa begins to get fragrant. Add the chopped kale and stir to combine. Add the water and bring to a boil. Reduce to a low simmer, cover, and cook for 12 minutes. Remove from heat and allow the quinoa to sit covered for another 10 minutes. Add the toasted almonds and serve.

Nutritional Analysis per Serving: calories 272, carbohydrates 33.2 g, fiber 5.1 g, protein 9.6 g, fat 12.1 g, cholesterol 0 mg, sodium 17 mg, calcium 110 mg.

FISH AND VEGETABLES IN PARCHMENT

Serves 4   Prep time: 5 minutes   Cook time: 20 minutes
Program: basic and advanced plans

- 1½ pounds fresh fish filet (best is haddock or cod)
- pinch of sea salt and freshly ground pepper
- 1 small fennel bulb, sliced into julienne strips
- 1 small leek, sliced into julienne strips
- 1 small carrot, sliced into julienne strips
- 4 stalks broccolini, sliced lengthwise
- 4 garlic cloves, crushed
- 1½ tablespoons extra virgin olive oil
- 4 slices of lemon
- ½ teaspoon fennel seeds, crushed

- 2 tablespoons white wine
- chopped fresh parsley for garnish

Preheat oven to 450°F. Cut parchment baking paper into eight pieces approximately twice the size of each piece of fish. Stack two pieces of parchment on top of an equal-size piece of aluminum foil.

Cut the fish into four pieces and season with salt and pepper to taste. On each parchment/aluminum stack, arrange one-quarter of the vegetables and garlic, then place one piece of the fish on top and drizzle some of the olive oil. Lay a slice of lemon on each piece of fish and sprinkle on a little of the fennel seed. Splash with white wine.

Fold the parchment and foil to enclose the fish and crimp the edges neatly to seal completely. Place the packets on a large baking sheet and bake for 20 minutes, until the parchment is puffed. Cut open the packets and garnish with parsley. Parchments can be placed directly on individual plates for service, or the fish and vegetables can be gently removed and placed on a serving platter. Serve with Pecan Wild Rice and Goji Berry Pilaf (see page 529).

Nutritional Analysis per Serving: calories 277, carbohydrates 11.8 g, fiber 3.4 g, protein 40.9 g, fat 6.9 g, cholesterol 94 mg, sodium 223 mg, calcium 95 mg.

PECAN WILD RICE AND GOJI BERRY PILAF

Serves 4   Prep time: 5 minutes   Cook time: 45 minutes
Program: basic plan only

- 1 tablespoon extra virgin olive oil
- ½ cup leeks, diced
- 1 carrot, diced
- 2 stalks celery, diced
- ¾ cup long-grain brown rice
- ¼ cup wild rice or wehani
- fresh herbs (we suggest rosemary and thyme)
- pinch of sea salt
- 2 cups water
- ⅓ cup dried goji berries
- ⅓ cup pecans, chopped and roasted
- chopped fresh parsley for garnish

Heat the olive oil in a medium pot over medium heat, and lightly sauté the leeks, carrots, and celery. Add the rice, herbs, and salt, and stir to combine. Add the water and bring to a boil. Cover and reduce to a simmer for 30 minutes until the rice is tender.

When the rice is done, add the goji berries and pecans, fluff, and serve with a sprinkle of fresh parsley.

Nutritional Analysis per Serving: calories 303, carbohydrates 45.3 g, fiber 4.1 g, protein 7.3 g, fat 11.1 g, cholesterol 0 mg, sodium 84 mg, calcium 65 mg.

TURKEY AND SPINACH MEAT LOAF

Serves 4   Prep time: 10 minutes   Cook time: 30 minutes
Program: basic and advanced plans

- 1½ cups pecans
- 1 pound lean ground organic turkey
- 10-ounce package frozen spinach, thawed and squeezed dry
- 2 eggs
- 1 tablespoon extra virgin olive oil
- ½ small onion, diced
- 1 teaspoon dried basil
- ¼ teaspoon sea salt
- pinch of black pepper

Preheat oven to 375°F. In a food processor, grind the raw pecans to a medium-fine texture. In a large mixing bowl, combine the ground pecans with the remaining ingredients. Mix well. Place into an oiled loaf pan and bake for 30 minutes. Remove from the oven and allow to cool for 5 minutes before serving. Serve with Millet Cauliflower Mash (see page 531) and Braised Greens with Red Onion and Sun-Dried Tomatoes (see page 532).

Nutritional Analysis per Serving: calories 418, carbohydrates 7.4 g, fiber 4.5 g, protein 24.7 g, fat 34.5 g, cholesterol 139 mg, sodium 255 mg, calcium 100 mg.

MILLET CAULIFLOWER MASH

Serves 4   Prep time: 5 minutes   Cook time: 30 minutes
Program: basic plan only

- 1 tablespoon extra virgin olive oil
- ½ small onion, diced
- ½ cup millet, rinsed
- 4 cups cauliflower, chopped
- 1 teaspoon dried sage or 1 tablepoon fresh sage
- 1½ cups water
- ¼ teaspoon sea salt
- chopped fresh parsley for garnish

In a medium saucepan over medium heat, heat the olive oil and sauté the onions until they start to brown. Add the millet, cauliflower, and sage and sauté 1 more minute. Add the water and bring to a boil, then add the salt. Cover, reduce heat, and simmer for 20 minutes, until the millet is soft. When done, blend with a potato masher. Sprinkle with the chopped parsley and serve.

Nutritional Analysis per Serving: calories 122, carbohydrates 19.5 g, fiber 3.8 g, protein 3.9 g, fat 3.6 g, cholesterol 0 mg, Sodium 121 mg, calcium 20 mg.

Braised Greens with Red Onion and Sun-Dried Tomatoes

Serves 4   Prep time: 5 minutes   Cook time: 10 minutes
Program: basic and advanced plans

- ½ red onion, sliced
- 2 tablespoons sun-dried tomatoes, sliced
- 4–6 cups thinly sliced greens (any combination of kale, chard, and collard greens works well)
- ½ cup water
- 1 tablespoon extra virgin olive oil
- splash of balsamic vinegar (optional)

Place the onion, tomatoes, and greens in a sauté pan with the water. Bring to a boil, then reduce to simmer on low until the greens are soft. Splash with olive oil and balsamic vinegar before serving.

Nutritional Analysis per Serving: calories 82, carbohydrates 10.6 g, fiber 2.1 g, protein 3.1 g, fat 4.0 g, cholesterol 0 mg, sodium 72 mg, calcium 120 mg.

Asian Tofu Snap Pea Stir-Fry with Sesame Peanut Sauce

Serves 4   Prep time: 5 minutes   Cook time: 10 minutes
Program: basic and advanced plans

- 1½ pounds firm tofu
- 2 tablespoons peanut butter
- 1 tablespoon white wine

- 1 tablespoon wheat-free tamari
- ½ tablespoon brown rice vinegar
- pinch of chili pepper flakes
- 1 tablespoon sesame seeds
- 1 tablespoon sesame oil
- 1 tablespoon ginger, minced
- 1 tablespoon garlic, minced
- 4 scallions, sliced, plus more for garnish
- 4 cups snap peas

Rinse the tofu and pat dry. Cut into medium cubes and set aside. To make the sauce, combine the peanut butter, wine, tamari, rice vinegar, chili pepper flakes, and sesame seeds in a small bowl, and mix until smooth.

In a wok or large sauté pan, heat the sesame oil, add the ginger, garlic, and scallions, and stir-fry for a minute, being careful not to burn. Add the tofu and sauté until the sides begin to brown. Add the snap peas and sauté 1 minute until tender. Add the sauce and cook for another minute. Serve immediately with Brown Rice (see page 534), garnished with extra scallions.

Nutritional Analysis per Serving: calories 346, carbohydrates 29.0 g, fiber 10.3 g, protein 25.2 g, fat 16.3 g, cholesterol 0 mg, sodium 319 mg, calcium 462 mg.

Brown Rice

*Serves 4   Prep time: 2 minutes   Cook time: 25 minutes
Program: basic plan only*

- 1 cup short-grain brown rice, rinsed
- 2 cups water
- pinch of sea salt

Place the rice in a medium saucepan. Cover with the water and bring to a boil. Reduce heat, add the salt, and cover. Simmer on low until the rice is tender and the water has evaporated. Serve immediately. Refrigerate leftovers in a sealed container. Brown rice will stay fresh for 5 days.

Nutritional Analysis per Serving: calories 172, carbohydrates 12 g, fiber 1.6 g, protein 3.6 g, fat 1.3 g, cholesterol 0 mg, sodium 44 mg, calcium 21 mg.

Mediterranean Shrimp

*Serves 6   Prep time: 10 minutes   Cook time: 5 minutes
Program: basic and advanced plans*

- 1 pound raw shrimp, peeled and deveined
- pinch of sea salt and pepper
- 2 tablespoons extra virgin olive oil
- 1 small red onion, sliced
- 2 tablespoons garlic, minced
- 2 cups grape tomatoes, halved
- 2 tablespoons fresh basil, thinly sliced

- ¼ cup kalamata olives, diced
- 4 cups baby spinach

Rinse the shrimp and pat dry. Season with the salt and pepper and set aside. In a large sauté pan, heat the olive oil on medium heat, add the onions and garlic, and sauté for 2–3 minutes until the onions lightly crisp. Add the tomatoes and sauté another minute. Add the shrimp and sear 1 minute on each side. Add the fresh basil and olives, combine, and remove from heat. Gently toss in the spinach to wilt and serve over Grilled Polenta (see below).

Nutritional Analysis per Serving: calories 144, carbohydrates 5.1 g, fiber 1.5 g, protein 17.2 g, fat 6.1 g, cholesterol 147 mg, sodium 277 mg, calcium 77 mg.

GRILLED POLENTA

Serves 4–6   Prep time: 5 minutes   Cook time: 1 hour (includes setting and grilling time)   Program: basic plan only

- 2 cups corn grits
- ½ teaspoon salt
- 6 cups water
- 2 tablespoons extra virgin olive oil

In a medium pot, combine the corn grits, salt, and water. Stir to remove any lumps and then slowly bring to a strong simmer. Continue to stir over medium-low heat until all the water is absorbed and the corn grits are soft, about 30 minutes.

Oil a 9 × 13-inch baking dish with 1 tablespoon of the olive oil. Pour the polenta into the pan and allow to set until cool, about 20 minutes. Once cooled, cut the polenta into squares.

To grill the polenta, heat a skillet on medium heat. Add the remaining olive oil. When the oil is hot, add the polenta squares and grill for 3 minutes on each side until crispy on the outside but still soft on the inside. Serve immediately or keep warm in the oven until ready to use.

Nutritional Analysis per Serving: calories 141, carbohydrates 30.0 g, fiber 2.9 g, protein 2.7 g, fat 1.5 g, cholesterol 0 mg, sodium 203 mg, calcium 10 mg.

BLACK BEAN SOUP

Serves 5–7   Prep time: 5 minutes   Cook time: 20–25 minutes   Program: basic and advanced plans

- 1 tablespoon extra virgin olive oil
- 1 tablespoon garlic
- 1 small onion, diced
- 1 tablespoon cumin
- 2 (15-ounce) cans black beans
- 2 cups water or vegetable stock
- 1 bay leaf
- 1½ tablespoons wheat-free tamari
- 1 tablespoon lemon juice
- chopped fresh cilantro for garnish

Heat the olive oil over medium heat in a soup pot. Add the garlic and onions, and cook until the onions are translucent. Add the cumin and sauté a few more minutes. Add the canned beans including their liquid, water or stock, and bay leaf. Bring to a boil, reduce heat, and simmer for 10–15 minutes. Add the tamari and lemon juice and simmer 1 minute more. Top with the cilantro. Serve with Toasted Cumin Rice (see below) and Garlic Kale and Cauliflower (see page 538).

Nutritional Analysis per Serving: calories 443, carbohydrates 77.7 g, fiber 18.8 g, protein 27.0 g, fat 3.9 g, cholesterol 0 mg, sodium 224 mg, calcium 176 mg.

Toasted Cumin Rice

Serves 4   Prep time: 5 minutes   Cook time: 35 minutes
Program: basic plan only

- 1 cup long-grain brown rice, rinsed
- ½ tablespoon cumin seeds
- 2 cups water
- Pinch sea salt

Preheat oven to 350°F. Spread the rice on a baking sheet, sprinkle the cumin seed on top, and toast in the oven for approximately 10 minutes. Turn occasionally to ensure even browning. Place the toasted rice and cumin with the water in a saucepan. Bring to a boil, add the salt, and then reduce heat, cover, and simmer until tender, about 20 minutes.

Nutritional Analysis per Serving: calories 175, carbohydrates 36.5 g, fiber 1.7 g, protein 3.7 g, fat 1.4 g, cholesterol 0 mg, sodium 45 mg, calcium 30 mg.

GARLIC KALE AND CAULIFLOWER

Serves 4   Prep time: 3 minutes   Cook time: 10 minutes
Program: basic and advanced plans

- 1 tablespoon extra virgin olive oil
- 1 tablespoon garlic, minced
- 2 cups cauliflower, small florets
- 6 cups Lacinato or Tuscan kale, chopped
- ½ cup water

Heat the oil in a sauté pan, then sauté the garlic and cauliflower on medium heat until the cauliflower starts to soften. Add the kale and water. Cover and steam until the kale is tender and the water evaporates, about 3–4 minutes.

Nutritional Analysis per Serving: calories 96, carbohydrates 13.4 g, fiber 3.3 g, protein 4.4 g, fat 4.1 g, cholesterol 0 mg, sodium 59 mg, calcium 165 mg.

SALMON PECAN CAKES

Makes 8 medium cakes   Prep time: 5 minutes   Cook time: 30 minutes   Program: basic and advanced plans

- 1 (7.5-ounce) can wild salmon
- 1¾ cups pecans
- 2 eggs

- 3 small scallions, chopped
- 1 small celery stalk, chopped
- 1 tablespoon extra virgin olive oil
- 1 tablespoon lime juice
- ½ teaspoon sea salt
- pinch of paprika

Preheat oven to 350°F. Drain the canned salmon. In a food processor, grind the pecans to a fine texture. Add the remaining ingredients and pulse to combine. Separate into 8 medium patties, place on a lightly oiled baking tray, and bake until golden, about 25–30 minutes. Top with Peach Chutney (see below) and serve with Sautéed Swiss Chard with Slivered Almonds (see page 540).

Nutritional Analysis per Serving: calories 251, carbohydrates 4.0 g, fiber 2.5 g, protein 9.5 g, fat 23.1 g, cholesterol 63 mg, sodium 151 mg, calcium 33 mg.

PEACH CHUTNEY

Makes approximately 8 servings   Prep time: 5 minutes
Cook time: 15 minutes   Program: basic plan only

- 4 fresh ripe peaches or 2 cups frozen peaches, peeled and diced
- 3 scallion shoots, chopped
- 1½ tablespoons extra virgin olive oil
- 2 tablespoons fresh cilantro
- 2 tablespoons fresh lime juice

- ½ teaspoon diced jalapeño peppers (or to taste)
- pinch of sea salt

Heat the peaches in a small saucepan over low-medium heat; if using fresh peaches, add 2 tablespoons of water to the pan. Add the scallions, olive oil, cilantro, lime juice, jalapeño, and salt. Cook on medium-low heat until the peaches are mushy. The mixture should not be a sauce; however, flavors should combine for about 12–15 minutes. Serve warm or cooled.

Nutritional Analysis per Serving: calories 44, carbohydrates 5.4 g, fiber 0.9 g, protein 0.6 g, Fat 2.7 g, cholesterol 0 mg, sodium 21 mg, calcium 9 mg.

Sautéed Swiss Chard with Slivered Almonds

Serves 4   Prep time: 3 minutes   Cook time: 10 minutes
Program: basic and advanced plans

- ¼ cup slivered almonds
- 1 tablespoon extra virgin olive oil
- 6 cups Swiss chard, chopped
- Pinch sea salt

Preheat oven to 350°F. Place the almonds on a baking tray and bake for 6–7 minutes, until lightly toasted.

In a sauté pan, heat the oil on medium heat. Add the Swiss chard and salt and continue to sauté until the chard is tender. Add the almonds and serve.

Nutritional Analysis per Serving: calories 74, carbohydrates 6.4 g, fiber 1.6 g, protein 2.2 g, fat 6.4 g, cholesterol 0 mg, sodium 154 mg, calcium 45 mg.

COCONUT CURRY CHICKEN AND VEGETABLES

Serves 4   Prep time: 10 minutes   Cook time: 25–30 minutes
Program: basic and advanced plans

- 2 tablespoons sesame oil
- 1 tablespoon mustard seeds
- 1 cup onion, chopped
- 1 tablespoon garlic, chopped
- 1 tablespoon curry powder
- pinch of cayenne pepper
- 2 large (or 4 small) chicken breasts, bone in
- ½ teaspoon sea salt
- 1 small carrot, diced
- 2 cups cauliflower, medium florets
- ½ green bell pepper, diced
- 1 apple, chopped
- 1 (13-ounce) can coconut milk
- 1½ cups frozen peas
- chopped fresh cilantro for garnish

In a large sauté pan, heat the sesame oil on medium heat. Add the mustard seeds and stir for 10 seconds until they start to pop; be careful not to burn them.

Immediately add the onions and garlic and sauté for 5 minutes until they begin to sweat. Add the curry and cayenne and stir to coat the onions. Add the chicken, sprinkle with ½ teaspoon of the salt, and sear on all sides. Add the carrots, cauliflower, and green pepper and cook 3–4 minutes. Add the apple, coconut milk, and remaining salt and simmer on low heat for 15–20 minutes until the chicken is cooked through. Add the peas and simmer 2–3 more minutes. Garnish with the cilantro and serve.

Nutritional Analysis per Serving: calories 565, carbohydrates 29.1 g, fiber 9.8 g, protein 34.9 g, fat 36.6 g, cholesterol 73 mg, sodium 618 mg, calcium 110 mg.

CORIANDER AND ALMOND-CRUSTED SCALLOPS

Serves 2   Prep time: 15 minutes   Cook time: 10 minutes
Program: basic and advanced plans

- 6 large scallops
- ½ cup white wine
- 2 pinches of sea salt
- ¼ cup raw almonds
- 1 tablespoon coriander seed
- pinch of black pepper
- ½ tablespoon grape seed oil
- 2 teaspoons balsamic vinegar

Preheat oven to 375°F. Remove the tough muscle from the scallops, rinse, and pat dry. Combine the wine and a pinch of salt and place the scallops in this marinade for 10 minutes. Meanwhile, place the almonds on a baking sheet and bake for 7–8 minutes. In a food processor, coarsely grind the coriander seed. Add the toasted almonds, another pinch of salt, and the pepper, and pulse to grind coarsely.

Remove the scallops from the marinade and coat each side with the almond mixture. Heat the oil in a skillet on medium-high heat, and grill the scallops for 2–3 minutes on each side. Splash with balsamic vinegar and serve immediately with Whipped Yams (see below) and Sautéed Spinach and Watercress (see page 544).

Nutritional Analysis per Serving: calories 228, carbohydrates 6.4 g, fiber 1.5 g, protein 17.7 g, fat 9.9 g, cholesterol 30 mg, sodium 383 mg, calcium 65 mg.

WHIPPED YAMS

Serves 4   Prep time: 5 minutes   Cook time: 20 minutes
Program: basic plan only

- 3 small to medium yams
- 2 tablespoons extra virgin olive oil
- pinch of sea salt

Wash the yams and place in a large pot. Cover with water and bring to a boil. Reduce to low and simmer for 15–20 minutes until the yams are soft yet not mushy. Remove the yams from the water and set aside to cool until you can handle them. Using a knife or your fingers, remove the skin. Remove the water from the pot and place the yams back in the pot, add the olive oil and salt, and mash with a fork or potato masher.

Nutritional Analysis per Serving: calories 137, carbohydrates 17.7 g, fiber 2.8 g, protein 1.7 g, fat 6.9 g, cholesterol 0 mg, sodium 89 mg, calcium 32 mg.

SAUTÉED SPINACH AND WATERCRESS

Serves 4   Prep time: 5 minutes   Cook time: 5 minutes
Program: basic and advanced plans

- 1 tablespoon extra virgin olive oil
- 2 cups fresh watercress
- 8 cups fresh spinach
- pinch of sea salt

In a large sauté pan, heat the olive oil on medium heat. Add the watercress and sauté until tender, about 3 minutes. Remove from heat and add the spinach to wilt. Season with the salt.

Nutritional Analysis per Serving: calories 46, carbohydrates 3.6 g, fiber 1.4 g, protein 2.1 g, fat 3.6 g, cholesterol 0 mg, sodium 113 mg, calcium 87 mg.

BRAISED LAMB AND POMEGRANATE MOLASSES OVER WHITE BEANS

Serves 4   Prep time: 30 minutes, including marinating time   Cook time: 20–25 minutes   Program: basic plan

- 2 tablespoons balsamic vinegar
- 1 tablespoon garlic
- 1 tablespoon Dijon mustard
- 4 lamb shanks
- 2 tablespoons extra virgin olive oil
- ½ small onion, diced
- 1 tablespoon garlic
- 2 tablespoons pomegranate molasses
- 1 bay leaf
- 1 tablespoon fresh or 1 teaspoon dried sage
- ¼ teaspoon sea salt
- 1 (15-ounce) can cannellini beans
- ¼ cup water or red wine
- ¼ cup fresh parsley
- ½ cup fresh pomegranate seeds, optional

In a large shallow dish, combine the vinegar, garlic, and mustard. Trim excess fat from the lamb and place in the dish, turning to cover with the marinade. Let stand for 30 minutes.

Meanwhile, heat the olive oil in a braising pan on medium heat. Add the onions and garlic and sauté until the onions begin to brown, about 8 minutes.

Add the lamb and sear on both sides. Pour the molasses over the lamb and continue to brown on both sides. Add the bay leaf, sage, salt, and beans with their liquid, and water or red wine. Simmer on low heat until the lamb is tender and the beans are heated through, about 15–20 minutes, depending on the thickness of the lamb and how well done you like it.

Garnish the lamb and beans with pomegranate seeds and parsley. Serve with Lemon Broccoli (see below).

Nutritional Analysis per Serving: calories 720, carbohydrates 74.1 g, fiber 27.0 g, protein 65.4 g, fat 18.2 g, cholesterol 128 mg, sodium 265 mg, calcium 230 mg.

LEMON BROCCOLI

Serves 4   Prep time: 2 minutes   Cook time: 5 minutes
Program: basic and advanced plans

- 1 tablespoon extra virgin olive oil
- 4 cups broccoli, large florets
- pinch of sea salt
- ½ lemon, cut into wedges

Heat the olive oil in a large sauté pan on medium heat. Add the broccoli, stirring constantly until it becomes tender. Add the salt. Serve with lemon wedges.

Nutritional Analysis per Serving: calories 64, carbohydrates 7.2 g, fiber 2.4 g, protein 2.5 g, fat 3.7 g, cholesterol 0 mg, sodium 88 mg, calcium 45 mg.

QUICK MEXICANA CHILI WITH QUINOA

Servings 8   Prep time: 5 minutes   Cook time: 25 minutes
Program: basic plan only

- 2 tablespoons extra virgin olive oil
- 1 small onion, diced
- 2 tablespoons garlic, diced
- 2 tablespoons chili powder
- 1 tablespoon ground cumin
- 1 tablespoon paprika
- ½ teaspoon chili flakes
- 1 teaspoon dried oregano
- 2 tablespoons tomato paste
- 1 tablespoon red wine or water
- ½ cup quinoa, rinsed
- ½ green bell pepper, seeds removed then diced
- 1 small zucchini, diced
- 1 (15-ounce) can black beans
- 1 (15-ounce) can pinto beans
- 4 cups water or vegetable stock
- 1 (8-ounce) can tomato sauce
- 1 teaspoon sea salt
- squeeze of fresh lime juice
- chopped fresh cilantro for garnish (optional)

In a large soup pot, heat the olive oil on medium heat. Add the onions and garlic and cook until they begin to sweat. Add the spices and continue to sauté for 2 more minutes. Add the tomato paste and sauté another minute. Deglaze with the water or wine, and then add the quinoa. Sauté until the quinoa is browned.

Add the green pepper and zucchini and sauté a few minutes until they begin to soften. Add the beans with their liquid, water or stock, tomato sauce, and salt. Bring to a boil, then reduce heat to low and simmer for 15 minutes. Garnish with the lime juice and cilantro. Serve with Baked Corn Tortilla Strips (see below).

Nutritional Analysis per Serving: calories 467, carbohydrates 79.8 g, fiber 19.2 g, protein 25.9 g, fat 6.2 g, cholesterol 0 mg, sodium 423 mg, calcium 176 mg.

BAKED CORN TORTILLA STRIPS

Serves 4   Prep time: 5 minutes   Cook time: 5 minutes
Program: basic plan only

- 1 tablespoon extra virgin olive oil
- 4 organic corn tortillas
- pinch of sea salt

Preheat oven to 375°F. Brush oil on both sides of the tortillas. Cut the tortillas into strips. Place on a baking sheet and bake for 5 minutes, until crispy. Sprinkle with salt immediately after removing from the oven.

Nutritional Analysis per Serving: calories 62,
carbohydrates 10.7 g, fiber 1.5 g, protein 1.4 g, fat 1.8 g,
cholesterol 0 mg, sodium 69 mg, calcium 21 mg.

LACINTO KALE WITH ROASTED SQUASH

Serves 4   Prep time: 5 minutes   Cook time: 30 minutes
Program: basic plan only

- 2 cups butternut squash, peeled and cubed
- ½ red onion, thinly sliced
- 2 tablespoons extra virgin olive oil
- pinch of sea salt
- 6 cups Lacinato or Tuscan kale, chopped
- ¾ cup water

Preheat oven to 375°F. Toss the cubed squash and
red onion with 1 tablespoon of the olive oil and salt.
Place in a baking pan and roast until the squash is
soft, about 25 minutes.

Heat a sauté pan on medium heat. Add the kale
and water and cook for a few minutes, then cover
with a lid to steam the kale. When the kale is tender
and the water has evaporated, add the roasted squash
and onions, top with the remaining olive oil, and serve.

Nutritional Analysis per Serving: calories 147,
carbohydrates 19.5 g, fiber 3.6 g, protein 4.2 g, fat 7.5 g,
cholesterol 0 mg, sodium 105 mg, calcium 186 mg.

GRILLED SALMON WITH CILANTRO MINT CHUTNEY

Serves 4   Prep time: 10 minutes   Cook time: 20 minutes
Program: basic and advanced plans

- 1½ pounds wild salmon
- 1 tablespoon extra virgin olive oil
- pinch of sea salt
- pinch of black pepper

FOR THE CHUTNEY

- 1 small bunch cilantro, including stems, rinsed
- 2 tablespoons fresh mint leaves, chopped
- 3 tablespoons extra virgin olive oil
- 1½ tablespoons garlic, minced
- pinch of sea salt
- 1 tablespoon fresh lemon or lime juice
- pinch of chili peppers flakes (optional)

Season the salmon with the olive oil, salt, and pepper. Set aside for 10 minutes.

Combine all the chutney ingredients in a blender. Blend until smooth and fragrant. Set aside.

Heat a griddle, grill, or grill pan on medium-high heat and place the fish on the grill, skin side down. Allow the salmon to cook until the skin is charred and the fish is almost cooked through. This will take about 15 minutes, depending on the thickness of the salmon. Turn the salmon over and grill a few more minutes, until the fish is fully cooked. Remove from heat and lay skin side up on a platter. Pull the skin off the salmon and flip back to serve. Spread chutney on top of the salmon. Serve with wedges of lemon or lime, White Bean and Corn Salad (see below), and Grilled Summer Vegetables (see pages 552–553).

Nutritional Analysis per Serving: calories 479, carbohydrates 1.9 g, fiber 0.5 g, protein 38.1 g, fat 34.6 g, cholesterol 107 mg, sodium 226 mg, calcium 43 mg.

WHITE BEAN AND CORN SALAD

Serves 4   Prep time: 10 minutes   Cook time: none
Program: basic plan only

- 1 (15-ounce) can cannellini or navy beans, drained
- 1 ear fresh-cooked corn, removed from cob, or ¾ cup frozen corn, thawed
- 1 small carrot, grated or diced
- 1 stalk celery, diced
- 1 tablespoon chopped fresh parsley

FOR THE DRESSING

- 3 tablespoons extra virgin olive oil
- 1½ tablespoons lemon juice
- 1 teaspoon ground cumin
- ½ teaspoon ground coriander
- ½ teaspoon sea salt
- chopped fresh cilantro to taste

Combine the beans, corn, carrots, celery, and parsley. Set aside.

Whisk together the dressing ingredients and fold into the salad.

NOTE: This salad can be eaten immediately or made ahead to let the flavors meld—it gets even better as it sits. Refrigerate leftovers.

Nutritional Analysis per Serving: calories 478, carbohydrates 71.4 g, fiber 27.7 g, protein 26.3 g, fat 11.5 g, cholesterol 0 mg, sodium 278 mg, calcium 185 mg.

GRILLED SUMMER VEGETABLES

Serves 4–6   Prep time: 1 hour and 5 minutes (includes marinating time)   Cook time: 15 minutes   Program: basic and advanced plans

- 1 bunch asparagus, trimmed
- 1 zucchini
- 1 summer squash
- 1 onion
- 1 red bell pepper
- ⅓ cup extra virgin olive oil
- pinch of sea salt
- pepper to taste

Wash the vegetables and cut into the preferred sizes and shapes. Place in a bowl. Toss with the olive oil, salt, and pepper. Cover and refrigerate; allow to sit for at least 1 hour.

Heat grill on medium-high heat and place the marinated vegetables on the grill, turning occasionally until the desired tenderness is achieved. You can also roast in an oven at 350 degrees. Baking time will depend on the size of the vegetables.

Nutritional Analysis per Serving: calories 143, carbohydrates 7.7 g, fiber 2.9 g, protein 2.7 g, fat 12.3 g, cholesterol 0 mg, sodium 49 mg, calcium 33 mg.

Tofu and Cashew Stir-Fry over Basmati Rice

Serves 4   Prep time: 10 minutes   Cook time: 10 minutes
Program: basic and advanced plans

- ½ head broccoli, stems included
- 1 pound firm tofu
- 1½ tablespoons sesame oil
- 1 tablespoon ginger, minced
- 2 garlic cloves, minced
- 1 large carrot, cut into matchsticks
- 1 cup bok choy, sliced
- 1 tablespoon wheat-free tamari
- 1 teaspoon toasted sesame oil
- 1 cup snow peas
- ¾ cup whole raw cashews
- 1 teaspoon hot sauce or 1 teaspoon hoisin sauce (optional)

Rinse the tofu and pat dry. Cut into cubes. Remove the broccoli stems from the florets. Cut the florets and set aside. Peel the stems and cut into matchsticks. Set aside. In a sauté pan, heat half of the sesame oil on medium heat. Add the ginger and garlic and stir. Immediately add the tofu and allow to brown on all sides. Remove the tofu from the pan and set aside.

Rinse and dry the sauté pan and heat the rest of the sesame oil. Add the carrots and broccoli stems and sauté until they start to soften. Add the bok choy and broccoli florets and continue to sauté. Add the tamari, sesame oil, and snow peas. Sauté until the snow peas just start to soften.

Add the tofu back to the stir-fry, along with the cashews. Heat through and serve with hot sauce or hoisin sauce.

NOTE: Omit the rice if you are on the advanced plan.

Nutritional Analysis per Serving: calories 354, carbohydrates 24.4 g, fiber 7.5 g, protein 18.3 g, fat 23.5 g, cholesterol 0 mg, sodium 601 mg, calcium 365 mg.

SUNDAY NIGHT BOUILLABAISSE

Serves 4   Prep time: 10 minutes   Cook time: 15 minutes
Program: basic and advanced plans

- 1½ tablespoons extra virgin olive oil
- 1 small onion, chopped
- 2 garlic cloves, chopped

- 2 medium tomatoes, diced
- 2 tablespoons fresh parsley, chopped
- 1 tablespoon fresh thyme, chopped
- 1 tablespoon fresh rosemary, chopped
- 1 bay leaf
- ½ teaspoon chili flakes
- 1 pound white fish (such as haddock or cod), cubed
- ½ pound shrimp, shelled and deveined
- 1 cup white wine
- 2 cups fish or vegetable stock
- ½ teaspoon sea salt
- pepper to taste
- ½ pound mussels, washed and debearded
- ½ pound small clams
- 1 lemon, cut into wedges
- chopped fresh parsley for garnish

In a large pot, heat the olive oil on medium heat. Add the onions and garlic and sauté a few minutes until the onions start to soften. Add the tomatoes, herbs, and chili flakes and sauté another few minutes. Lay the fish, then the shrimp, on top of the vegetables.

Add the white wine, stock, salt, and pepper, and bring to a boil. Reduce heat to low, cover, and simmer for 4 minutes. Add the clams, cover, and simmer until the clams start to open, about 5 minutes. Then add the mussels and simmer another 3 minutes until the mussels and clams open fully and the fish is firm.

Ladle into bowls and top with the lemon wedges, fresh parsley, and pepper to taste.

Nutritional Analysis per Serving: calories 371, carbohydrates 15.6 g, fiber 2.0 g, protein 48.5 g, fat 9.3 g, cholesterol 190 mg, sodium 826 mg, calcium 107 mg.

GENERAL TIPS

- Before shopping for your weekly menu:
  1. Clean out any old perishable foods from your refrigerator and determine if you can substitute something you already have for something on the shopping list.
  2. Decide which items you'd like to make a double batch of to freeze for future use. Items that are great for freezing include soups and stews, burgers, meat loaf, rice dishes, and sauces.
  3. If you have leftovers that cannot be successfully frozen, look ahead and plan where in your week you will use them.
- Make sure you have plenty of storage containers. Pyrex and glass work best to preserve flavors.
- Offer to do a food exchange with a friend—each person makes a double batch of a different recipe, sharing half. This way if you both cook on Monday, neither needs to cook on Tuesday. Plus this

creates a wonderful connection with a friend or neighbor!

- As you put away your groceries, take an extra few minutes to arrange your cupboards and refrigerator to reflect the order in which items will be used. It is helpful to have containers for all refrigerated items that go with a particular meal to be stored together and labeled.
- Post your weekly menu on the refrigerator, noting any prep to be done for the following days.
- Look over the week's menu and see what items you can make ahead of time. Examples are roasting nuts and seeds; making a sauce, chutney, or pesto; or toasting grains.
- Plan which meals you can cook the night before or make in a Crock-Pot, such as soups, stews, or grains.

Make Your Own Salad Bar!

Many of the meals in this book would be complemented nicely by a big green salad. To help ease preparation, start your week with setting up your own salad bar fixings.

- Wash and cut veggies into convenient salad-size bits and store in sealed Pyrex containers all in one location in your refrigerator. Cut enough for two to three days and repeat throughout the week as needed. Add different veggies at least twice a week for freshness and variety.

- Store items not requiring refrigeration in small glass jars on a single shelf. Toasted and raw nuts and seeds stay fresh for weeks when sealed in glass jars.

For a simple dressing, top salads with a little extra virgin olive oil and a splash of your favorite vinegar or squeeze of lemon. Fresh herbs add great flavor and help reduce the need for heavy dressings.

Note: Salad bar fixings are not included in the weekly shopping lists. Pick a variety from the items below to add to your list each week. This list also includes leftovers that can easily be incorporated into a salad.

Refrigerated items:

- Arugula
- Spinach
- Mixed greens
- Cucumber
- Bell peppers: red, green, yellow
- Sprouts: pea shoots, clover, broccoli, etc.
- Tomatoes: grape, cherry
- Carrots
- Beets
- Red onions
- Scallions

- Parcooked and cooled broccoli florets
- Parcooked and cooled cauliflower florets
- Fresh herbs, such as parsley, cilantro, and dill
- Pomegranates
- Fresh figs
- Blueberries
- Raspberries
- Apples (don't cut these ahead of time)
- Avocados (don't cut these ahead of time)
- Hard-boiled eggs
- Canned chickpeas (open and drained)
- Canned salmon or sardines
- Leftover grains (toss with a little sesame or olive oil before refrigerating)
- Leftover roasted asparagus or cooked greens
- Cooked and cooled edamame

Nonrefrigerated items:

- Toasted or raw seeds: sunflower, pumpkin, sesame, flax, etc.
- Toasted or raw nuts: almonds, walnuts, pecans, cashews, etc.
- Dried goji berries
- Extra virgin olive oil
- Vinegars: balsamic, apple cider, wine, etc.
- Fresh-ground pepper
- Dried oregano and basil

WEEK 1 SHOPPING LIST

Seasonings	Dry Goods	Produce
☐ Extra virgin olive oil	☐ Wild rice (2 cups)	☐ 2 small red onions
☐ Sesame oil	☐ Short-grain brown rice (2 cups)	☐ 4 small yellow onions
☐ Wheat-free tamari (natural soy sauce)	☐ Long-grain rice (2¼ cups)	☐ 1 head garlic
☐ Rice wine vinegar	☐ Quinoa (1 cup)	☐ 1 piece ginger
☐ White cooking wine	☐ Millet (½ cup)	☐ 4 bunches of greens — choose from kale, chard, collards
☐ Balsamic vinegar	☐ Dry French lentils (1 cup)	☐ Celery
☐ Apple cider vinegar	☐ Cannellini beans (1 can)	☐ 6 small carrots
	☐ Black beans (3 cans)	☐ 1 small fennel bulb
Herbs (dried)	☐ Dry split peas (1 cup)	☐ 2 small leeks
☐ Basil	☐ Raw walnuts (⅔ cup)	☐ 2 bunches broccoli, broccolini, or broccoli rabe
☐ Bay leaf	☐ Sesame seeds (1 small container)	☐ 2 red bell peppers
☐ Sage	☐ Raw pecans (3¼ cups)	☐ 2 bunches scallions
☐ Thyme	☐ Goji berries (⅓ cup)	☐ 1 cauliflower
	☐ Corn grits or premade polenta (2 cups)	☐ 1 small winter squash
Spices	☐ Natural peanut butter	☐ 1 small green cabbage
☐ Black pepper	☐ Kalamata olives	☐ Snap peas (4 cups)
☐ Cayenne pepper	☐ Sun-dried tomatoes (½ cup)	☐ Baby spinach (4 cups)
☐ Ground cumin	☐ Tomato paste	☐ Arugula (4 cups)
☐ Cumin seed	☐ Capers	☐ Cherry or grape tomatoes (2 pints)
☐ Fennel seed	☐ Canned salmon (two 7.5-ounce cans)	☐ 1 avocado
☐ Chili powder		
☐ Paprika		
☐ Sea salt		

Perishable and Frozen Foods	Fresh Herbs and Fruits
☐ 14 eggs	☐ 1 bunch basil
☐ 4 bone-in chicken breasts	☐ 1 bunch Italian parsley
☐ ¼ pound boneless, skinless chicken	☐ 1 bunch cilantro
☐ 1 pound shrimp	☐ 1 bunch rosemary
☐ 1½ pounds white fish	☐ 1 bunch thyme
☐ 1 pound ground organic turkey	☐ 1 jalapeño pepper
☐ 2 pounds firm tofu	☐ Chili peppers
☐ 10 ounces frozen spinach	☐ 2 lemons
☐ 10 ounces frozen peas	☐ 2 limes
☐ 10 ounces frozen peaches	

WEEK 2 SHOPPING LIST

Seasonings	Dry Goods	Produce
In addition to what will be left over from last week:	☐ Coconut milk (one 15-ounce can)	☐ 2 red bell peppers
☐ Mustard seed	☐ Pinto beans (two 15-ounce cans)	☐ 1 green bell pepper
☐ Curry powder	☐ Cannellini beans (two 15-ounce cans)	☐ 2 bunches scallions
☐ Coriander	☐ Red lentils (1¼ cups)	☐ 1 cup bok choy
	☐ Quinoa (½ cup)	☐ 2 ripe avocadoes
	☐ Short brown rice (1¾ cups)	☐ 1 pint grape or cherry tomatoes
	☐ Dijon mustard (small bottle)	☐ 6 ripe tomatoes
	☐ Stoneground mustard (small bottle)	☐ 5 yellow onions
	☐ Vegenaise (small jar)	☐ 1 red onion
	☐ Sun-dried tomatoes (¼ cup)	☐ 2 heads garlic
	☐ Tomato sauce (one 8-ounce can)	☐ 1 cup snow peas
	☐ Whole cashews (¾ cup)	☐ 1 bunch kale
	☐ Raw almonds (¾ cup)	☐ 1 bunch collard greens
		☐ 1 head celery
		☐ 6 carrots
		☐ 1 small turnip
		☐ 4 cups arugula
		☐ 8 cups spinach
		☐ 1 head Romaine lettuce
		☐ 1 bunch watercress
		☐ 2 bunches asparagus
		☐ 2 zucchini
		☐ 1 yellow squash
		☐ 1 head broccoli
		☐ 3 yams
		☐ 1 small butternut squash

Perishable Foods

- ☐ 10 eggs
- ☐ 1 pound peeled, deveined shrimp
- ☐ 6 large scallops
- ☐ 1 pound white fish
- ☐ 1.5 pounds wild salmon
- ☐ 1 pound mussels
- ☐ 1 pound very small clams
- ☐ 4 bone-in chicken breasts
- ☐ 1 pound ground turkey
- ☐ ½ pound boneless, skinless chicken breast
- ☐ 4 lamb shanks
- ☐ one 10-ounce pack frozen peas and corn
- ☐ 1 pound firm tofu
- ☐ 4 organic tortillas

Fresh Herbs and Fruits

- ☐ 1 bunch basil
- ☐ 1 bunch Italian parsley
- ☐ 1 bunch cilantro
- ☐ 1 bunch rosemary
- ☐ 1 bunch thyme
- ☐ 1 bunch sage
- ☐ 1 jalapeño pepper
- ☐ 2 lemons
- ☐ 2 limes
- ☐ 1 apple
- ☐ 1 pomegranate

Acknowledgments

The opportunity to write a book is both a gift and a burden. In this case, its virtues are often borrowed, and its errors entirely my own. Writing it was a journey supported by the vast community I find myself living in and exploring with wonder.

I am indebted to all the scientists who have worked thanklessly to understand the mysteries of the human body, and all my patients who trusted me, then worked with me to find a solution to their health struggles when they could not find answers through the current medical paradigm. They taught me more than they realized.

My agent, Richard Pine, has guided this book from the beginning with patience, clarity, insight, and an uncommon directness, as usual in his understated, loving way. Tracy Behar, my editor, and all my friends and supporters at Little, Brown saw the possibility of a new solution to our health care crisis.

Acknowledgments

My publicist, Bruce Bobbins, and his team at DKC helped me clarify the message and get it heard. Thanks especially to my UltraTeam: Spencer Smith, Anne McLaughlin, Shibani Subramanya, Daffnee Cohen, Rachel Goldstein, and Bernie Plishtin, who make it possible for me to do the work I love every day.

My thanks extend to well over a hundred people, not all of whom, unfortunately, I can name here. You know who you are—thank you, thank you, thank you. I must mention a few special people who have inspired, helped, and supported me: Jeffrey Bland, who cracked open my world fifteen years ago (it has never been the same); Sidney Baker, one of the greatest unrecognized and original thinkers of our time; my friends and co-faculty at the Institute for Functional Medicine—Laurie Hoffman, David Jones, and the many unnamed who just make it happen there. And all those who have supported me from the beginning with their time and money to launch the future of medicine: the Bitzers, the Musses, Maja Hoffmann and Stanley Buchthal, Adelaide Gomer, Alicia Wittink, Ritchie Scaife, the Baldridges, the Nevzlins, Damon Giglio, Donna Karan, Daphne Barak, and so many more.

And without friendship and my whole community I couldn't do what I do—thank you for being there even when I am not—and for those unnamed.

Again, you know who you are: Marc David, David and Zea Piver, Michael and Lisa Bronner, Michael Lerner, Colby and Dena Lewis, Jonathan and Michelle Kalman, Dan and Ditte Ruderman, Paul and Andrea DeBotton, Andy and Lisa Corn, David Ludwig, Alberto Villoldo and Marcela Lobos, and the list goes on and on. And a special thanks to Hillary, Bill, Chelsea, and Marc, who have supported this work and helped to build a better future for all of us.

To my co-creators of medicine's transformation, who have touched me and continue to create seismic shifts in our way of thinking and living, thank you: Dean Ornish, Mehmet C. Oz, James Gordon, Andrew Weil, Deepak Chopra, Christiane Northrup, Daniel and Tara Goleman, Jon Kabat-Zinn, Leo Galland, David Perlmutter, Frank Lipman, Patrick Hanaway, Robert Hedaya, Joel Evans, David Eisenberg, Bethany Hayes, David Jones, Tracy Gaudet, Kenneth Pelletier, Peter Libby, and Martha Herbert. And a special thanks to Arianna Huffington for providing a place for the truth to be told.

Thank you, Rick Warren, and all my friends at Saddleback for believing in and making real the possibility of getting healthy together.

Without the support of my team at the Ultra-Wellness Center, where I do my real work of seeing patients, I couldn't begin to do anything else. You are my foundation and at the core of my life. Your

contributions wash over me daily; thank you for showing up and believing.

Lastly, and most importantly, my family has put
up with the dangers of my passion (early mornings,
late nights, and too many absences to remember). I
could not have done this without all your love and
belief in what I am doing. Thank you Pier, Rachel,
Misha, Thor, Ace, Ruth, Richard, Saul, Jesse, Car-
rie, Ben, Sarah, Paul, Lauren, Jake, and Zachary. It is
for you and because of you that I wake up every day
grateful and joyful.

Resources

As promised, here is a list of resources for finding high-quality food, living clean and green, relaxing, locating a practitioner of functional medicine in your area, and pursuing optimal health.

FURTHER READING AND RESOURCES FROM MARK HYMAN, MD

Mark Hyman, MD's Websites

www.drhyman.com
www.bloodsugarsolution.com
www.takebackourhealth.org
www.ultramind.com

The UltraWellness Center

45 Walker Street
Lenox, MA 01240
(413) 637-9991
www.ultrawellnesscenter.com

Our team of experienced functional medicine physicians, nutritionists, nurses, and health coaches guide you through diet and lifestyle modifications, as well as specialized testing, nutritional supplementation, and medications.

The UltraMind Solution

www.bloodsugarsolution.com/ultramind-solution
Whether you suffer from a mood disorder, neurological problems, difficulty with attention, or just low energy and a little brain fog, this six-week program will help you heal your brain by fixing your body first.

The UltraMind Solution PBS Special

www.bloodsugarsolution.com/ultramind-dvd
Learn about the seven key systems that are at the root of all broken brains, and what you can do to live a vibrantly healthy life.

Six Weeks to an UltraMind

www.bloodsugarsolution.com/six-weeks-to-ultramind
This dynamic self-coaching program provides you with a combination of audio, video, and printed materials that make incorporating the UltraMind program into your life as simple as possible.

UltraCalm

www.bloodsugarsolution.com/ultracalm
Are you stressed out? Do you suffer from anxiety, obsessive-compulsive disorders, or panic attacks? In

this audio program, I walk you through steps you can take to help you resolve stress and anxiety. It includes guided visualizations, breathing exercises, tips on nutrition and detoxification, and more.

UltraMetabolism

www.bloodsugarsolution.com/ultrametabolism
This book promises to reprogram your body to automatically lose weight by turning on the messages of weight loss and health and turning off the messages of weight gain and disease.

The UltraMetabolism PBS Special

www.bloodsugarsolution.com/ultrametabolism-dvd
This two-hour special brings the secrets and steps of the UltraMetabolism program home.

The UltraMetabolism Cookbook

www.bloodsugarsolution.com/ultrametabolism-cookbook
This book provides 200 recipes to put the UltraMetabolism program into overdrive. They are also great for *The Blood Sugar Solution*.

The UltraSimple Diet

www.bloodsugarsolution.com/ultrasimple-diet
This simple seven-day program provides you with the tools you need to treat the two primary underlying factors of weight gain—toxins and inflammation—and lose not only weight but many of your chronic health symptoms.

The UltraSimple Challenge

www.bloodsugarsolution.com/ultrasimple-challenge
- **DVD Coaching Program.** Two DVDs include information on why and how the program works, the science behind it, daily motivational and instructional videos, and a special section on how to keep the weight *off* and the health *on* for good.
- **7-Day Action Plan Guide.** This includes meal plans, shopping lists, recommended supplements, exercises and relaxation techniques, daily check-lists, food logs, a journal, and progress trackers.
- **Online Support Community.** Connect with other people on the program and share your experiences. Community support is a critical factor in making long-term changes.

The UltraThyroid Solution

www.bloodsugarsolution.com/ultrathyroid
Learn the seven steps that will help you comprehensively address your low-functioning thyroid and heal from this potentially devastating disorder.

UltraPrevention

www.bloodsugarsolution.com/ultraprevention
This includes an innovative program that shatters the myths of today's "fix the broken parts" medicine.

Five Forces of Wellness

www.bloodsugarsolution.com/5forces
Learn about the five imbalances that lead to disease

and how you can turn them into the five forces of wellness instead.

The Detox Box

www.bloodsugarsolution.com/detoxbox
Designed to remove toxins and allergens, boost immunity, and restore energy, this box, which includes CDs, flash cards, and a quick-start guide, gives you everything you need to complete a safe, effective, and medically informed detoxification program at home.

Nutrigenomics

www.bloodsugarsolution.com/nutrigenomics
Find out which foods you can use to leverage your body's natural ability to heal itself.

TOOLS FOR HEALTHY LIVING, YOGA, AND RELAXATION

There are many wonderful resources available to help you activate the relaxation response and reduce stress. Below is a selection of some of the best CDs, lifestyle products (such as biofeedback tools), and at-home saunas.

CDs and DVDs

Best of Stress Management Kit

James Gordon, MD
www.bloodsugarsolution.com/best-of-stress-management

In plain language, this teaches you the science of stress and relaxation and how to choose the stress management techniques that are right for you.

Mindfulness Meditation Practice CDs

Jon Kabat-Zinn
www.bloodsugarsolution.com/mindfulness-meditation
Dr. Kabat-Zinn provides guided meditations that take you into deep relaxation and healing through exercises that cultivate mindfulness of breath, body sensations, sounds, and meditations on loving kindness.

Health Journeys

www.bloodsugarsolution.com/healthjourneys
Resources for self-healing, including guided imagery tapes.

Natural Journeys

www.bloodsugarsolution.com/naturaljourneys
DVDs on Pilates, yoga, tai chi, fitness, meditation, and self-healing.

Kripalu Center for Yoga and Health

www.bloodsugarsolution.com/kripalu
Many CDs and DVDs to support health and relaxation.

Biofeedback Tools

Journey to Wild Divine

www.bloodsugarsolution.com/wilddivine

A biofeedback computer game that brings deep relaxation.

emWave

www.bloodsugarsolution.com/emwave
From the developers of HeartMath, a personal hand-held device that allows you to retrain your nervous system and reduce stress. It also connects to your computer and comes with many exercises that help soothe your mind and heart.

Saunas for Detoxification

Sunlighten Saunas

www.bloodsugarsolution.com/sunlighten
My preferred source of infrared saunas.

High-Tech Health

www.bloodsugarsolution.com/hightechhealth
Another good source of infrared saunas.

Tracking Your Weight and Blood Pressure

Wi-Fi Body Scale and Blood Pressure Monitor

www.bloodsugarsolution.com/withings
The remarkable Wi-Fi Body Scale allows you to effortlessly and automatically track and graph your weight and BMI, access it from your smartphone or web browser at any time, and share it with your social network and our nutrition and health coaches.

Designed specifically for IOS devices, the Wi-Fi Blood Pressure Monitor connects to your iPhone, iPad, or iPod touch and instantly provides a precise measurement of your blood pressure.

CLEAN AND GREEN

Home Products

The following products are helpful in reducing your toxic load and keeping your home clean and green.

Green Home

www.bloodsugarsolution.com/greenhome
An online department store and resource for all your green living needs, where you can find up-to-date, credible information to help you make decisions about how to improve the quality of your life.

Gaiam

www.bloodsugarsolution.com/gaiam
Gaiam provides information, goods, and services to customers who value the environment, a sustainable economy, healthy lifestyles, alternative health care, and personal development.

H3Environmental Corporation

www.bloodsugarsolution.com/h3environmental
The "H3" in H3Environmental refers to the three homes we inhabit: the home within ourselves, the literal home we live in, and our home on the planet.

H3Environmental provides healthy, sophisticated, elegant home products as well as valuable practical healthy-home information.

EcoChoices Natural Living Store

www.bloodsugarsolution.com/ecochoices
Environmentally friendly products for the home.

Allergy Buyers Club

www.bloodsugarsolution.com/allergybuyersclub
This organization specializes in allergy relief products and education on the control and prevention of allergies, sinusitis, and asthma. Its best-in-class products are natural, green, and hypoallergenic, perfect for a clean, healthy home free of pollutants.

Lifekind

www.bloodsugarsolution.com/lifekind
Lifekind provides information and products to help reduce your daily exposure to hazardous chemicals. It offers safe, certified organic alternatives to products made with unhealthy and toxic ingredients.

Water Filters

Custom Pure

www.bloodsugarsolution.com/custompure
Custom Pure offers a variety of filtration systems. Its trained professionals will help you select the right equipment, install it properly, and maintain it for optimum performance.

Air Filters

AllerAir

www.bloodsugarsolution.com/allerair
AllerAir is dedicated to offering you the safest, most effective air-cleaning technology available. It carries more than a hundred models to meet any air purification need.

Nontoxic Household Cleaning Products

Seventh Generation

www.bloodsugarsolution.com/seventhgeneration
Seventh Generation is the nation's leading brand of household and personal care products that help protect human health and the environment.

Ecover

www.bloodsugarsolution.com/ecover
In a unique ecological factory, Ecover produces washing and cleaning products in an ecological, economic, and socially responsible way.

Life Without Plastic

www.bloodsugarsolution.com/lifewithoutplastic
LWP is an Internet-based retailer offering customers around the world nonplastic alternatives to everyday products such as water bottles, food storage containers, and children's dishes, bottles, and cups.

Clean Cosmetics

Cosmetic Safety Database

www.bloodsugarsolution.com/cosmeticdatabase
This website provides the findings of the Environmental Working Group's six-month investigation into the health and safety of more than 10,000 personal care product ingredients.

The Campaign for Safe Cosmetics

www.bloodsugarsolution.com/safecosmetics
A coalition whose goal is to pass legislation requiring the health and beauty industry to phase out the use of chemicals that are known toxins.

Natural Cosmetics

The following companies produce clean cosmetics.

Dr. Hauschka Skin Care

www.bloodsugarsolution.com/drhauschka

Sophyto Organics

www.bloodsugarsolution.com/sophytoorganics

Avalon Cosmetics

www.bloodsugarsolution.com/avalonorganics

Evan Healy Skincare

www.bloodsugarsolution.com/evanhealy

Sumbody Skincare

www.bloodsugarsolution.com/sumbody

FOOD RESOURCES

You'll find a vast array of organic foods; home care, health care, kitchenware, and pet care products; as well as other valuable resources at these sites.

Organic Essentials

The Organic Pages

www.bloodsugarsolution.com/theorganicpages
According to their website, the Organic Trade Association (OTA) presents The Organic Pages™ to provide users with a quick, easy way to find certified organic products, producers, ingredients, supplies, and services offered by OTA members, as well as items of interest to the entire organic community.

Organic Provisions

www.bloodsugarsolution.com/orgfood
Organic Provisions is a convenient new way of choosing a wide array of quality natural foods and products right from your home.

Organic Planet

www.bloodsugarsolution.com/organic-planet
Organic Planet is a leading supplier of natural and organic food ingredients.

Sun Organic Farm

www.bloodsugarsolution.com/sunorganicfarm
Sun Organic Farm provides a direct source for online ordering of a wide variety of organic foods.

Produce

Earthbound Farms

www.bloodsugarsolution.com/earthboundfarm
Fresh, packaged organic produce.

Maine Coast Sea Vegetables

www.bloodsugarsolution.com/seaveg
A variety of sea vegetables, including some organically certified types.

Organic Frozen and Canned Foods

Cascadian Farm

www.bloodsugarsolution.com/cfarm
A great source of organic frozen fruit and vegetables for those in a hurry.

Stahlbush Island Farms, Inc.

www.bloodsugarsolution.com/stahlbush
An excellent source of sustainably grown frozen berries.

Pacific Foods

www.bloodsugarsolution.com/pacificfoods

Pacific Foods carries high-quality soups, broths, nut milk, hemp milk, and more.

Imagine Foods

www.bloodsugarsolution.com/imaginefoods
A high-quality purveyor of delicious organic soups.

Meat, Poultry, Eggs, and Dairy

Eat Wild

www.bloodsugarsolution.com/eatwild
Grass-fed meat and dairy products.

Organic Valley

www.bloodsugarsolution.com/organicvalley
Organic meats, dairy, eggs, and produce from more than 600 member-owned organic farms.

Peaceful Pastures

www.bloodsugarsolution.com/peacefulpastures
Grass-fed and grass-finished meat, poultry, and dairy products.

Applegate Farms

www.bloodsugarsolution.com/applegatefarms
Packaged poultry, meat, and deli products.

Pete and Gerry's Organic Eggs

www.bloodsugarsolution.com/peteandgerrys
Organic omega-3 eggs.

Stonyfield Farm

www.bloodsugarsolution.com/stonyfield
Certified organic dairy products and soy yogurt.

Fish

Vital Choice Seafood

www.bloodsugarsolution.com/vitalchoice
A selection of fresh, frozen, and canned wild salmon, sardine, black cod, and small halibut.

EcoFish, Inc.

www.bloodsugarsolution.com/ecofish
Environmentally responsible seafood products and information.

Crown Prince Natural

www.bloodsugarsolution.com/crownprince
Wild-caught, sustainably harvested, specialty canned seafood.

SeaBear

www.bloodsugarsolution.com/seabear
Wild salmon jerky for a convenient snack.

Nuts, Seeds, and Oils

Barlean's Organic Oils

www.bloodsugarsolution.com/barleans
Organic oils and ground flaxseeds.

Omega Nutrition

www.bloodsugarsolution.com/omeganutrition
A variety of organic oils, and flax and hemp seed products.

Spectrum Naturals

www.bloodsugarsolution.com/spectrumorganic
An extensive line of high-quality oils, vinegars, flax products, and culinary resources.

Maranatha

www.bloodsugarsolution.com/worldpantry
Organic nut and seed butters.

Once Again Nut Butter

www.bloodsugarsolution.com/onceagainnutbutter
Organic nut and seed butters.

Beans and Legumes

Eden Foods

www.bloodsugarsolution.com/edenfoods
A complete line of organic dried and canned beans.

Westbrae Natural

www.bloodsugarsolution.com/westbrae
A full variety of organic beans and vegetarian products (soups, condiments, pastas, etc.).

ShariAnn's Organic

www.bloodsugarsolution.com/shariannsorganic
Organic beans, refried beans, soups, and more.

Grains

Arrowhead Mills

www.bloodsugarsolution.com/arrowheadmills
Organic grains, including many gluten-free choices.

Lundberg Family Farms

www.bloodsugarsolution.com/lundberg
Organic grains and gluten-free items, such as wild rice.

Hodgson Mill, Inc.

www.bloodsugarsolution.com/hodgsonmill
A complete line of whole grains, including many gluten-free grains.

Shiloh Farms

www.bloodsugarsolution.com/shilohfarms
Organic whole grains, sprouted grains, and gluten-free items.

Spices, Seasonings, Sauces, Soups, and Such

Spice Hunter

www.bloodsugarsolution.com/spicehunter
A complete line of organic spices.

Frontier Natural Products Co-Op

www.bloodsugarsolution.com/frontiernaturalbrands
An extensive line of organic spices, seasonings, baking flavors and extracts, dried foods, teas, and culinary gadgets.

Rapunzel Pure Organics

www.bloodsugarsolution.com/rapunzel
A great selection of seasonings such as Herbamare, made with sea salt and organic herbs.

Seeds of Change

www.bloodsugarsolution.com/seedsofchange
Organic tomato sauces, salsas, and more.

Edward and Sons Trading Co.

www.bloodsugarsolution.com/edwardandsons
An extensive line of vegetarian organic food products, including miso, sauces, brown rice crackers, etc.

Flavorganics

www.bloodsugarsolution.com/flavorganics
A full product line of certified organic pure flavor extracts.

Beverages

Nondairy, Gluten-Free Beverages

Westbrae WestSoy

www.bloodsugarsolution.com/westsoy
Unsweetened soy milk.

Imagine Foods (Soy Dream)

www.bloodsugarsolution.com/tastethedream
Soy and rice milk and ice creams.

White Wave

www.bloodsugarsolution.com/silksoymilk
Silk soy milk beverage.

WholeSoy & Co.

www.bloodsugarsolution.com/wholesoyco
Unsweetened soy yogurt.

Organic Herbal Teas

Mighty Leaf Tea

www.bloodsugarsolution.com/mightyleaf
Artisan-crafted loose teas in biodegradable pouches.

Choice Organic Teas

www.bloodsugarsolution.com/choiceorganicteas
Organic fair-trade teas.

Yogi Tea

www.bloodsugarsolution.com/yogitea
Medicinal herbal teas.

Numi Tea

www.bloodsugarsolution.com/numitea
According to their website, Numi inspires well-being
of mind, body, and spirit through the simple art of tea.

Water

The best water filters are reverse osmosis filters. While they can be more expensive, the investment is worth it as they remove more toxins from your water supply. If your budget won't allow reverse osmosis filters, Brita is a good alternative.

Reverse-Osmosis Filters

www.bloodsugarsolution.com/h2odistributors

Brita Filters

www.bloodsugarsolution.com/brita

NUTRITIONALLY ORIENTED DOCTORS AND ORGANIZATIONS

The following are resources for doctors who can help you work through many of the protocols in this book.

You can visit our team at **The UltraWellness Center** in Lenox, Massachusetts. Go to www .ultrawellnesscenter.com or call (413) 637-9991 for more information on how to make a personal appointment with Dr. Hyman and his specialized team of doctors, nurses, and nutritionists. You can also use the resources listed below to find additional recommendations.

The Institute for Functional Medicine (IFM)

www.functionalmedicine.org
I am the chairman of the board of IFM, a 501c3 nonprofit whose mission is to serve the highest expression of individual health through widespread adoption of functional medicine as the standard of care.

American Board of Holistic Medicine

www.holisticboard.org
The goal of the ABIHM is to establish standards of care in the application of the body of knowledge encompassed by integrative holistic medicine, so that these concepts can be fully integrated into medical practices, education, health planning, and research.

American Academy of Environmental Medicine

www.aaem.com
The mission of the American Academy of Environmental Medicine is to promote optimal health through prevention, and safe and effective treatment of the causes of illness by supporting physicians and other professionals in serving the public through education about the interaction between humans and their environment.

American College for Advancement in Medicine

www.acam.org
An educational organization training physicians and health care providers in integrative and functional

medicine, with specialization in detoxification and chelation.

LABORATORIES FOR SPECIALIZED TESTING

You can get the tests outlined in this program through the following labs. Work with a doctor trained in integrative or functional medicine to get the tests you need.

Quest Diagnostics

www.bloodsugarsolution.com/questdiagnostics
A resource for most conventional laboratory testing needs.

LabCorp

www.bloodsugarsolution.com/labcorp
Most conventional laboratory testing is available here.

LipoScience

www.bloodsugarsolution.com/liposcience
Innovative nuclear medicine spectroscopy for the assessment of lipid particle size and improved accuracy in assessing cardiovascular risk factors. This test is also done through LabCorp.

IGeneX

www.bloodsugarsolution.com/igenex
Specialized testing for detecting chronic infections (such as Lyme disease) with PCR technology.

Doctor's Data

www.bloodsugarsolution.com/doctorsdata
Experts in testing for heavy metal toxicity and other nutritional and metabolic disorders.

Metametrix

www.bloodsugarsolution.com/metametrix
Leaders in nutritional and metabolic testing.

Genova Diagnostics

www.bloodsugarsolution.com/genovadiagnostics
Offering genetic, functional, metabolic, and nutritional testing.

Immuno Laboratories

www.bloodsugarsolution.com/TheRightFoodForYou
IgG food-sensitivity testing.

Medical Diagnostic Laboratories

www.bloodsugarsolution.com/mdlab
Advanced infection testing.

DiagnosTechs

www.bloodsugarsolution.com/diagnostechs
Saliva testing for adrenal function, stress hormones, and more.

Prometheus Labs

www.bloodsugarsolution.com/prometheuslabs
Testing for gluten and celiac disease.

Notes

Introduction

1. Garber AJ, et al. Diagnosis and management of pre-diabetes in the continuum of hyperglycemia: when do the risks of diabetes begin? A consensus statement from the American College of Endocrinology and the American Association of Clinical Endocrinologists. *Endocr Pract.* 2008 Oct;14(7):933–46.

2. DECODE Study Group, European Diabetes Epidemiology Group. Is the current definition for diabetes relevant to mortality risk from all causes and cardiovascular and noncardiovascular diseases? *Diabetes Care.* 2003 Mar;26(3):688–96.

Chapter 1. A Hidden Epidemic: The United States of Diabetes

1. Lin SX, Pi-Sunyer EX Prevalence of the metabolic syndrome among US middle-aged and older adults with and without diabetes—a preliminary analysis of the NHANES 1999–2002 data. *Ethn Dis.* 2007 Winter;17(1):35–39.

2. http://www.who.int/mediacentre/news/releases/ 2007/pr61/en/index.html.

3. Chan JC, et al. Diabetes in Asia: epidemiology, risk factors, and pathophysiology. *JAMA*. 2009 May 27;301(20):2129–40. Review.

4. http://apps.nccd.cdc.gov/DDTSTRS/FactSheet.aspx (National Diabetes Fact Sheet 2007).

5. http://www.cdc.gov/diabetes/statistics/cvd/fig5 .htm.

6. Lakka HM, et al. The metabolic syndrome and total and cardiovascular disease mortality in middle-aged men. *JAMA*. 2002 Dec 4;288(21): 2709–16.

7. Ott A, et al. Diabetes mellitus and the risk of dementia: The Rotterdam Study. *Neurology*. 1999 Dec 10;53(9):1937–42.

8. Key T, Reeves GK, Spencer EA. Symposium 1: Overnutrition: consequences and solutions for obesity and cancer risk. *Proc Nutr Soc*. 2009 Dec 3:1–5.

9. Targher G, Day CP, Bonora E. Risk of cardiovascular disease in patients with nonalcoholic fatty liver disease. *N Engl J Med*. 2010 Sep 30;363(14):1341– 50. Review.

10. Pan A, et al. Bidirectional association between depression and type 2 diabetes mellitus in women. *Arch Intern Med*. 2010 Nov 22;170(21):1884–91.

11. Emerging Risk Factors Collaboration et al. Diabetes mellitus, fasting glucose, and risk of cause-specific death. *N Engl J Med*. 2011 Mar 3;364(9): 829–41.

12. Huang ES, Basu A, O'Grady M, Capretta JC. Projecting the future: diabetes population size and related costs for the U.S. *Diabetes Care.* 2009 Dec;32(12):2225–29.

13. Seligman HK, Schillinger D. Hunger and socioeconomic disparities in chronic disease. *N Engl J Med.* 2010 Jul 1;363(1):6–9.

14. Yach D, Hawkes C, Gould CL, Hofman KJ. The global burden of chronic diseases: overcoming impediments to prevention and control. *JAMA.* 2004 Jun 2;291(21):2616–22.

15. Ibid.

Chapter 2. The Real Causes of Diabesity

1. Action to Control Cardiovascular Risk in Diabetes Study Group, Gerstein HC, et al. Effects of intensive glucose lowering in type 2 diabetes. *N Engl J Med.* 2008 Jun 12;358(24):2545–59.

2. Chen L, et al. Reduction in consumption of sugar-sweetened beverages is associated with weight loss: the PREMIER trial. *Am J Clin Nutr.* 2009 May; 89(5):1299–306.

3. Bhashyam S, et al. Aging is associated with myocardial insulin resistance and mitochondrial dysfunction. *Am J Physiol Heart Circ Physiol.* 2007 Nov; 293(5):H3063–71.

4. Ryan AS. Insulin resistance with aging: effects of diet and exercise. *Sports Med.* 2000 Nov;30(5): 327–46. Review.

5. Gaziano JM, et al. Fasting triglycerides, high-density lipoprotein, and risk of myocardial infarction. *Circulation*. 1997 Oct 21;96(8):2520–25.

Chapter 3. Seven Myths About Obesity and Diabetes That Keep Us Sick

1. McCarthy MI. Genomics, type 2 diabetes, and obesity. *N Engl J Med*. 2010 Dec 9;363(24):2339–50. Review.
2. Rappaport SM. Implications of the exposome for exposure science. *J Expo Sci Environ Epidemiol*. 2011 Jan;21(1):5–9.
3. Lichtenstein P, et al. Environmental and heritable factors in the causation of cancer—analyses of cohorts of twins from Sweden, Denmark, and Finland. *N Engl J Med*. 2000 Jul 13;343(2):78–85.
4. Olshansky SJ, et al. A potential decline in life expectancy in the United States in the 21st century. *N Engl J Med*. 2005 Mar 17;352(11):1138–45.
5. Bibbins-Domingo K, et al. Adolescent overweight and future adult coronary heart disease. *N Engl J Med*. 2007 Dec 6;357(23):2371–79.
6. Diabetes Prevention Program Research Group, Knowler WC, et al. 10-year follow-up of diabetes incidence and weight loss in the Diabetes Prevention Program Outcomes Study. *Lancet*. 2009 Nov 14;374(9702):1677–86.
7. Lim EL, et al. Reversal of type 2 diabetes: normalisation of beta cell function in association with decreased pancreas and liver triacylglycerol. *Diabetologia*. 2011 Oct;54(10):2506–14.

8. Henry B, Kalynovskyi S. Reversing diabetes and obesity naturally: a NEWSTART lifestyle program. *Diabetes Educ.* 2004 Jan-Feb;30(1):48–50, 55–56, 58–59.

9. Jessani S, et al. Should oral glucose tolerance testing be mandatory following acute myocardial infarction? *Int J Clin Pract.* 2007 Apr;61(4):680–83.

10. Khaw KT, et al. Association of hemoglobin A1c with cardiovascular disease acute mortality in adults: the European prospective investigation into cancer in Norfolk. *Ann Intern Med.* 2004 Sep 21;141(6):413–20.

11. Yaffe K, et al. The metabolic syndrome, inflammation, and risk of cognitive decline. *JAMA.* 2004 Nov 10;292(18):2237–42.

12. de la Monte SM, Wands JR. Alzheimer's disease is type 3 diabetes — evidence reviewed. *J Diabetes Sci Technol.* 2008 Nov;2(6):1101–13.

13. Stein JL, Jack CR Jr, Weiner MW, Toga AW, Thompson PM; Cardiovascular Health Study; ADNI. Obesity is linked with lower brain volume in 700 AD and MCI patients. *Neurobiol Aging.* 2010 Aug;31(8):1326–39.

14. http://www.acpm.org/LifestyleMedicine.htm.

15. Haffner SM, et al. Mortality from coronary heart disease in subjects with type 2 diabetes and in nondiabetic subjects with and without prior myocardial infarction. *N Engl J Med.* 1998;339: 229–34.

16. The NAVIGATOR Study Group. Effect of nateglinide on the incidence of diabetes and cardiovascular

events. *N Engl J Med.* 2010. Apr 22;362(16): 1463–76.

17. The NAVIGATOR Study Group. Effect of valsartan on the incidence of diabetes and cardiovascular events. *N Engl J Med.* 2010. Apr 22;362(16):1477–90.

18. The ACCORD Study Group. Effects of combination lipid therapy in type 2 diabetes mellitus. *N Engl J Med.* 2010. Apr 29;362(17):1563–74.

19. Taylor F, et al. Statins for the primary prevention of cardiovascular disease. *Cochrane Database Syst Rev.* 2011 Jan 19:CD004816.

20. Abramson J, Wright JM. Are lipid-lowering guidelines evidence-based? *Lancet.* 2007 Jan 20;369 (9557):168–89.

21. Sirvent P, Mercier J, Lacampagne A. New insights into mechanisms of statin-associated myotoxicity. *Curr Opin Pharmacol.* 2008 Jun;8(3):333–38.

22. Kuncl RW. Agents and mechanisms of toxic myopathy. *Curr Opin Neurol.* 2009 Oct;22(5):506–15. PubMed PMID: 19680127.

23. Tsivgoulis G, et al. Presymptomatic Neuromuscular Disorders Disclosed Following Statin Treatment. *Arch Intern Med.* 2006;166:1519–24.

24. Preiss D, et al. Risk of incident diabetes with intensive-dose compared with moderate-dose statin therapy: a meta-analysis. *JAMA.* 2011 Jun 22;305 (24):2556–64.

25. The BARI 2D Study Group. A randomized trial of therapies for type 2 diabetes and coronary artery disease. *N Engl J Med.* 2009 Jun 11;360:2503.

26. Newman MF, et al. Neurological Outcome Research Group and the Cardiothoracic Anesthesiology Research Endeavors Investigators. Longitudinal assessment of neurocognitive function after coronary-artery bypass surgery. *N Engl J Med.* 2001 Feb 8;344(6):395–402.

27. Saliba J, Wattacheril J, Abumrad NN. Endocrine and metabolic response to gastric bypass. *Curr Opin Clin Nutr Metab Care.* 2009 Sep;12(5):515–21. Review.

28. Sturm W, et al. Effect of bariatric surgery on both functional and structural measures of premature atherosclerosis. *Eur Heart J.* 2009 Aug;30(16): 2038–43.

Chapter 4. Food Addiction: Fixing Your Brain Chemistry

1. Gearhardt AN, Corbin WR, Brownell KD. Preliminary validation of the Yale Food Addiction Scale. *Appetite.* 2009;52(2):430–36.

2. Gearhardt A, et al. Food addiction, an examination of the diagnostic criteria for dependence. *J Addict Med.* 2009;3:1–7.

3. Colantuoni C, Schwenker J, McCarthy P, et al. Excessive sugar intake alters binding to dopamine and mu-opioid receptors in the brain. *Neuroreport.* 2001;12(16):3549–52.

4. Volkow, ND, Wang, GJ, Fowler, JS, et al. "Nonhedonic" food motivation in humans involves dopamine in the dorsal striatum and methylphenidate amplifies this effect. *Synapse.* 2002;44(3): 175–80.

5. Malik VS, Schulze MB, Hu FB. Intake of sugar-sweetened beverages and weight gain: a systematic review. *Am J Clin Nutr.* 2006 Aug;84(2):274–88. Review.

6. Brownell KD, et al. The public health and economic benefits of taxing sugar-sweetened beverages. *N Engl J Med.* 2009 Oct 15;361(16):1599–605. Epub 2009 Sep 16.

7. Wang YC, et al. Impact of change in sweetened caloric beverage consumption on energy intake among children and adolescents. *Arch Pediatr Adolesc Med.* 2009 Apr;163(4):336–43.

8. Ludwig DS, Peterson KE, Gortmaker SL. Relation between consumption of sugar-sweetened drinks and childhood obesity: a prospective, observational analysis. *Lancet.* 2001;357:505–8.

9. Ellenbogen SJ, et al. Effects of decreasing sugar-sweetened beverage consumption on body weight in adolescents: a randomized, controlled pilot study. *Pediatrics.* 2006;117:673–80.

10. Schulze MB, et al. Sugar-sweetened beverages, weight gain, and incidence of type 2 diabetes in young and middle-aged women. *JAMA.* 2004; 292(8):927–34.

11. Palmer JR, et al. Sugar sweetened beverages and incidence of type 2 diabetes mellitus in African American women. *Arch Intern Med.* 2008;168(14):1487–92.

12. Fung TT, et al. Sweetened beverage consumption and risk of coronary heart disease in women. *Am J Clin Nutr.* 2009;89(4):1037–42.

13. Malik VS, Schulze MB, Hu FB. Intake of sugar-sweetened beverages and weight gain: a systematic review. *Am J Clin Nutr.* 2006;84(2):274–88.

14. Wang YC, et al. Impact of change in sweetened caloric beverage consumption on energy intake among children and adolescents. *Arch Pediatr Adolesc Med.* 2009;163(4):336–343.

15. Dennis EA, et al. Water consumption increases weight loss during a hypocaloric diet intervention in middle-aged and older adults. *Obesity.* 2010 Feb;18(2):300–7.

16. Forshee RA, Anderson PA, Storey ML. Sugar-sweetened beverages and body mass index in children and adolescents: A metaanalysis. *Am J Clin Nutr.* 2008:87:1662–71.

17. Lesser LI, et al. Relationship between funding source and conclusion among nutrition-related scientific articles. *PLoS Med.* 2007 Jan;4(1):e5.

18. http://consumerfreedom.com/about.cfm.

19. Swithers SE, Davidson TL. A role for sweet taste: calorie predictive relations in energy regulation by rats. *Behav Neurosci.* 2008;122(1):161–73.

20. Lenoir M, et al. Intense sweetness surpasses cocaine reward. *PLoS One.* 2007;2(1):e698.

21. Ludwig DS. Artificially sweetened beverages: cause for concern. *JAMA.* 2009 Dec 9;302(22):2477–78.

Chapter 5. How Big Food, Big Farming, and Big Pharma Are Killing Us

1. http://www.theatlantic.com/life/archive/2011/04/new-federal-guidelines-regulate-junk-food-ads-for-kids/238053/.
2. Nestle M. Food marketing and childhood obesity—a matter of policy. *N Engl J Med.* 2006 Jun 15;354(24):2527–29.
3. http://www.cspinet.org/new/200709171.html.
4. Kahneman DA. Perspective on judgment and choice: mapping bounded rationality. *Am Psychol.* 2003 Sep;58(9):697–720. Review.
5. Barry CL, et al. Obesity metaphors: how beliefs about the causes of obesity affect support for public policy. *Milbank Q.* 2009 Mar;87(1):7–47.

Chapter 6. Functional Medicine: A New Approach to Reverse This Epidemic

1. Snyderman R, Williams RS. Prospective medicine: the next health care transformation. *Acad Med.* 2003 Nov;78(11):1079–80.
2. Nelson RA, Bremer AA. Insulin resistance and metabolic syndrome in the pediatric population. *Metab Syndr Relat Disord.* 2010 Feb;8(1):1–14.
3. Silverstein JH, Rosenbloom AL. Type 2 diabetes in children. *Curr Diab Rep.* 2001 Aug;1(1):19–27. Review.
4. The Textbook of Functional Medicine. Institute of Functional Medicine, 2005.

Chapter 7. Understanding the Seven Steps

1. Choi HK, Willett W, Curhan G. Fructose-rich beverages and risk of gout in women. *JAMA*. 2010 Nov 24;304(20):2270–78.

Chapter 8. Step 1: Boost Your Nutrition

1. Gillis L, Gillis A. Nutrient inadequacy in obese and non-obese youth. *Can J Diet Pract Res*. 2005 Winter;66(4):237–42.
2. Cordain L, et al. Origin and evolution of the Western diet: health implications for the 21st century. *Am J Clin Nutr*. 2005;8(2):341–54. Review.
3. United States Department of Agriculture. Agriculture Factbook Chapter 2: Profiling Food Consumption in America. 2001. Accessed online (http://www.usda.gov/factbook/chapter2.pdf).
4. Dufault R, et al. Mercury from chlor-alkali plants: measured concentrations in food product sugar. *Environ Health*. 2009 Jan 26;8:2.
5. Bray GA, Nielsen SJ, Popkin BM. Consumption of high-fructose corn syrup in beverages may play a role in the epidemic of obesity. *Am J Clin Nutr*. 2004 Apr;79(4):537–43. Review.
6. Eaton SB, Konner M. Paleolithic nutrition: a consideration of its nature and current implications. *N Engl J Med*. 1985 Jan 31;312(5):283–89. Review.
7. Robson AA. Preventing diet induced disease: bioavailable nutrient-rich, low-energy-dense diets. *Nutr Health*. 2009;20(2):135-66. Review.

8. Chandalia M, et al. Beneficial effects of high dietary fiber intake in patients with type 2 diabetes mellitus. *N Engl J Med*. 2000 May 11;342(19):1392–98.

9. Reis JP, et al. Vitamin D status and cardiometabolic risk factors in the United States adolescent population. *Pediatrics*. 2009 Sep;124(3):e371–79.

10. A scientific review: the role of chromium in insulin resistance. *Diabetes Educ*. 2004;Suppl:2–14. Review.

11. Lau FC, Bagchi M, Sen CK, Bagchi D. Nutrigenomic basis of beneficial effects of chromium(III) on obesity and diabetes. *Mol Cell Biochem*. 2008 Oct;317(1–2):1–10. *Epub*. 2008 Jul 18. Review.

12. Chaudhary DP, Sharma R, Bansal DD. Implications of magnesium deficiency in type 2 diabetes: A review. *Biol Trace Elem Res*. 2010 May;134(2):119–29.

13. Masood N, et al. Serum zinc and magnesium in type-2 diabetic patients. *J Coll Physicians Surg Pak*. 2009 Aug;19(8):483–86.

14. Albarracin CA, et al. Chromium picolinate and biotin combination improves glucose metabolism in treated, uncontrolled overweight to obese patients with type 2 diabetes. *Diabetes Metab Res Rev*. 2008 Jan-Feb;24(1):41–51.

15. Flachs P, et al. Cellular and molecular effects of n-3 polyunsaturated fatty acids on adipose tissue biology and metabolism. *Clin Sci*. 2009 Jan;116(1):1–16. Review.

16. Shay KP, et al. Alpha-lipoic acid as a dietary supplement: molecular mechanisms and therapeutic potential. *Biochim Biophys Acta*. 2009 Oct;1790 (10):1149–60.

17. Ornish D, et al. Changes in prostate gene expression in men undergoing an intensive nutrition and lifestyle intervention. *Proc Natl Acad Sci U S A.* 2008 Jun 17;105(24):8369–74.

18. Kallio P, et al. Dietary carbohydrate modification induces alterations in gene expression in abdominal subcutaneous adipose tissue in persons with the metabolic syndrome: the FUNGENUT Study. *Am J Clin Nutr.* 2007 May;85(5):1417–27.

19. Salsberg SL, Ludwig DS. Putting your genes on a diet: the molecular effects of carbohydrate. *Am J Clin Nutr.* 2007 May;85(5):1169–70.

20. Giugliano D, Esposito K. Mediterranean diet and metabolic diseases. *Curr Opin Lipidol.* 2008 Feb; 19(1):63–68. Review.

21. Reis JP, et al. Vitamin D status and cardio-metabolic risk factors in the United States adolescent population. *Pediatrics.* 2009 Sep;124(3): e371–79.

22. Chaudhary DP, Sharma R, Bansal DD. Implications of magnesium deficiency in type 2 diabetes: A review. *Biol Trace Elem Res.* 2010 May;134(2): 119–29.

23. Poh Z, Goh KP. Current update on the use of alpha lipoic acid in the management of type 2 diabetes mellitus. *Endocr Metab Immune Disord Drug Targets.* 2009 Dec;9(4): 392–98.

24. Kligler B, Lynch D. An integrative approach to the management of type 2 diabetes mellitus. *Altern Ther Health Med.* 2003 Nov-Dec;9(6):24–32; quiz 33. Review.

25. Kelly GS. Insulin resistance: lifestyle and nutritional interventions. *Altern Med Rev.* 2000 Apr; 5(2):109–32. Review.
26. Kreisberg J. Learning from organic agriculture. *Explore.* 2006 Sep-Oct;2(5):450–52. Review.
27. Fairfield KM, Fletcher RH. Vitamins for chronic disease prevention in adults: scientific review. *JAMA.* 2002 Jun 19;287(23):3116–26. Review.

Chapter 9. Step 2: Regulate Your Hormones

1. Maratou E, et al. Studies of insulin resistance in patients with clinical and subclinical hypothyroidism. *Eur J Endocrinol.* 2009 May;160(5): 785–90.
2. Ayturk S, et al. Metabolic syndrome and its components are associated with increased thyroid volume and nodule prevalence in a mild-to-moderate iodine-deficient area. *Eur J Endocrinol.* 2009 Oct; 161(4):599–605.
3. Golden SH. A review of the evidence for a neuroendocrine link between stress, depression and diabetes mellitus. *Curr Diabetes Rev.* 2007 Nov;3(4):252–59. Review.
4. Van Cauter E, et al. Impact of sleep and sleep loss on neuroendocrine and metabolic function. *Horm Res.* 2007;67 Suppl 1:2–9.
5. Garruti G, et al. Adipose tissue, metabolic syndrome and polycystic ovary syndrome: from pathophysiology to treatment. *Reprod Biomed Online.* 2009 Oct;19(4):552–63.

6. Chavarro JE, et al. Diet and lifestyle in the prevention of ovulatory disorder infertility. *Obstet Gynecol.* 2007 Nov;110(5):1050–58.

7. Chavarro JE, et al. Use of multivitamins, intake of B vitamins, and risk of ovulatory infertility. *Fertil Steril.* 2008 Mar;89(3):668–76.

8. Rhodes ET, et al. Effects of a low-glycemic load diet in overweight and obese pregnant women: a pilot randomized controlled trial. *Am J Clin Nutr.* 2010 Dec;92(6):1306–15.

9. Zitzmann M. Testosterone deficiency, insulin resistance and the metabolic syndrome. *Nat Rev Endocrinol.* 2009 Dec;5(12):673–81.

Chapter 10. Step 3: Reduce Inflammation

1. Deng Y, Scherer PE. Adipokines as novel biomarkers and regulators of the metabolic syndrome. *Ann NY Acad Sci.* 2010 Nov;1212(1):E1–E19.

2. Sedghizadeh PP, et al. Celiac disease and recurrent aphthous stomatitis: a report and review of the literature. *Oral Surg, Oral Med, Oral Pathol, Oral Radiol, and Endod.* 2002 Oct;94(4):474–78. Review.

3. Freeman MP, et al. Omega-3 fatty acids: evidence basis for treatment and future research in psychiatry. *J Clin Psychiatry.* 2006 Dec;67(12):1954–67. Review.

4. Vasquez, A. The clinical importance of vitamin D (cholecalciferol): a paradigm shift with implications for all healthcare providers, *Altern Ther Health Med.* 2004 Sep–Oct;10(5):28–36.

5. Holick, M. Vitamin D: importance in the prevention of cancers, type 1 diabetes, heart disease and osteoporosis. *Am J Clin Nutr.* 2004;79:362–71.

6. Wilkins CH, et al. Vitamin D deficiency is associated with low mood and worse cognitive performance in older adults. *Am J Geriatr Psychiatry.* 2006 Dec;14(12):1032–40.

7. Mischoulon D, Raab MF. The role of folate in depression and dementia. *J Clin Psychiatry.* 2007;68 Suppl 10:28–33. Review.

8. Penninx BW, et al. Vitamin B(12) deficiency and depression in physically disabled older women: epidemiologic evidence from the Women's Health and Aging Study. *Am J Psychiatry.* 2000 May;157(5): 715–21.

9. Almeida C, et al. Subclinical hypothyroidism: psychiatric disorders and symptoms. *Rev Bras Psiquiatr.* 2007 Jun;29(2):157–59.

10. Smith RN, et al. A low-glycemic-load diet improves symptoms in acne vulgaris patients: a randomized controlled trial. *Am J Clin Nutr.* 2007 Jul;86(1): 107–15.

11. Koponen H, et al. Metabolic syndrome predisposes to depressive symptoms: a population-based 7-year follow-up study. *J Clin Psychiatry.* 2008 Feb; 69(2):178–82.

12. Ludvigsson JF, et al. Coeliac disease and risk of mood disorders—a general population-based cohort study. *J Affect Disord.* 2007 Apr;99(1–3):117–26. Epub 2006 Oct 6.

13. Ch'ng CL, Jones MK, Kingham JG. Celiac disease and autoimmune thyroid disease. *Clin Med Res.* 2007 Oct;5(3):184–92. Review.

14. Wilders-Truschnig M, et al. IgG antibodies against food antigens are correlated with inflammation and intima media thickness in obese juveniles. *Exp Clin Endocrinol Diabetes.* 2008 Apr;116(4): 241–45.

15. Pradhan AD, et al. C-reactive protein, interleukin 6, and risk of developing type 2 diabetes mellitus. *JAMA.* 2001 Jul 18;286(3):327–34.

16. Wilders-Truschnig M, et al. IgG antibodies against food antigens are correlated with inflammation and intima media thickness in obese juveniles. *Exp Clin Endocrinol Diabetes.* 2008 Apr;116(4):241–45.

17. Pelsser, et al. Effects of a restricted elimination diet on the behaviour of children with attention-deficit hyperactivity disorder (INCA study): a randomised controlled trial. *Lancet.* 2011;377:494–503.

18. Cortese S, Morcillo Peñalver C. Comorbidity between ADHD and obesity: exploring shared mechanisms and clinical implications. *Postgrad Med.* 2010 Sep; 122(5):88–96. Review.

19. Rubio-Tapia A, et al. Increased prevalence and mortality in undiagnosed celiac disease. *Gastroenterology.* 2009 Jul;137(1):88–93.

20. Ludvigsson JF, et al. Small-intestinal histopathology and mortality risk in celiac disease. *JAMA.* 2009 Sep 16;302(11):1171–78.

21. Sapone A, et al. Divergence of gut permeability and mucosal immune gene expression in two

gluten-associated conditions: celiac disease and gluten sensitivity. *BMC Med.* 2011 Mar 9;9:23.

22. Catassi C, Fasano A. Celiac disease diagnosis: simple rules are better than complicated algorithms. *Am J Med.* 2010 Aug;123(8):691–93.

23. Atkinson RL. Viruses as an etiology of obesity. *Mayo Clin Proc.* 2007 Oct;82(10):1192–98. Review.

24. Navas-Acien A, et al. Arsenic exposure and prevalence of type 2 diabetes in US adults. *JAMA.* 2008 Aug 20;300(7):814–22.

25. Jones OA, Maguire ML, Griffin JL. Environmental pollution and diabetes: a neglected association. *Lancet.* 2008 Jan 26;371(9609):287–88.

26. Munhoz CD, et al. Stress-induced neuroinflammation: mechanisms and new pharmacological targets. *Braz J Med Biol Res.* 2008 Dec;41(12):1037–46. Review.

27. Smith JK, et al. Long-term exercise and atherogenic activity of blood mononuclear cells in persons at risk of developing ischemic heart disease. *JAMA.* 1999 May 12;281(18):1722–27.

28. Church TS, et al. Reduction of C-reactive protein levels through use of a multivitamin. *Am J Med.* 2003 Dec 15;115(9):702–7.

Chapter 11. Step 4: Improve Your Digestion

1. Larsen N, et al. Gut microbiota in human adults with type 2 diabetes differs from non-diabetic adults. *PLoS One.* 2010 Feb 5;5(2):e9085.

2. Tsai F, Coyle WJ. The microbiome and obesity: is obesity linked to our gut flora? *Curr Gastroenterol Rep.* 2009 Aug;11(4):307–13. Review.

3. Bäckhed F, Ding H, Wang T, Hooper LV, Koh GY, Nagy A, Semenkovich CF, Gordon JI. The gut microbiota as an environmental factor that regulates fat storage. *Proc Natl Acad Sci U S A.* 2004 Nov 2;101(44):15718–23.

4. Cani PD, et al. Metabolic endotoxemia initiates obesity and insulin resistance. *Diabetes.* 2007 Jul; 56(7):1761–72.

Chapter 12. Step 5: Maximize Detoxification

1. Jones OA, Maguire ML, Griffin JL. Environmental pollution and diabetes: a neglected association. *Lancet.* 2008 Jan 26;371(9609):287–88.

2. http://www.ewg.org/reports/bodyburden2/news release.php.

3. Lang IA, et al. Association of urinary bisphenol A concentration with medical disorders and laboratory abnormalities in adults. *JAMA.* 2008 Sep 17;300(11): 1303–10.

4. Lee DH, et al. A strong dose-response relation between serum concentrations of persistent organic pollutants and diabetes: results from the National Health and Examination Survey 1999–2002. *Diabetes Care.* 2006 Jul;29(7):1638–44.

5. Navas-Acien A, Silbergeld EK, Pastor-Barriuso R, Guallar E. Arsenic exposure and prevalence of type

2 diabetes in US adults. *JAMA.* 2008 Aug 20; 300(7):814–22.

6. Fujiyoshi PT, Michalek JE, Matsumura F. Molecular epidemiologic evidence for diabetogenic effects of dioxin exposure in U.S. Air Force veterans of the Vietnam War. *Environ Health Perspect.* 2006 Nov; 114(11):1677–83.

7. Chen JQ, Brown TR, Russo J. Regulation of energy metabolism pathways by estrogens and estrogenic chemicals and potential implications in obesity associated with increased exposure to endocrine disruptors. *Biochim Biophys Acta.* 2009 Jul;1793(7): 1128–43. Review.

8. Hyman M. Systems biology, toxins, obesity, and functional medicine. *Altern Ther Health Med.* 2007 Mar–Apr;13(2):S134–39. Review.

9. Remillard RB, Bunce NJ. Linking dioxins to diabetes: epidemiology and biologic plausibility. *Environ Health Perspect.* 2002 Sep;110(9):853–38. Review.

10. Griffin JL, Scott J, Nicholson JK. The influence of pharmacogenetics on fatty liver disease in the wistar and kyoto rats: a combined transcriptomic and metabonomic study. *J Proteome Res.* 2007 Jan; 6(1):54–61.

Chapter 13. Step 6: Enhance Energy Metabolism

1. Hampton T. Mitochondrial defects may play role in the metabolic syndrome. *JAMA.* 2004 Dec 15; 292(23):2823–24.

2. Petersen KF, et al. Impaired mitochondrial activity in the insulin-resistant offspring of patients with type 2 diabetes. *N Engl J Med.* 2004 Feb 12; 350(7):664–71.

3. Henriksen EJ, Diamond-Stanic MK, Marchionne EM. Oxidative stress and the etiology of insulin resistance and type 2 diabetes. *Free Radic Biol Med.* 2011 Sep 1;51(5):993–99.

4. Thomas DE, Elliott EJ, Naughton GA. Exercise for type 2 diabetes mellitus. *Cochrane Database Syst Rev.* 2006 Jul 19;3:CD002968. Review.

5. Fontana L. The scientific basis of caloric restriction leading to longer life. *Curr Opin Gastroenterol.* 2009 Mar;25(2):144–50. Review.

6. Valerio A, D'Antona G, Nisoli E. Branched-chain amino acids, mitochondrial biogenesis, and health-span: an evolutionary perspective. *Aging.* 2011 May;3(5):464–78.

7. http://www.ultrawellness.com/blog/resveratrol.

Chapter 14. Step 7: Soothe Your Mind

1. Holt RI, et al. Hertfordshire Cohort Study Group. The relationship between depression and diabetes mellitus: findings from the Hertfordshire Cohort Study. *Diabet Med.* 2009 Jun;26(6): 641–48.

2. Pan A, et al. Bidirectional association between depression and type 2 diabetes mellitus in women. *Arch Intern Med.* 2010 Nov 22;170(21): 1884–91.

Chapter 15. Start the Journey

1. Dufault R, et al. Mercury from chlor-alkali plants: measured concentrations in food product sugar. *Environ Health.* 2009 Jan 26;8:2.

Chapter 16. Harness the Power of Community

1. Boltri JM, et al. Diabetes prevention in a faith-based setting: results of translational research. *J Public Health Manag Pract.* 2008;14(1):29–32.
2. Knowler WC, et al. Reduction in the incidence of type 2 diabetes with lifestyle intervention or metformin. *N Engl J Med.* 2002;346 (6):393–403.
3. Diabetes Prevention Program Research Group, et al. 10-year follow up of diabetes incidence and weight loss in the Diabetes Prevention Program Outcomes Study. *Lancet.* 2009 Nov 14;374(9702):1677–86.
4. Ilanne-Parikka P, et al. Finnish Diabetes Prevention Study Group. Effect of lifestyle intervention on the occurrence of metabolic syndrome and its components in the Finnish Diabetes Prevention Study. *Diabetes Care.* 2008 Apr;31(4):805–7.
5. Look AHEAD Research Group, Wing RR. Long-term effects of a lifestyle intervention on weight and cardiovascular risk factors in individuals with type 2 diabetes mellitus: four-year results of the Look AHEAD trial. *Arch Intern Med.* 2010 Sep 27; 170(17):1566–75.
6. United Health Center for Health Reform and Modernization, The United States of Diabetes. November 2010 (www.unitedhealthgroup.com/reform).

Chapter 17. Take a Measure of Yourself

1. Schneider HJ, et al. The predictive value of different measures of obesity for incident cardiovascular events and mortality. *J Clin Endocrinol Metab.* 2010 Apr;95(4):1777–85.

Chapter 19. Week 1: Eat Your Medicine: Nutrition Basics

1. Ebbeling CB, Leidig MM, Feldman HA, Lovesky MM, Ludwig DS. Effects of a low-glycemic load vs low-fat diet in obese young adults: a randomized trial. *JAMA.* 2007 May 16;297(19):2092–102.
2. Larsen TM, et al. Diet, Obesity, and Genes (Diogenes) Project. Diets with high or low protein content and glycemic index for weight-loss maintenance. *N Engl J Med.* 2010 Nov 25;363(22):2102–13.
3. Campbell TC. A study on diet, nutrition and disease in the People's Republic of China. Part I. *Bol Asoc Med P R.* 1990 Mar;82(3):132–34.
4. Campbell TC. A study on diet, nutrition and disease in the People's Republic of China. Part II. *Bol Asoc Med P R.* 1990 Jul;82(7):316–18. Review.
5. Jiang R, et al. Nut and peanut butter consumption and risk of type 2 diabetes in women. *JAMA.* 2002 Nov 27;288(20):2554–60.
6. Fung TT, et al. Dietary patterns, meat intake, and the risk of type 2 diabetes in women. *Arch Intern Med.* 2004 Nov 8;164(20):2235–40.
7. Arya F, et al. Differences in postprandial inflammatory responses to a 'modern' v. traditional meat meal: a preliminary study. *Br J Nutr.* 2010 Sep;104(5):724–28.

8. Luopajärvi K, et al. Enhanced levels of cow's milk antibodies in infancy in children who develop type 1 diabetes later in childhood. *Pediatr Diabetes.* 2008 Oct;9(5):434–41.

9. Frisk G, et al. A unifying hypothesis on the development of type 1 diabetes and celiac disease: gluten consumption may be a shared causative factor. *Med Hypotheses.* 2008;70(6):1207–9.

10. de Kort S, Keszthelyi D, Masclee AA. Leaky gut and diabetes mellitus: what is the link? *Obes Rev.* 2011 Jun;12(6)449–500.

11. Hoppe C, et al. High intakes of milk, but not meat, increase s-insulin and insulin resistance in 8-year-old boys. *Eur J Clin Nutr.* 2005;59:393–98.

12. Liljeberg EH, Bjorck I. Milk as a supplement to mixed meals may elevate postprandial insulinanemia. *Eur J Clin Nutr.* 2001;55:994–99.

Chapter 20. Week 2: Optimize Metabolism with Nutritional Supplements

1. Kelly GS. Insulin resistance: lifestyle and nutritional interventions. *Altern Med Rev.* 2000 Apr;5(2):109–32. Review.

2. Nikooyeh B, et al. Daily consumption of vitamin D- or vitamin D + calcium–fortified yogurt drink improved glycemic control in patients with type 2 diabetes: a randomized clinical trial. *Am J Clin Nutr.* 2011 Apr;93(4):764–71.

3. Ou HY, et al. Interaction of BMI with vitamin D and insulin sensitivity. *Eur J Clin Invest.* 2011 Nov;41(11):1195–1201.

4. Woods MN, et al. Effect of a dietary intervention and n-3 fatty acid supplementation on measures of serum lipid and insulin sensitivity in persons with HIV. *Am J Clin Nutr.* 2009 Dec;90(6): 1566–78.

5. Okuda Y, et al. Long-term effects of eicosapentaenoic acid on diabetic peripheral neuropathy and serum lipids in patients with type II diabetes mellitus. *J Diabetes Complications.* 1996 Sep-Oct;10(5): 280–87.

6. Singh U, Jialal I. Alpha-lipoic acid supplementation and diabetes. *Nutr Rev.* 2008 Nov;66(11):646–57. Review.

7. Davì G, Santilli F, Patrono C. Nutraceuticals in diabetes and metabolic syndrome. *Cardiovasc Ther.* 2010 Aug;28(4):216–26. Review.

8. Larrieta E, et al. Pharmacological concentrations of biotin reduce serum triglycerides and the expression of lipogenic genes. *Eur J Pharmacol.* 2010 Oct 10; 644(1-3):263–68.

9. Kirkham S, et al. The potential of cinnamon to reduce blood glucose levels in patients with type 2 diabetes and insulin resistance. *Diabetes Obes Metab.* 2009 Dec;11(12):1100–13.

10. Fenercioglu AK, et al. The effects of polyphenol-containing antioxidants on oxidative stress and lipid peroxidation in type 2 diabetes mellitus without complications. *J Endocrinol Invest.* 2010 Feb; 33(2):118–24.

11. Vuksan V, et al. Beneficial effects of viscous dietary fiber from Konjacmannan in subjects with the

insulin resistance syndrome: results of a controlled metabolic trial. *Diabetes Care.* 2000 Jan;23(1):9–14.

12. Sood N, Baker WL, Coleman CI. Effect of glucomannan on plasma lipid and glucose concentrations, body weight, and blood pressure: systematic review and meta-analysis. *Am J Clin Nutr.* 2008 Oct;88(4):1167–75. Review.

13. Minich DM, Bland JS. Dietary management of the metabolic syndrome beyond macronutrients. *Nutr Rev.* 2008 Aug;66(8):429–44. Review.

14. Pipe EA, et al. Soy protein reduces serum LDL cholesterol and the LDL cholesterol HDL cholesterol and apolipoprotein B: apolipoprotein A-I ratios in adults with type 2 diabetes. *J Nutr.* 2009 Sep; 139(9):1700–6.

15. Yajima H, et al. Bitter acids derived from hops, activate both peroxisome proliferator-activated receptor alpha and gamma and reduce insulin resistance. *J Biol Chem.* 2004 Aug 6;279(32):33456–62.

16. Krawinkel MB, Keding GB. Bitter gourd (Momordica Charantia): a dietary approach to hyperglycemia. *Nutr Rev.* 2006 Jul;64(7 Pt 1):331–37. Review.

17. Kanetkar P, Singhal R, Kamat M. Gymnema sylvestre: a Memoir. *J Clin Biochem Nutr.* 2007 Sep; 41(2):77–81.

18. Hasani-Ranjbar S, et al. The efficacy and safety of herbal medicines used in the treatment of hyperlipidemia; a systematic review. *Curr Pharm Des.* 2010;16(26):2935–47.

19. Katan MB, et al. Efficacy and safety of plant stanols and sterols in the management of blood choles-

terol levels. *Mayo Clin Proc.* 2003 Aug;78(8):965–78. Review.

20. Houston MC. Nutrition and nutraceutical supplements in the treatment of hypertension. *Expert Rev Cardiovasc Ther.* 2010 Jun;8(6):821–33. Review.

21. Walker AF, et al. Hypotensive effects of hawthorn for patients with diabetes taking prescription drugs: a randomised controlled trial. *Br J Gen Pract.* 2006 Jun;56(527):437–43.

22. Tai MW, Sweet BV. Nattokinase for prevention of thrombosis. *Am J Health Syst Pharm.* 2006 Jun 15;63(12):1121–23.

23. Kasim M, et al. Improved myocardial perfusion in stable angina pectoris by oral lumbrokinase: a pilot study. *J Altern Complement Med.* 2009 May; 15(5):539–44.

24. Diabetes Prevention Program Research Group, et al. 10-year follow-up of diabetes incidence and weight loss in the Diabetes Prevention Outcomes Study. *Lancet.* 2009 Nov 14;374(9702):1677–86.

25. Hyman MA. The failure of risk factor treatment for primary prevention of chronic disease. *Altern Ther Health Med.* 2010 May–Jun;16(3):60–63. Review.

26. Taylor AJ, et al. Extended-release niacin or ezetimibe and carotid intima-media thickness. *N Engl J Med.* 2009 Nov 26;361(22):2113–22.

27. Preiss D, et al. Risk of incident diabetes with intensive-dose compared with moderate-dose statin therapy: a meta-analysis. *JAMA.* 2011 Jun 22; 305(24):2556–64.

Chapter 21. Week 3: Relax Your Mind, Heal Your Body

1. Grossniklaus DA, et al. Biobehavioral and psychological differences between overweight adults with and without waist circumference risk. *Res Nurs Health.* 2010 Dec;33(6):539–51.
2. Galvin JA, et al. The relaxation response: reducing stress and improving cognition in healthy aging adults. *Complement Ther Clin Pract.* 2006 Aug; 12(3):186–91.

Chapter 22. Week 4: Fun, Smart Exercise

1. Jorge ML, et al. The effects of aerobic, resistance, and combined exercise on metabolic control, inflammatory markers, adipocytokines, and muscle insulin signaling in patients with type 2 diabetes mellitus. *Metabolism.* 2011 Sep;60(9):1244–52.
2. Goodpaster BH, et al. Effects of diet and physical activity interventions on weight loss and cardiometabolic risk factors in severely obese adults: a randomized trial. *JAMA.* 2010 Oct 27;304(16): 1795–802.
3. Rosen RC, et al. Erectile dysfunction in type 2 diabetic men: relationship to exercise fitness and cardiovascular risk factors in the Look AHEAD trial. *J Sex Med.* 2009 May;6(5):1414–22.
4. Church TS, et al. Effects of aerobic and resistance training on hemoglobin A1c levels in patients with type 2 diabetes: a randomized controlled trial. *JAMA.* 2010 Nov 24;304(20):2253–62. Erratum in: *JAMA.* 2011 Mar 2;305(9):892.

Chapter 23. Week 5: Live Clean and Green

1. Galletti PM, Joyet G. Effect of fluorine on thyroidal iodine metabolism in hyperthyroidism. *J Clin Endocrinol Metab.* 1958 Oct;18(10):1102–10.

2. Xanthis A, et al. Advanced glycosylation end products and nutrition — a possible relation with diabetic atherosclerosis and how to prevent it. *J Food Sci.* 2007 Oct;72(8):R125–29.

3. Dolan M, Rowley J. The precautionary principle in the context of mobile phone and base station radiofrequency exposures. *Environ Health Perspect.* 2009 Sep;117(9):1329–32.

4. Volkow ND, et al. Effects of cell phone radiofrequency signal exposure on brain glucose metabolism. *JAMA.* 2011 Feb 23;305(8):808–13.

5. Genuis SJ. Fielding a current idea: exploring the public health impact of electromagnetic radiation. *Public Health.* 2008 Feb;122(2):113–24.

Chapter 24. Week 6: Personalize the Program

1. Persky VW, et al. Effect of soy protein on endogenous hormones in postmenopausal women. *Am J Clin Nutr.* 2002 Jan;75(1):145–53. Erratum in: *Am J Clin Nutr.* 2002 Sep;76(3):695.

2. Galletti PM, Joyet G. Effect of fluorine on thyroidal iodine metabolism in hyperthyroidism. *J Clin Endocrinol Metab.* 1958 Oct;18(10):1102–10.

3. Schellenberg R. Treatment for the premenstrual syndrome with agnus castus fruit extract: prospective, randomised, placebo controlled study. *BMJ.* 2001 Jan 20;322(7279):134–37.

4. Estruch R. Anti-inflammatory effects of the Mediterranean diet: the experience of the PREDIMED study. *Proc Nutr Soc.* 2010 Aug;69(3):333–40.

5. Church TS, Earnest CP, Wood KA, Kampert JB. Reduction of C-reactive protein levels through use of a multivitamin. *Am J Med.* 2003 Dec 15; 115(9):702–7.

6. Cani PD, Delzenne NM. The role of the gut microbiota in energy metabolism and metabolic disease. *Curr Pharm Des.* 2009;15(13):1546–58. Review.

7. Cecchini M, LoPresti V. Drug residues stored in the body following cessation of use: impacts on neuroendocrine balance and behavior—use of the Hubbard sauna regimen to remove toxins and restore health. *Med Hypotheses.* 2007;68(4):868–79.

8. Beever R. The effects of repeated thermal therapy on quality of life in patients with type II diabetes mellitus. *J Altern Complement Med.* 2010 Jun; 16(6):677–81.

9. Kamenova P. Improvement of insulin sensitivity in patients with type 2 diabetes mellitus after oral administration of alpha-lipoic acid. *Hormones.* 2006 Oct–Dec;5(4):251–58.

10. Wu G, et al. Arginine metabolism and nutrition in growth, health and disease. *Amino Acids.* 2009 May;37(1):153–68.

11. El-Ghoroury EA, et al. Malondialdehyde and coenzyme Q10 in platelets and serum in type 2 diabetes mellitus: correlation with glycemic control. *Blood Coagul Fibrinolysis.* 2009 Jun;20(4): 248–51.

12. Sadruddin S, Arora R. Resveratrol: biologic and therapeutic implications. *J Cardiometab Syndr.* 2009 Spring;4(2):102–6. Review.

13. Jiang WJ. Sirtuins: novel targets for metabolic disease in drug development. *Biochem Biophys Res Commun.* 2008 Aug 29;373(3):341–44. Epub 2008 Jun 23. Review.

14. Solerte SB, et al. Nutritional supplements with oral amino acid mixtures increases whole-body lean mass and insulin sensitivity in elderly subjects with sarcopenia. *Am J Cardiol.* 2008 Jun 2;101(11A): 69E–77E.

15. Yin J, Zhang H, Ye J. Traditional Chinese medicine in treatment of metabolic syndrome. *Endocr Metab Immune Disord Drug Targets.* 2008 Jun;8(2): 99–111. Review.

16. Xie JT, Mchendale S, Yuan CS. Ginseng and diabetes. *Am J Chin Med.* 2005;33(3):397–404. Review.

Chapter 27. Get Healthy Together: Creating a Social Movement

1. http://www.yaleruddcenter.org.

2. http://online.wsj.com/article/SB1244768040263 08603.html.

3. http://bostonreview.net/BR35.3/angell.php.

4. Adams KM, Kohlmeier M, Zeisel SH. Nutrition education in U.S. medical schools: latest update of a national survey. *Acad Med.* 2010 Sep;85(9): 1537–42.

5. http://www.acpm.org/LifestyleMedicine.htm.

About the Author

Mark Hyman, MD, has dedicated his career to identifying and addressing the root causes of chronic illness through a groundbreaking whole-systems-medicine approach known as functional medicine. He is a family physician, a four-time *New York Times* bestselling author, and an internationally recognized leader in his field. Through his private practice, education efforts, writing, research, advocacy, and public-policy work, he strives to improve access to functional medicine and to widen the understanding and practice of it, empowering others to stop managing symptoms and instead treat the underlying causes of illness, thereby also tackling our chronic-disease epidemic.

Dr. Hyman is chairman of the Institute for Functional Medicine and was awarded its 2009 Linus Pauling Award for Leadership in Functional Medicine. He is on the board of directors of the Center for Mind-Body Medicine and a faculty member of its

Food As Medicine training program. He is also on the board of advisers of Mehmet Oz's HealthCorps, which tackles the obesity epidemic by "educating the student body" in American high schools about nutrition, fitness, and mental resilience. He is a volunteer for Partners in Health, with whom he worked immediately after the earthquake in Haiti and continues to help rebuild the country's health care system. He was featured on *60 Minutes* for his work there.

Dr. Hyman has testified before the White House Commission on Complementary and Alternative Medicine and has consulted with the Surgeon General on diabetes prevention. He has testified before the Senate Working Group on Health Care Reform on functional medicine and participated in the White House Forum on Prevention and Wellness in June 2009. Dr. Hyman was nominated by Senator Tom Harkin for the President's Advisory Group on Prevention, Health Promotion, and Integrative and Public Health, a 25-person group to advise the administration and the new National Council on Prevention, Health Promotion and Public Health. With Drs. Dean Ornish and Michael Roizen, Dr. Hyman crafted and helped to introduce the Take Back Your Health Act of 2009 into the United States Senate, to provide for reimbursement of lifestyle treatment of chronic disease. He continues to work in Washington on health reform, recently testifying before a Congressional hearing on Functional Medicine, nutrition, and the use of dietary supplements.

Through his work with corporations, church groups, and government entities, such as CIGNA, the Veterans Administration, Google, and Saddleback Church, he is helping to improve health outcomes and reduce costs around the world. He initiated and is a key participant in the ongoing development of a faith-based initiative that enrolled over 14,000 people at Saddleback Church in a healthy lifestyle program and research study. In recognition of his efforts, he was recently awarded the Council on Litigation Management's 2010 Professionalism Award, citing individuals who have demonstrated leadership by example in the highest standard of their profession. He also received the American College of Nutrition 2009 Communication and Media Award for his contribution to promoting better understanding of nutrition science. He has been featured on *The Dr. Oz Show, 60 Minutes, Larry King Live,* CNN, and MSNBC.

Dr. Hyman is founder and medical director of The UltraWellness Center in Lenox, Massachusetts, where he directs a team of physicians, nutritionists, and nurses who utilize a comprehensive approach to health. Before starting his practice, he was co–medical director at Canyon Ranch Lenox, one of the world's leading health resorts. While at Canyon

Ranch, he coauthored the *New York Times* bestseller *UltraPrevention: The 6-Week Plan That Will Make You Healthy for Life* (Scribner)—winner of the Books for a Better Life Award honoring the best self-improvement books each year. He has since written *UltraMetabolism: The Simple Plan for Automatic Weight Loss* and a companion public television special. His latest book and PBS special, *The UltraMind Solution*, a comprehensive approach for addressing the causes of mental illness and cognitive disorders, was released in December 2008.

Dr. Hyman graduated with a B.A. from Cornell University and magna cum laude from the Ottawa University School of Medicine. He completed his residency at the University of San Francisco's program in Family Medicine at the Community Hospital of Santa Rosa.

Please join him in helping us all take back our health at www.drhyman.com, follow him on twitter @markhymanmd, and see him on Facebook at face book.com/drmarkhyman.